ELECTRONIC TECHNIQUES IN ANAESTHESIA AND SURGERY

By the same author:
Principles of Electronics in Medical Research (2nd edition)
Physics Applied to Anaesthesia (2nd edition)

Electronic Techniques in Anaesthesia and Surgery

Second Edition

D. W. Hill
M.Sc., Ph.D., F.Inst.P., F.I.E.E.

Reader in Medical Physics, Research Department of Anaesthetics, Royal College of Surgeons of England, and Institute of Basic Medical Sciences, University of London

Butterworths

ENGLAND: BUTTERWORTH & CO. (PUBLISHERS) LTD.
                  LONDON: 88 Kingsway, W.C.2B 6AB
AUSTRALIA: BUTTERWORTHS PTY. LTD.
                  SYDNEY: 586 Pacific Highway, 2067
                  MELBOURNE: 343 Little Collins Street, 3000
                  BRISBANE: 240 Queen Street, 4000
CANADA: BUTTERWORTH & CO. (CANADA) LTD.
                  TORONTO: 14 Curity Avenue, 374
NEW ZEALAND: BUTTERWORTHS OF NEW ZEALAND LTD.
                  WELLINGTON: 26-28 Waring Taylor Street, 1
SOUTH AFRICA: BUTTERWORTH & CO. (SOUTH AFRICA) LTD.
                  DURBAN: 152-154 Gale Street

First Edition Published 1970
Second Edition Published 1973

Suggested U.D.C. Number 621·389-79:616-098
Suggested Additional Numbers 616-7
                              615.475

ISBN 0 407 16401 4

*Printed in Gt. Britain at
the St. Ann's Press, Park Road, Altrincham*

Contents

Preface to the Second Edition xi

Preface to the First Edition xii

1—Recording systems for physiological signals 1

The choice of a recording system—Encountered signals—Patient monitoring—The impedance matching of the components of a monitoring or recording system—Pre-amplifiers—Performance requirements for recording system amplifiers—Transistorized ECG pre-amplifier—Phonocardiographic pre-amplifiers and microphones—Pre-amplifiers for use with resistive and reactive transducers—Chopper-type pre-amplifiers—Carrier-type pre-amplifiers—Parametric amplifiers—The provision of a low-level output from the final amplifier—Display systems—Cathode-ray tube displays—Double-beam displays—Multi-trace displays—Storage oscilloscopes—Recorder displays—Rapid response recorders—Pen-arm and hot-stylus recorders—Moving-coil pen motors—Moving-iron pen motors—Ultra-violet and photographic recorders—Characteristics of galvanometers—Characteristics of pencil galvanometers—Frequency response of pen motors—The role of friction—Linearity aspects of galvanometer and pen motor recorders—Error-correction system for pen recorders—The ink-jet recorder—Behaviour of the writing mass of fluid—Tangent error in the ink-jet recorder—Slow-response recorders—Strip or roll chart recorders—Circular-chart recorders—Recording inks—Potentiometric recorders—X-Y recorders—Orders of instruments—The zero-order instrument—The first-order instrument—The second-order instrument—Criteria for the faithful reproduction of a physiological quantity—Amplitude distortion—Frequency response—Phase distortion—Transient response—Step function testing—Poor low-frequency response—Poor high-frequency response—Stimulators for nerve and muscle—The use of computers in patient monitoring—Terms commonly encountered in computing.

2—Pressure transducers and myographs 70

Pressure transducers—Variable capacitance transducers—Variable inductance transducers—The optical de-focusing pressure manometer—Linear variable-differential transformer pressure transducers—Strain gauges—Silicon bonded strain gauges—Silicon-diaphragm pressure transducers—Mercury strain gauges—Unbonded strain gauge transducers—Catheter-tip pressure transducers—Manometer calibration systems—Resonance effects with needles and catheters—The use of small diameter catheters—The display of systolic, diastolic and mean arterial pressure from a pressure transducer—The site of pressure measurement —The recording of central venous pressure—Physical aspects of electromanometry—Further comparison of the electromanometer with the mass-spring analogue—Frequency response of the transducer-catheter system—Adjustment of the damping—Isometric myographs—Cardiac force and blood vessel stress transducers—Indirect methods for measuring and recording arterial blood pressure—The sphygmomanometer—Automated sphygmomanometer—Double-cuff methods for indirect blood pressure recording—The oscillotonometer—Automatic double-cuff methods—The accuracy of indirect blood pressure recording methods—Finger-cuff systems for recording systolic pressure only.

3—The measurement of gas flow, volume and respiratory rate   **108**

The pneumotachograph—The integrating pneumotachograph—Other applications of integrators—The measurement of respiratory rate—The use of a thermistor probe—The use of a spring-loaded switch—The use of an impedance pneumograph—Dry displacement gas meters—Correction factors for dry gas meters—Electrical impedance pneumographs—Calibration of impedance pneumographs—Applications of impedance pneumographs—Spirometry—The frequency response of spirometers—The application of spirometry to anaesthesia—The Wright respirometer.

4—The measurement of blood flow   **134**

Electromagnetic blood flowmeters—The d.c. field flowmeter—A.C. field flowmeters—The zero flow adjustment—The size of the flow head —Calibration of electromagnetic blood flowmeters—Applications of electromagnetic blood flowmeters—Catheter tip velometer—Thermal-type blood flowmeters—The thermal dilution blood flowmeter—Thermal conductivity blood flowmeters—Ultrasonic blood flowmeters —The Doppler shift ultrasonic blood flowmeter—Other applications of ultrasonic techniques to surgery—Venous occlusion plethysmography —The use of a water-filled plethysmograph—The capacitance plethysmograph—The mercury-in-rubber strain gauge plethysmograph—Electrical impedance plethysmography—The use of an air-filled plethysmograph—Thin-film resistance thermometers.

5—Recording electrodes   **171**

Desirable characteristics of electrodes—Reversible electrodes—Silver/silver chloride electrodes—Polarization over-voltage—ECG electrodes—Electrode jellies and creams—Types of adhesive chest electrodes for monitoring—Other forms of ECG electrode—Impedance electrodes—EEG electrodes—Electrodes for electromyography—The measurement of the contact impedance of recording electrodes—Effects of a high electrode contact impedance on the electrocardiogram—Equivalent circuits for the electrode-tissue interface—Garments for use with electrodes and transducers.

6—Gas and vapour analysis   **196**

Paramagnetic oxygen analysers—Thermal conductivity gas analysers—Infra-red gas analysers—The ultra-violet halothane meter—Gas analysis by the measurement of refractive index—The gas-discharge nitrogen meter—Mass spectrometers—Quadrupole mass spectrometers—Gas chromatography—The flame ionization detector—The electron capture detector—The thermal conductivity detector or katharometer—The preparation of standard gas and vapour mixtures.

7—Electrode systems for measuring the pH and oxygen and carbon dioxide tensions of blood   **224**

Membrane potential—The Nernst equation—Electrode systems for measuring pH of body fluids—The pH-sensitive glass electrode—The calomel reference electrode—pH meters—Buffer solutions for use in blood pH measurements—The temperature coefficient of blood and the effect upon it of the acid-base state—The carbon dioxide electrode—Calibration of a CO_2 electrode—Handling of blood samples for the CO_2 electrode—Effects of temperature changes on the CO_2 electrode—P_{CO_2} electrode read-out—Dynamic response of the CO_2 electrode—The use of a CO_2 electrode to estimate the CO_2 content of whole blood—Cation electrodes—Polarographic electrodes for the measurement of the oxygen tension of blood—The Clark electrode—The use of an oxygen electrode to measure the oxygen content of whole blood—Polarographic electrodes for the measurement of tissue oxygen tensions—Fuel cells—Catheter-type oxygen electrodes—Computer programs.

8—The measurement of cardiac output by indicator dilution methods and impedance measurements   **257**

Principles of the indicator dilution method—The use of dye dilution methods—Calibration of the dye densitometer—Cardiac output computers—The estimation of beat-by-beat changes in stroke volume—The use of a radioactive indicator—The analysis of double peaked radiocardiograms—The thermal dilution technique for the estimation of cardiac output—The measurement of cardiac output by an electrical impedance technique—Accuracy of cardiac output determinations by the impedance method—Origins of the impedance changes associated with cardiac activity—The use of transthoracic impedance measurements for the early detection of pulmonary oedema—Rheoencephalography.

9—Defibrillators   **288**

A.C. defibrillators—D.C. defibrillators—Synchronized d.c. defibrillators—Double square pulse defibrillators—Checking d.c. defibrillator performance—The concept of delivered energy—Routine inspection of d.c. defibrillators.

10—Cardiac pacemakers and bladder and anal stimulators 297

Implanted circuits—Electrode arrangements for use with cardiac pacemakers—Pacemaker systems for short-term pacing—Pacemaker systems for long-term pacing—External pacemakers—Implanted pacemakers—External rate control for implanted pacemakers—Atrial-triggered pacemakers—On-demand pacemakers—Cardiac pacemaker circuits—Electrolytic disintegration of pacemaker electrodes—Electrical hazards with cardiac pacemakers—Reliability of pacemakers—Bio-electric energy sources for cardiac pacemakers—Developments in power sources for cardiac pacemakers—Implanted electronic stimulators for the treatment of urinary incontinence—The use of implanted stimulators to induce micturition in cases of neurogenic bladder—The use of an electronic pessary to control stress incontinence and urgency in women—Choice of material for pessary electrodes—The use of an anal plug—Some other clinical applications of implanted circuits.

11—Surgical diathermy apparatus and electrical safety precautions in the operating room 327

Surgical diathermy units—Spark-gap surgical diathermy sets—Thermionic valve diathermy sets—Burns from diathermy sets—Electrical interference from diathermy sets—The use of screened rooms—Electrical safety precautions with patient monitoring apparatus—The use of an earth-free mains supply—The use of monitoring apparatus and surgical diathermy in the presence of explosive anaesthetic agents—The use of surgical diathermy on patients using cardiac pacemakers.

12—Oximeters, densitometers and colorimeters 346

Principles of optical absorption—The use of a monochromatic densitometer in colorimetry—The basic theory of oximetry—The effect of scattering upon the transmission of light through blood—Dichromatic transmission oximeters—Dichromatic densitometers for dye dilution curve recording—Theory of the reflection oximeter—Ear oximeters—Transmission oximeters—The use of an oximeter as a densitometer in dye dilution studies—Fibre optic oximeters and densitometers—Combined fibre optic oximeter and pressure transducer.

13—The measurement of body temperature 365

Resistance thermometers—Thermistors—Metal resistance thermometers—Thermistor endoradiosondes—Thermocouples—Laws of thermocouples—The law of the homogeneous circuit—The law of intermediate metals—The law of intermediate temperatures—Silicon diode temperature sensors—The construction of clinical temperature probes—The measurement of temperatures during hypothermia.

14—Counting equipment for use with radioactive isotopes 376

Radioactive isotopes—Energies of alpha and beta particles and gamma radiation—The absorption of beta particles—The interaction of gamma radiation with matter—The curie—Radiation detectors—Ionization—The d.c. ionization chamber—The use of a guard ring—Operating regions of ionization chambers—Proportional counters—Geiger counters—The operation of Geiger counters—Dead time—Miniature Geiger counters—Scintillation counters—Adjustment of a scintillation counter—Liquid scintillation counters—Semiconductor detectors—Choice of a counter—Beta particles—Gamma rays—Coincidence counting—Counting a mixture of two isotopes with a scintillation counter—The counting of gamma-emitting isotopes *in vivo*—The radioisotope scanner—The gamma camera—Radiological protection equipment—Film badges—Quartz fibre electroscope—Radiation monitors—Statistics of counting.

Index   **411**

Preface to the Second Edition

Three years have passed since the first edition of this book appeared. During this time a steady consolidation has occurred of the use of electronic techniques in surgery and anaesthesia. This has been reflected in the increased size of the second edition which has arisen from the inclusion of new topics such as computers and the addition of a considerable number of additional references.

Although it is impossible to be active in all aspects of the subject, the book very largely reflects my own experiences. This has been made possible by the wholehearted co-operation afforded by my colleagues on the staff of the Research Department of Anaesthetics at the Royal College of Surgeons of England and the St. Peter's Group of Hospitals. Especial thanks are due to the staffs of the Physiology Department, Baylor College of Medicine, Houston, Texas and of the Anesthesiology Department, University of Chicago Hospitals, who have allowed me to participate in their research programmes and gain a valuable insight into American technology. Teaching experience at the College and St. Thomas's Hospital has continued to provide an incentive to explain instrumentation techniques to clinicians and a wider view of the state of the art has come from my service as joint editor of the journal *Medical & Biological Engineering*.

For all of this, and for the continuing assistance and support of the staff of the Medical Division of Butterworths, I am deeply grateful.

D. W. HILL

Preface to the First Edition

The opportunity to collect the material for this book arose in the course of preparing lectures on Medical Physics and Clinical Measurement techniques for the new course provided by the Royal College of Surgeons of England for the Primary examination for the Fellowship in Anaesthesia.

While the needs of candidates for this examination have been borne in mind, additional material has been incorporated which it is hoped will make the book of interest both to surgeons and anaesthetists. Information has been obtained from many sources, and every effort has been made to acknowledge these in the text. The field to be covered is large and wherever possible references have been given so that readers interested in particular topics can readily gain information.

The chapters on cardiac pacemakers, bladder and anal stimulators, defibrillators and surgical diathermy have been included as the use of this apparatus will all impinge on measurements made in patients.

The writer takes this opportunity of expressing his thanks to his colleagues in the Research Department of Anaesthetics, Royal College of Surgeons, the Institute of Basic Medical Sciences and the Institute of Urology for their co-operation and encouragement in the use of a large number of measurement techniques. Professor J. P. Payne has kindly made available laboratory facilities and provided a great deal of stimulation.

D. W. HILL

1–Recording Systems for Physiological Signals

THE CHOICE OF A RECORDING SYSTEM

A recording system of some kind normally forms the heart of the measuring equipment used during anaesthesia and surgery, or in physiological experiments. Some of the quantities to be measured, such as the electrical activity of the heart (ECG), exist in an electrical form. This type of signal has then to be picked up by means of suitably chosen and sited electrodes, amplified, processed if necessary and displayed. Other quantities, such as blood pressure, oxygen saturation and cardiac output, have to be transduced (or transformed) into a corresponding electrical signal which can then be treated as before. Table 1.1 lists some commonly encountered signals.

Encountered signals

The range of possible transducers is wide, and these will be discussed in detail in later chapters. Obviously, to be able to follow the dependency of one quantity upon another is of importance, and hence it is essential to have available a versatile recording system so that several combinations of signal can be displayed. This is normally achieved by the use of a number of recording channels, each consisting of a pre-amplifier, main amplifier and display. Each channel may have its own power supply, or a common power supply may be used. The former arrangement minimizes interactions between the various channels. The main amplifiers are identical for each channel, but the pre-amplifiers are designed to have the appropriate characteristics for the particular quantity to be measured on that channel. Thus one would expect to have an EEG pre-amplifier, ECG pre-amplifier, phonocardiograph pre-amplifier, a strain gauge pre-amplifier, a temperature pre-amplifier and a general-purpose voltage pre-amplifier to name some of the versions.

1

TABLE 1.1

TYPICAL BIO-ELECTRIC SIGNALS

Signal	Approximate frequency range (Hz)	Typical amplitude	Electrodes used
Electrocardiogram (ECG)	0·1— 100	1 mV	Limb and chest
Electroencephalogram (EEG)	0·5— 70	50 μV	Scalp
Electromyogram (EMG)	10 — 70	100 μV	Skin
	3 —5000	1 mV	Needle
Electro-oculogram (EOG)	d.c.— 120	0·5 mV	Skin
Electroretinogram (ERG)	d.c.— 20	0·5 mV	Corneal

TYPICAL NON-ELECTRIC VARIABLES

Arterial blood pressure	d.c.—20 Hz	Unbonded wire strain gauge, Bonded semiconductor strain gauge, Capacitance, Differential transformer ⎫ pressure transducers ⎬
Phonocardiography	40—2000 Hz	Crystal or moving coil microphones
Force (isometric)	d.c.—100 Hz	⎰ Bonded wire strain gauge ⎱ Bonded semiconductor strain gauge
Displacement (isotonic)	d.c.—100 Hz	Photoelectric or strain gauge transducers
Respiration	0·1—5 Hz	⎰ Nasal thermistor probe ⎱ Impedance system ⎱ Microswitch
Temperature	d.c.—1 Hz	Thermistor or thermocouple

The choice of display will depend very much upon the application and inevitably upon the financial support available. For some work, a physically small one- or two-channel recorder may be necessary in order that the whole equipment may be mounted on a compact trolley which can be wheeled into the operating room or taken in a hurry to the medical intensive care unit in the small hours of the morning. In contrast, in a physiology laboratory mobility may not be so essential, but versatility will be. This requirement can be covered by using a rack mounted system on castors and providing a range of pre-amplifiers.

For experimental work, a paper chart record is essential together with a means of indicating the paper speed and signalling events of interest. This is usually supplemented with a multi-channel cathode ray tube display and by the use of a frequency modulation analogue tape recorder. The latter facility is mandatory when subsequent off-line analysis is to be performed by means of a digital computer.

Two chart recorders can be useful; one fast response recorder is used to display waveforms such as the arterial blood pressure, ECG, EEG and phonocardiogram; the second, with a slower paper speed and response, can provide an indication of trends in body temperature, oxygen tension and the display of cardiac output curves.

Patient monitoring

For the monitoring of individual patients during surgery, or in intensive or coronary care units, simple cathode ray tube displays are used to show the ECG and arterial blood pressure waveforms with an indication of the heart rate. For monitoring several patients in an intensive or coronary care unit a bar-graph display of the heart rates, temperatures and respiratory rates may be provided on a television raster type cathode ray tube. The display can be readily switched to show tracings of the analogue ECG and blood pressure signals when required. This may be to check for the presence of arrhythmias or clotting of a blood pressure cannula. Quantities such as the mean arterial blood pressure, heart rate and temperature are often shown on conventional meters or in-line digital displays. Facilities are provided for connecting a recorder. It is often desirable to be able to 'freeze' an analogue waveform on the oscilloscope screen, perhaps to check if there is a significant degree of S–T segment depression of the ECG or to observe the position of the dichrotic notch in an arterial blood pressure waveform. One solution is to use a storage type cathode ray tube display or to make use of an endless tape loop cassette. In the latter case, the analogue signal is played on to the tape loop which after storing 3 seconds of signal would normally erase it and carry on recording another 3 seconds. If an alarm condition is detected, such as a sudden drop in heart rate or a run of ectopic beats, then the contents of the tape loop are automatically dumped on to a chart recorder which continues to record whilst the alarm condition is still in force. In this way, both the alarm condition and the events leading up to it are available for inspection. This facility is particularly useful in coronary care units.

There is no universal solution to the choice of a recording system, each user having to decide on the best compromise in the light of his particular requirements. A concise account of the requirements to be met by a physiological recording system is that of Smale (1967).

Currently, a great deal of effort is being put into the exploration of non-invasive techniques for the monitoring of quantities such as a patient's cardiac output and cerebral function. Possibilities for cardiac output include the monitoring of blood flow through the aortic arch by means of an ultrasonic Doppler shift technique and the use of electrical impedance methods. Prior *et al.* (1971) have described a compact system for monitoring cerebral activity. An EEG signal is picked up from a pair of silver–silver chloride electrodes over the parietal regions on both sides of the head. The cerebral function monitor then selects only those signal frequencies in the range 2–15 Hz and displays the total activity (integral) in this band on a slow speed recorder with a chart speed in the range 2·5–9 cm per hour in contrast with the 1080 cm per hour used for conventional EEG recordings.

The impedance matching of the components of a monitoring or recording system

To some extent, a patient monitoring system or a physiological recording system can be thought of as a chain of 'black boxes'. In order to obtain an optimum power transfer between boxes it is necessary that the output impedance of a box is similar to the input impedance of the next box; in many cases, it is not required to transfer a significant amount of power, but to ensure that the output voltage of a particular 'box' is little attenuated by the addition of the next box. Similarly the connection of an amplifier to a transducer should not significantly load the transducer. It is very helpful if a 'box' can have a high value of input impedance and a low value of output impedance. This is usually achieved with, for example, operational amplifiers. Transducers with a high value of internal impedance, such as crystal microphones and dry electrodes, will require to be fed into a field effect transistor input stage having a high input impedance. On the other hand, low impedance devices, such as moving coil meters and solenoids, will need to be fed from a low output impedance emitter follower stage. When selecting the building blocks for a complete system, in addition to gains and bandwidths, careful consideration must be given to the interaction of the various input and output impedances.

Pre-amplifiers

Amplifiers designed for use with bio-electric potentials such as the electrocardiogram, electroencephalogram and electromyogram are invariably of the 'balanced' type. That is to say, three input terminals are provided. One is arranged to be at a fixed potential, while the other two 'live' terminals receive anti-phase input signals. This is the well-known push-pull action, one live terminal going positive as the other goes negative and vice versa. This type of amplifier is also known as a differential amplifier, since it will only respond to voltage differences existing between its live terminals. It can usually be arranged that unwanted signals such as those picked up from the mains wiring of the room fall on each of the live terminals in phase (or in step). Within limits, the amplifier will not respond to such signals. By suitably siting the recording electrodes, it can be arranged that the wanted signals arrive at the live terminals in anti-phase (or out of step), and these signals are then amplified. The ratio of the gain for anti-phase signals to the gain for in-phase signals is known as the rejection ratio for the amplifier and may be as high as five hundred thousand to one.

Each stage of a differential amplifier consists of a pair of active elements (valves or transistors). This is an excellent arrangement in regard to stability of the amplifier's gain and for minimizing baseline drifts, that is drifts occurring in the amplifiers' output level when the input signal amplitude is maintained at zero. Matched pairs of valves or transistors can be used, and in the case of transistors these can be mounted on a common heat sink. Changes in temperature and supply voltages tend to affect each side of the amplifier equally. The amplifier output, which is the difference in the signal level between the two sides is minimally affected.

Special purpose amplifiers, such as chopper-type d.c. amplifiers may have single-sided inputs, that is one live input terminal and one reference terminal. The majority of the amplifiers encountered in medical and biological work will, however, be of the balanced type. These amplifiers can be used with single-sided inputs, by joining one live input terminal to the reference terminal, and placing the input signal between their junction and the other live input terminal.

For most applications, the pre-amplifiers can be mounted in a cabinet along with the main amplifiers and display. When very low-level input signals have to be handled, or when interference is high, it may be advantageous to have the pre-amplifier(s) situated close to the recording site and separated from the main recorder.

Performance requirements for recording system amplifiers

The main amplifier of each recording channel is normally of the push-pull d.c. coupled type. With some types of final amplifier a maximum sensitivity of 10 mV/cm deflection of the output device is possible, but with other designs, in order to achieve this figure, a stage of d.c. amplification in a pre-amplifier is needed. The input impedance should be of the order of 5 MΩ between each live input terminal and earth, and the in-phase rejection ratio should be of the order 500 : 1 or better. The frequency response of the amplifier will normally extend from d.c. to 3 dB down at several thousand Hz. This range can only be utilized by using a cathode-ray tube display, or a 'pencil galvanometer' in conjunction with an ultra-violet or visible light beam. In other cases, the upper frequency limit is set by the characteristics of the galvanometer system. For an ink-jet recorder the response will be practically linear from d.c. to 500 Hz but for hot-stylus and ink-writing recorders it is normally not better than 100 Hz. However, hot-stylus recorders are available with a frequency response which is 10 per cent down at 150 Hz with a deflection of 17 mm.

Recording channels for the ECG, EEG and EMG are normally a.c. coupled in order to eliminate baseline shifts arising from slow potential changes occurring due to polarization effects at the recording electrodes. An ECG pre-amplifier designed to precede the main amplifier just described would have a fixed time constant of 2 seconds, and similar input impedances and in-phase rejection ratio to the main amplifier. Means will also be provided for balancing the amplifier and for injecting a standard 1 mV signal into the amplifier input for calibration purposes. After this, individual designs may vary considerably. The ECG pre-amplifier Type EMT 13 for the Swedish Mingograf system employs a fixed gain of 30 and is preceded by an ECG input unit containing a lead selector switch and an emitter-follower input circuit for the right and left arm and left leg electrodes. Other pre-amplifiers such as the Sanborn ECG pre-amplifier will provide for both an a.c. and a d.c. input and a coarse and fine attenuator. Whether the d.c. input is provided in the pre-amplifier or the main amplifier, it is certainly most convenient to be able to use two or three of the available channels for both ECG and general-purpose recording.

The requirements for both EEG and EMG can often be combined into a single pre-amplifier. The pre-amplifier must firstly offer a higher gain than that required for ECG work alone. If the maximum gain of the ECG channel is 0·25 mV/cm, that of the EEG channel would be 10 μV/cm., and when used for EMG recording 30 μV/cm. Secondly, the pre-amplifier must provide means for altering the time constant of the coupling circuits, and also means for altering the upper and lower limits of the frequency response curve. A rejection ratio for in-phase signals of the order of 1,000 : 1 is required.

For EEG work a choice of time constants would be available of

6

0·03, 0·1, 0·3 and 1 second to set the low-frequency response of the amplifier. A high-frequency loss filter can be inserted to give an additional loss of 15 per cent at 15, 25 or 75 Hz, with a slope of 6 dB per octave above the set frequency.

For EMG work, the frequency response of the amplifier is defined in terms of its 3 dB points. At the upper and lower frequencies corresponding to the 3 dB points, the gain of the amplifier is reduced to 0·7 of the maximum value which occurs for the centre frequencies of the response curve. The normal 3 dB points for an EMG amplifier would be 20 and 5,000 Hz. By means of a filter the low-frequency response can be reduced so that the lower 3 dB point becomes 80 Hz and similarly by inserting a second filter the upper 3 dB point can be reduced to 500 Hz.

This type of high-gain biological amplifier finds a number of other applications, for example in recording electro-oculograms and electroretinograms, (Shackel 1967). It is normally provided with a means for generating either a 1 mV or 1 μV calibration signal.

If a photographic or ink-jet recorder is available with a frequency response out to at least 500 Hz, it makes sense to combine the requirements for EMG, ECG and EEG recording into a single universal amplifier. This might have switched steps of gain from 20 micro-volts to 2 milli-volts per centimetre deflection; d.c. coupling can be used or various low-frequency time constants extending to 5 seconds, whilst the upper Band-pass frequency can be extended from 15 to 700 Hz. Such an amplifier could be used to record smooth muscle EMGs from the bladder with a 5 seconds time constant and a 30 Hz upper frequency, whilst with a 0·05 seconds time constant and a 500 Hz upper frequency it could be used to record striated muscle EMGs from the perineum or urethral sphincters.

With some amplifiers, provision may be made to switch in an optional twin-tee 'notch' filter to eliminate residual mains hum. For many purposes this is a useful facility, but the filter can introduce distortion if the signal contains spikes or transients (Gibson, Gibson and Hirsch, 1970).

Transistorized ECG pre-amplifier

Modern practice in biological amplifier design is shown in the ECG pre-amplifier Type EMT13 by the Elema–Schonander company of Stockholm, shown in *Figure 1.1*. The input stage consists of a matched pair of silicon planar transistors Q_1, Q_2 operated with a very low collector-current of 0·11 μA in order to produce an input impedance of more than 100 MΩ on either side of earth. Input resistors R_1 and R_2 together with capacitor C_1 form a low-pass filter. The d.c. input current of the amplifier is less than 9×10^{-10} A which minimizes polarization effects at the electrodes. In order to achieve minimum loading of the input stage, the second stage consists of a matched pair of field-effect transistors Q_3 and Q_4 Negative feedback is provided via resistors R_5 and R_6 and the amplifier balance can be set up by potentiometer R_8. The voltage gain of the pre-amplifier is 30 and the noise voltage referred to the input is less than 6 μV over the frequency band d.c. to 70 Hz. The maximum permissible d.c. input voltage is 400 mV.

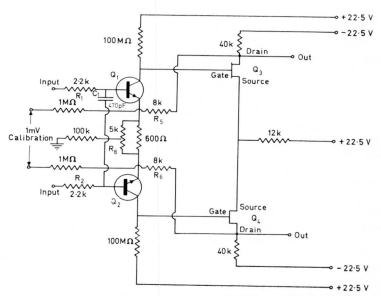

Figure 1.1. ECG pre-amplifier Type EMT13. (Reproduced by courtesy of Elema-Schonander)

Phonocardiographic pre-amplifiers and microphones

For the accurate recording of heart sounds, a low-frequency moving-coil microphone is commonly used in conjunction with an audio-frequency amplifier fitted with a set of filters so that a number of discrete frequency bands may be recorded. Other arrangements may use either an air-conduction or a direct-conduction microphone. The latter may be constructed on the lines of an acceleration-type vibration pick-up or utilize a mass coupled to the chest wall. Typically, the amplifier would provide five switched ranges having the following centre frequencies: 25–50, 100–200 and 500 Hz. Van Vollenhoven *et al.* (1969) give details of the frequency analysis of heart murmurs, whilst Van Vollenhoven and Wallenburg (1970) describe the calibration of microphones for phonocardiography. Holdack, Luisada and Lieda (1965) discuss the standardization of techniques for recording phonocardiograms whilst Ertel *et al.* (1966) give details of stethoscope acoustics.

The phonocardiogram presents difficulties during patient monitoring as it is easily upset by movement of the patient or by attendants handling the thorax. Nevertheless, it provides an extremely useful source of timing signals in relation to the heart valve movements. For example, a knowledge of the occurrence of the first and second heart sounds is invaluable in calculating stroke volume by the electrical impedance method. An electro-static microphone can be used feeding into a pre-amplifier having switched gains of 35 and 47 dB, and two filter positions giving a frequency response 3 dB down at either 80 or 250 Hz. Obviously, the display system fed by the amplifier channel must be capable of responding to these frequencies. Normally, an ink-jet or ultra-violet recorder would be used. A modulation system is now often used in conjunction with ink or hot-stylus galvanometers. The output from a direct conduction microphone is passed through an equalizing circuit and then rectified and integrated in order to obtain its envelope signal. This amplitude modulates a carrier frequency; the resulting modulated signal is displayed on the pen galvanometer. This system should have a frequency response covering 20–600 Hz. It is usable for clinical diagnoses, but is not reliable for time and amplitude measurements or accurate waveform analysis. Continental European phonocardiograph amplifiers use filters having frequency ranges based upon the specifications of Maas and Weber. Although possessing a good low-frequency response, moving-coil microphones are bulky, so a small crystal microphone fitted with a suction cup may be preferred. The frequency response of the microphone and phonocardiographic pre-amplifier might be split into three bands to cover the range 20–2,000 Hz. The maximum gain of the pre-amplifier could be 100 with an input voltage range of 100 μV to 50 mV peak with a noise level referred to the input less than 5μV peak to peak, and an input impedance greater than 2 MΩ.

9

PRE-AMPLIFIERS FOR USE WITH RESISTIVE AND REACTIVE TRANSDUCERS

Chopper-type pre-amplifiers

Resistive elements alone are employed in a number of transducers, such as strain gauge myographs, unbonded strain gauge pressure transducers and temperature sensors such as thermistors and wire-coil resistance thermometers. It is possible to use all these devices as arms of a d.c. Wheatstone bridge circuit, the output of the bridge, which may be only a few microvolts in the case of an unbonded strain gauge, being measured with a sensitive chopper-type d.c. amplifier. In this arrangement an electronic switch or 'chopper' regularly interrupts the input signal, converting it into a form of a.c. This is then amplified with a stable a.c. amplifier and converted back to d.c. by synchronous rectification at the amplifier output. The result is a stable, drift-free, d.c. amplifier. Its frequency response depends upon the value of the chopping frequency. This type of amplifier would also be suitable for use with a thermocouple. The output voltage from the amplifier is displayed on a meter or pen galvanometer. The chopper amplifier is usually incorporated in a self-balancing potentiometric recorder when a large (10-inch) chart width is required, the balancing time often being about 1 second. A greater flexibility is obtained if an X – Y potentiometric recorder is available. Two chopper-type potentiometric recorder movements are fitted to this type of recorder, each moving the recording pen in one of two mutually perpendicular axes. A sensitivity of 50 μV per inch deflection is obtainable. An X – Y recorder is convenient for use with d.c. excited semi-conductor strain gauge transducers, particularly for the plotting of pressure-flow and pressure-volume loops. It should be remembered that not only is a stable amplifier required for use with a d.c. excited bridge, but that the d.c. supply to the bridge must also be stable. Changes in the excitation of the bridge will be reflected in corresponding output voltage changes.

The use of resistive strain gauge bridges and pressure transducers enables a versatile pen-recording system to be constructed around a high-gain d.c. chopper-type amplifier. Each recording channel can be standardized on one of these pre-amplifiers feeding a power amplifier for driving the pen motor. The pre-amplifier for each channel is preceded by the appropriate input 'coupler' module which conditions the signal into a suitable form for the pre-amplifier to accept. This is the system adopted in the Beckman Type S–11 Dynograph direct-writing recorder, *Figure 1.2*.

Differential signals fed into the chopper pre-amplifier (Type 481B) are passed through an input attenuator to a mechanical chopper, S_1, running at 400 Hz. The resulting amplitude-modulated signal is fed through a transformer having a centre-tapped primary winding into the five-stage direct-coupled amplifier. The input transformer carries two secondary windings. The larger secondary winding is selected when sensitivity ranges of 0·5 mV/cm pen deflection to 50 mV/cm or 5 V/cm to 50 V/cm are required. The output from the smaller secondary winding is one hundredth of that provided by the larger winding, and is selected for sensitivities in the range 100 mV/cm to 2 V/cm. The closed-loop gain of the amplifier is controlled by varying the amount of negative feedback obtained

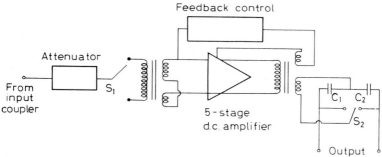

Figure 1.2. Beckman Type S-11 Dynograph direct writing recorder pre-amplifier.
(Reproduced by courtesy of Beckman Instruments)

from a winding of the output transformer of the amplifier. The feedback is applied in series with the input signal at the secondary winding of the input transformer. The other secondary winding of the output transformer has its two ends connected alternatively across a pair of capacitors C_1 and C_2 in series by means of a second mechanical chopper, S_2. This output chopper is synchronized with the input chopper. The chopper action allows the capacitors to charge in series and reproduce the original input signal in its now amplified form. The synchronizing of the output chopper with the input chopper causes the voltage developed across the two capacitors to possess the same phase and wave shape as did the original input signal.

The basic chopper pre-amplifier is complete with an input attenuator and calibrated gain control. Comparatively simple input coupler units can then be used with the pre-amplifier. For example, the a.c./d.c. input coupler enables either an input signal comprising

11

both a.c. and d.c. portions to be amplified or only the a.c. or the d.c. portion to be selected. A variable attenuation of either the high-frequency or the low-frequency components of the signal is available.

When a high input impedance is required an electrometer input coupler is available. Applications include the use of the chopper-pre-amplifier with high-impedance voltage sources such as glass pH electrodes, micro-electrodes and low-capacity crystal transducers. The electrometer input stage uses two sub-miniature electrometer valves in a push-pull arrangement set to have a stage gain of unity, so as not to affect the calibrated gain control of the main pre-amplifier. The input impedance is approximately 10^{10} Ω, with a maximum sensitivity of 0·5 mV/cm. The frequency response is flat within $\pm$ 10 per cent from d.c. to 150 Hz.

For use with resistive strain gauges, the strain-gauge input coupler unit has fine and coarse balancing controls for adjusting a full strain gauge bridge, a pair of matched resistors being available in the coupler to complete a full bridge if only two strain gauges are in use. In addition to a sensitivity control and polarity reversal switch, a calibration control provides a simulated load for setting up a known calibration. For a typical four-arm active bridge using 120 Ω gauges having gauge factors of 2 and a bridge excitation voltage of 2 V, the maximum strain deflection sensitivity obtainable with the input coupler and pre-amplifier is 1 microinch/inch/cm. The frequency response is again flat within $\pm$ 10 per cent from d.c. to 150 Hz.

Carrier-type pre-amplifiers

At audio frequencies, the impedance of a transducer such as a differential transformer consists of a resistive part and an inductive part, while that of a capacitance manometer is mainly capacitive with a small resistive component. Gauges such as these, having a reactive component, need to be operated in an a.c. bridge. This has two balance controls, one for the reactive and one for the resistive component of the gauge impedance. In the case of either a.c. or d.c. bridges, the effect to be observed can be arranged to alter the characteristics of either two or four of the bridge arms. In the case of a 'half-bridge' two of the arms are 'active' while the other two are fixed resistors. The two active elements are placed in opposite arms of the bridge, so that any effects on them due to changes in the ambient conditions will tend to cancel. A bridge having four active arms is known as a 'full' bridge. For this technique, comprehensive physiological recording systems provide 'carrier pre-amplifiers'. The pre-amplifier contains a fixed frequency oscillator generating perhaps 5 V at 3,000 Hz. This output is used to energize a strain gauge bridge or differential transformer. A pair of resistive ratio arms is brought out on terminals for use in completing the bridge when a 'half bridge' arrangement is in use. The output from the bridge consists of an amplitude-modulated signal at the carrier frequency. This is then amplified in the pre-amplifier and rectified in a phase-sensitive rectifier. The combination is known as a carrier amplifier/demodulator. A typical output would be $\pm$ 2 V d.c. for a 250 μV bridge output. The resulting d.c. output signal is then fed into the normal main amplifier of the recording channel. Coarse and fine gain controls are provided together with two balancing controls and a zero control. Normally, the company selling the carrier pre-amplifier will recommend a particular type of pressure transducer to go with it. When used with this type of gauge, a calibration control is usually provided. This unbalances the bridge by an amount equivalent to the application of 100 mmHg pressure to the transducer. Of course, a carrier pre-amplifier can equally well be used with a resistive strain gauge transducer such as an unbonded strain gauge or semi-conductor strain gauge.

For many purposes, the following combination of pre-amplifiers is satisfactory; two general-purpose voltage pre-amplifiers having the choice of both a.c. and d.c. differential inputs, two ECG pre-amplifiers, and two carrier pre-amplifiers. The ECG pre-amplifiers should also have provision for d.c. inputs. Spare pre-amplifiers can be obtained as required, for example, a third ECG pre-amplifier for vector cardiography, a phonocardiograph pre-amplifier and one or more EEG amplifiers. A versatile physiological recording system is essential for any serious attempt at clinical measurement. Its choice demands care, since the cost is likely to lie in the range £1,500 to £3,500.

Parametric amplifiers

It has been seen that the advent of silicon planar transistors has enabled transistor amplifier input stages to be designed with input impedances of the order of megohms and having noise levels referred to the input of only a few microvolts. These are differential amplifiers and they will respond only to voltage differences existing between their 'live' input terminals. However, if the input stage is direct coupled then the maximum voltage that can be applied between either of the inputs and the indifferent terminal is only a few hundred millivolts. If this is exceeded, then damage can be caused to the transistors. When a parametric type of amplifier is used, it is possible for the maximum in-phase voltage that can be applied to be 500 V. In an extreme case, even if the patient happened to be at the mains voltage potential, if such an amplifier were connected to him it would not break down to earth and allow a dangerous current to flow.

In a parametric amplifier, the input stage is an a.c. bridge, the input signal voltage being arranged to unbalance the bridge. The resulting out-of-balance voltage is then amplified and synchronously rectified. The principle of operation can be followed by reference to *Figure 1.3*, which shows the circuit diagram of an amplifier due to P. Styles. Transistor Q_1 is in a 20 kHz Colpitts oscillator which energizes the a.c. bridge and also provides a reference signal for the synchronous rectifier. The differential input to the amplifier is isolated from the rest of the circuitry via the insulation resistance of transformers T_1 and T_2 and the 0·1 μF capacitors. Two of the arms of the a.c. bridge are resistive, the other two comprising the reverse biased Zener diodes D_1 and D_2. Because they are arranged to be reverse biased, these diodes have a high reverse resistance. They also have an associated capacitance whose value is dependent on the voltage placed across them. The reverse bias would be of the order 1 V and the maximum input signal 250 mV. The application of the input voltage alters the diode capacities and unbalances the bridge, which has previously been balanced by means of VR_1. The output signal from T_1 is amplified by the three stage amplifier Q_2, Q_3, Q_4, VR_2 acting as a gain control. A portion of the output from the Colpitt's oscillator is fed to transistor Q_5 which supplies the synchronous rectifiers Q_6, Q_7, Q_8 and Q_9. The input impedance is better than 100 MΩ, and the maximum input signal is 250 mV. The maximum output voltage is greater than 1 V the sensitivity being better than 1 V output for 10 mV input. The temperature coefficient referred to the input is less than 25 μV per degree centigrade change in the ambient temperature. Current practice is to use a four-arm bridge having a reverse biased voltage-dependent capacitive silicon diode in each arm. The bridge is energized via a transformer at 200 kHz, a fifth diode rectifying the 200 kHz signal to provide the 1 V reverse bias voltage for the diodes. The floating input to the amplifier has an input impedance of more than 100 MΩ in parallel with a capacity of 800 pF. It can tolerate an in-phase voltage of 500 V applied to the input. The in-phase rejection ratio is greater than 15,000 : 1. When this amplifier is used with the Mingograf ink-jet recorder, the maximum sensitivity is 10 mV d.c. input for a 1 cm deflection on the chart when a 35 mm jet length is used.

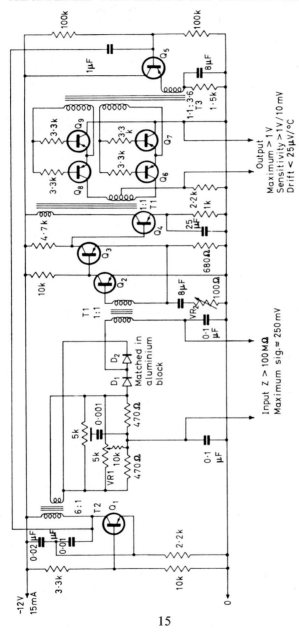

Figure 1.3. Schematic diagram of a parametric amplifier

THE PROVISION OF A LOW-LEVEL OUTPUT FROM THE FINAL AMPLIFIER

It is now common practice to run a frequency-modulation tape recorder in parallel with one or more of the recording channels. A frequency modulation system is able to handle signals with frequencies down to d.c. and would normally work with input signals lying within 1 V of earth. The primary aim of most physiological recording systems is to produce an output tracing on a chart or cathode-ray tube. In the case of a transistorized amplifier feeding a galvanometer, the amplifier supply lines are likely to be of the order of $\pm$ 24 V. In this case, it can be arranged to follow the output stage with a direct coupled 'compressor' stage, that is, one with a push-pull input and single-sided output. The stage is fitted with a gain control to vary the amplitude of the output signal, and a control for setting the output level at earth potential or at a predetermined voltage difference from earth. This arrangement is most useful when it is desired to transmit signals from the physiological recording system over a telephone line link using a frequency modulation arrangement. It should be remembered that the output voltage level of the compressor stage will be dependent on the balance setting for the final amplifier. This should previously be adjusted to the condition for which it will be used during recording before the compressor stage is set up. The problems of obtaining a suitable output voltage to feed into frequency modulation devices were much more acute in the older valve physiological recorders, where the mean potential of the output galvanometer coils might be 380 V with respect to earth.

DISPLAY SYSTEMS

Having achieved a satisfactory amplification of the physiological signal it is normally necessary to display its variation with time or in relation to some other quantity. In the author's experience it is most desirable to have available some form of direct writing system, so that the analogue tracings are immediately available for inspection. In order to save running through a lot of recording paper, it is usual to have a cathode-ray tube monitor working in parallel with the recorder. The paper drive can then be started only when events of particular interest need to be recorded. Even if a frequency modulation tape recorder is available, a direct writing recorder is still required in order to play back the tape on to it for a visible chart record.

Cathode-ray tube displays

The principle of the cathode-ray tube is shown in *Figure 1.4*. This is an electrostatic tube. The 'electron gun' and deflection plates are mounted inside a highly evacuated glass envelope, normally having a flat face for measurement purposes. The cathode of the electron gun produces a supply of electrons which are accelerated by means of a high potential of several thousand volts maintained between the cathode and the final anode of the electron gun. The anode system of the electron gun forms an electrostatic lens in order that the electron beam can be brought to a point focus on the

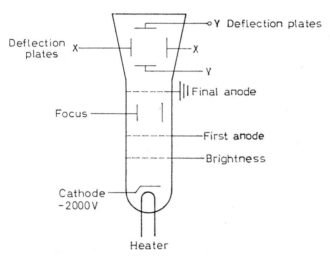

Figure 1.4. Schematic diagram of an electrostatic deflection cathode-ray tube

flat screen of the tube. The screen is coated with a uniform layer of a phosphor. This glows with light when it is struck by the stream of electrons. Within limits, the brightness of the image is proportional to the rate at which electrons strike the screen. The brightness control of the oscilloscope adjusts the grid voltage of the electron gun, and thus affects the number of electrons leaving the gun per unit time. In order to produce a sharply focused spot of light on the screen, for a given brightness setting, both the focus and astigmatism controls must be carefully adjusted. The focus control affects the focal length of the gun's electron lens by altering the voltage applied

17

to the second anode of the gun. The astigmatism control adjusts the mean voltage of each pair of deflection plates so that it is as near as possible that of the gun's final anode. If this is not so, a low power cylindrical lens is formed between the deflection plates and the final anode. This results in an aberration of the image on the screen, known as astigmatism. The presence of astigmatism is shown by the fact that the spot cannot be simultaneously focused in both the horizontal and vertical planes. When a cathode-ray tube is required to produce a detailed display, careful attention must be given to producing the optimum spot size in relation to the brilliance setting. The combination of spot size and brilliance markedly affects the exposure setting if an oscilloscope camera is used. A good example of this occurs in the gamma camera display used to visualize the concentration of a gamma-ray-emitting isotope such as Chlormerodrin (^{197}Hg) in the kidneys.

With a conventional cathode-ray tube, the e.h.t. (extra high tension) voltage applied across the gun in order to accelerate the beam of electrons towards the screen is of the order 2,000–3,000 V for a 4–6-inch screen diameter tube. It is generated either by half-wave rectification from the instrument's mains transformer, or by an audiofrequency oscillator feeding a step-up transformer, the oscillator frequency being of the order 10–15 kHz, and voltages in excess of 10 kV can be generated for use with cathode-ray tubes having a length along the diagonal of a rectangular face of 17 inches or more. A transistorized switching system and step-up transformer is used in portable oscilloscopes powered from 6- or 12-V batteries to develop the cathode-ray tube accelerating potentials. Electrostatic cathode-ray tubes of the type so far described are adequate for the smaller type of display (up to a 6-inch screen diameter) of physiological variables. There is no stringent requirement for a fast writing speed of the spot of light on the tube face forming the image.

This is not the case when the waveforms of switching circuits, or pulses developed from nuclear detectors have to be examined. The sharply rising wavefronts require a high writing speed and at the same time a high brilliance of the spot in order to provide a clearly visible tracing. These two requirements are mutually conflicting in a conventional cathode-ray tube. The higher accelerating voltage needed to produce a bright spot produces a 'stiffer' beam of electrons, that is, one which needs a higher deflection voltage in the direction of the X and Y axes. The problem is overcome in a post-deflection acceleration (P.D.A.) tube. In this arrangement, the main acceleration of the beam is performed after the X and Y deflections have been performed. A modern 5-inch screen diameter P.D.A. tube may have an accelerating voltage of 10 kV and yet achieve a deflection sensitivity of 25 V/inch. One design of a P.D.A. tube, due to Hewlett Packard Ltd., is that of *Figure 1.5*. A linear vertical deflection of 6 cm is possible at high frequencies. This is obtained by the use of a curved, high-transmission mesh electrode situated at the exit side of the deflection region. The mesh develops a spherical equi-potential electric field which increases the sensitivity of the tube, as well as reducing defocusing of the beam and preventing stray illumination of the screen. A thin aluminium film laid down on the

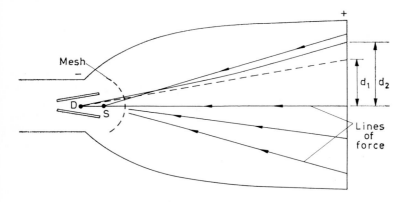

D — Centre of deflection
S — Centre of curvature of mesh
d_1 — Deflection without P.A. field
d_2 — Deflection with radial P.A. field

Figure 1.5. Post-deflection cathode-ray tube. (Reproduced by courtesy of Hewlett Packard Ltd.)

inner surface of the phosphor enhances the brilliancy of the trace. This film acts as a mirror to reflect the inward-directed component of the phosphor light which otherwise would be absorbed in the interior of the tube. The inner face of the glass screen carries a graticule marking which is visible against the phosphor. In this way parallax in reading the spot deflection against the graticule due to the thickness of the glass is avoided. The screen face of the tube consists of a flat glass plate which is welded on to the rest of the tube during manufacture. The flat face allows accurate deflection

19

measurements to be made. The outer face of the glass screen is slightly roughened to reduce glare and reflection.

For general-purpose laboratory use, Hewlett Packard recommend their Type P31 phosphor. This glows blue-green when excited by electron impact, the light decaying with a light-green afterglow. The low-level persistence time of the phosphor is 500 ms, that is, the time taken for the afterglow to fall to 10 per cent of its initial brightness. For medical work, their blue-white P7 phosphor is used. This has a 3-second yellow afterglow. Other manufacturers produce phosphors with afterglows of 10 seconds or more, but these are more susceptible to burning from a stationary or slowly moving spot.

Double beam displays

Although single-beam cathode-ray tube oscilloscopes have their application, a double-beam oscilloscope is particularly useful, for example, in comparing the waveform of an evoked potential with a reference timing signal. A suitable switching technique enables one cathode-ray tube to be shared between two or more input channels. In one system, the outputs from two pre-amplifiers are displayed on alternative timebase sweeps. This method is convenient for high-frequency signals. Owing to the lower timebase speeds, a flicker would arise with this arrangement when showing low-frequency signals. For these, a 'chopping' technique is used, the cathode-ray tube sampling each input at a high rate (40 kHz to 1 MHz). The choice of these two input arrangements is provided on expensive high-frequency oscilloscopes with bandwidths of 10 MHz or more.

The cost of two wide-bandwidth Y amplifiers is high, but feasible for the limited-bandwidth low-frequency amplifiers required for medical signal inputs. Here the cathode-ray tube has two independent electron guns and two separate Y channels. This arrangement is valuable when it is required to display 'loop' figures. Then the timebase is stopped, and one signal applied to the Y axis and the other to the X axis. The resulting figure traced out on the oscilloscope screen shows the interaction of the X and Y signals. Examples of this technique occur in the display of vector cardiograph loops and pressure-volume loops in respiratory mechanics studies. For loop studies, it is usual to disconnect one of the two Y amplifiers and connect it on to the X axis. The two Y amplifiers are of identical construction, so that the phase-shift characteristics of the X and Y axes are now equal. If the phase-shift characteristics were not equal, this could in itself give rise to a loop figure. A true double-beam oscilloscope with Y amplifiers each having a maximum gain of

50 μV/cm over a bandwidth of d.c. to 200 kHz is of considerable value in a medical electronics laboratory.

Multi-trace displays

In a number of patient-monitoring applications, apart from general laboratory use, it is necessary to have three or four traces available on a cathode-ray tube screen. Using a cathode-ray tube having a single electron gun, it is possible to produce multiple traces in two ways. Firstly, by using a beam switch system. Each input channel has associated with it a certain value of 'Y shift' so that the timebase deflection corresponding to it is located at a certain height on the tube face. The channels are sampled in sequence, and thus each is displayed at its appropriate level on the cathode-ray tube face. The switching rate might be 100 kHz, which would be adequate to display four 1 kHz signals.

A more flexible approach is to use a vertical raster display, the number of available channels being limited only by the width available for each on the tube face. One version of this arrangement is that of Mable and Stone (1965). The advantage of the raster technique lies in the fact that it lends itself to the use of magnetic deflection coils and standard television tubes modified to have a long-persistence phosphor screen. Beam switching techniques are not suited for use in electromagnetic scan coils having appreciable inductance. In *Figure 1.6*, taken from Mable and Stone (1965), is shown a block diagram of the raster system. Four channels are available, each commencing with a long-tail pair differential amplifier having the option of a.c. or d.c. input coupling (*Figure 1.7*). The maximum sensitivity is one volt for 4 cm deflection. A positive or negative synchronizing signal may be taken off the left- or right-hand collectors as desired. RV_5 provides a means of unbalancing the stage to give the desired Y shift. From the collector of Tr_2 an amplified version of the input signal is d.c. coupled to Tr_3-Tr_4. These transistors form a Schmitt voltage comparator relating the d.c. (Y shift+signal) voltage of a particular channel to the ramp voltage produced by the sawtooth waveform raster generator running at 20 kHz. As the amplitude of the ramp voltage rises, Tr_3 is normally on until the ramp voltage and (Y-shift voltage+signal) of the channel coincide. Then regeneration via C_6 switches Tr_3 off and Tr_4 on. Resetting of the Schmitt comparator occurs during the ramp flyback, Tr_3 staying off until the ramp flyback. Thus each channel is unblanked from its lowest excursion on the Y-shift setting

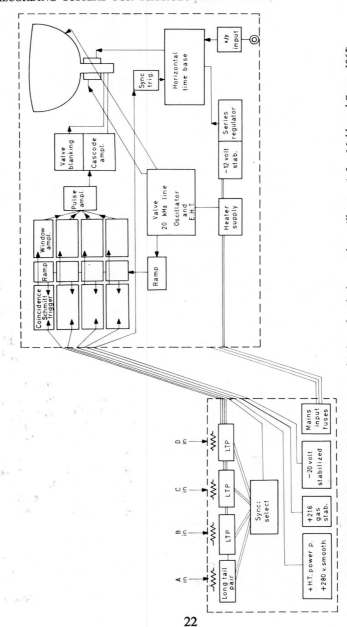

Figure 1.6. Block diagram of a raster-type multi-channel cathode-ray tube oscilloscope (after Mable and Stone, 1965)

22

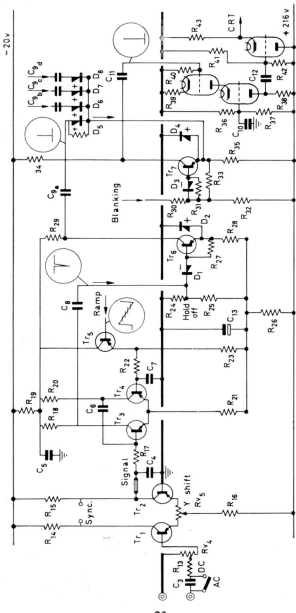

Figure 1.7. Input pre-amplifier for use with raster-type cathode-ray tube oscilloscope (after Mable and Stone, 1965)

23

to the top of the screen. In addition to the vertically rising ramp generator, a conventional slow-speed time base is provided for the X axes of all the channels.

Commercial forms of this type of raster display currently use either 8·5- or 19-inch diagonal, 110 degree scanning-angle cathode-ray tubes fitted with a phosphor having a 50-seconds persistence. Up to 12 channels can be provided. At the maximum channel sensitivity a signal of 2 V amplitude will fill the whole screen. The power supplies and channel pre-amplifiers are mounted in a separate case, close to the patient or experiment. The cathode-ray tube can then be mounted at a convenient height for viewing from a distance if desired. This system is often found in cardiac catheterization rooms. It is useful to have available at least 8 traces, so that some can be used to generate baselines.

Storage oscilloscopes

Many occasions arise when it would be desirable to be able to 'capture' the image shown on a cathode ray tube timebase sweep for subsequent detailed inspection. Many transient conditions come to mind, for example a cardiac arrhythmia on an ECG trace. The original storage oscilloscopes were based upon the use of a storage type of cathode ray tube. One type, known as a direct-view bistable storage tube, utilizes a secondary emission principle. The construction of the tube is illustrated in *Figure 1.8*. The normal writing electron gun bombards the phosphor screen with a beam of high-speed electrons. The impinging beam writes the trace on the screen and also dislodges large numbers of secondary electrons from the screen. As a result, the written surface where the waveform is traced out loses electrons and becomes negatively charged. By making use of the flood-guns, it is possible to store the image on the screen. The flood-guns flood the whole area of the phosphor with low-velocity electrons. These electrons strike the unwritten portions of the screen but do not release many secondary electrons. Hence these areas merely collect electrons until they become sufficiently negatively charged to ensure that no more electrons are attracted. The latent, positively charged, image attracts flood-gun electrons at such a velocity that each entering primary electron dislodges sufficient secondary electrons to hold the image positively charged. Thus, the continued attraction of electrons to the trace regions keeps these glowing, whilst the unwritten areas do not attract electrons and remain dark. In addition to the general viewing of transient phenomena, storage oscilloscopes are widely used to build up the image from a gamma camera used for visualizing the distribution *in vivo* of gamma emitting radioisotopes, and for alpha-numeric displays driven by digital computers.

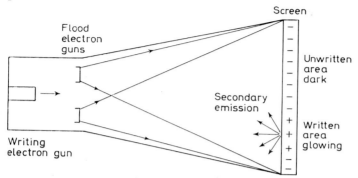

Figure 1.8. Schematic arrangement of a direct-view bistable storage cathode ray tube. (Reproduced by courtesy of Tektronix Ltd.)

Currently, storage cathode ray tube oscilloscopes are being replaced by oscilloscopes utilizing shift register type recycling internal stores. The input to this type of device might consist of a wide band d.c.—3 MHz amplifier giving a sensitivity of 10 mV to 50 V full-scale. The output from the amplifier is fed into a 5 MHz 8-bit analogue-to-digital converter connected to an 8-bit × 1024 word metal oxide silicon transistor shift register memory. When a trigger signal is received by the storage oscilloscope, the converter starts sampling and the selected portion of the input waveform is held in the store. A variable time delay may be inserted between the trigger pulse and the start of the sampling process. After the total of 1024 samples have been stored, the oscilloscope automatically scans through its store and, via a digital-to-analogue converter, displays the store contents on its cathode ray tube screen. The store contents can also be output to a paper tape punch or directly input into an associated digital computer. By using a suitable timing train of external pulses, samples can be automatically taken and displayed on command or at regular intervals of time.

Recorder displays

Although frequency-modulation tape recorders and cathode-ray tube displays may be available, a time always arises when it becomes necessary to have a written record of the physiological variables of interest. These can be broadly divided into two main groups; rapidly

25

changing quantities or signals that contain high-frequency components, and slowly varying quantities in which there are no high-frequency components. The first group will include the ECG, EMG and EEG and arterial blood pressures. The second group includes quantities such as body temperature, respiratory rate and integrated heart rate. Before discussing the more commonly encountered types of recorder in detail, it would be as well to list the main types.

(1) Recorders using moving-coil or moving-iron pen motors (galvanometers) fitted with ink pens or heated styli.

(2) Recorders using galvanometer movements where pressure-sensitive paper is employed in conjunction with a bar which periodically presses the stylus down on to the paper.

(3) Recorders using galvanometer movements carrying mirrors. A beam of visible or ultra-violet light is reflected on to a light-sensitive paper.

(4) Recorders using galvanometer movements carrying glass jets from which ink is squirted on to a roll of absorbent paper.

(5) Null-balance or potentiometric recorders operated by continuously balancing the input d.c. voltage against a reference voltage.

(6) X–Y recorders.

In the first five types of recorder the input variable(s) is (are) plotted against time on the continuously moving recording medium. The X axis of the recorder is calibrated in terms of time. In an X–Y recorder, however, the pen-carriage is moved under the control of a second input voltage in the X direction. Some versions of X – Y recorders also contain a ramp generator which can be switched on to the X axis to provide a timebase.

Rapid response recorders

Pen-arm and hot-stylus recorders

For many purposes, a four-channel recorder having a frequency response from 0 to 80 or 100 Hz over a four-centimetre deflection for each channel will suffice. Ink recorders offer the advantage of a good contrast tracing with the use of cheap recording paper. Although inky fingers are a nuisance, with care, little trouble is experienced with ink as a recording medium. The tip of the pen traces out an arc on the recording chart as the galvanometer deflects and a distorted trace results. For many purposes this is acceptable in the interests of cheapness, but care must be taken to measure times along the axis of the undeflected position of each pen. The problems of relating times of events of tracings on different channels in curvilinear co-ordinates are illustrated in *Figure 1.9*. Some makes of pen recorder, such as those by Brush, utilize a mechanical linkage to convert the curvilinear motion of the galvanometer coil into a rectilinear deflection.

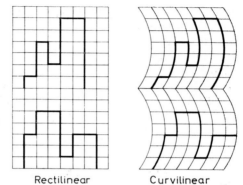

Figure 1.9. Curvilinear and rectilinear recordings

Rectilinear   Curvilinear

The production of 'rectilinear' recordings is assured by the use of a hot stylus deflecting over a knife-edge placed at right angles to the direction of motion of the chart (*Figure 1.10*). The hot stylus at the end of the galvanometer arm burns off the white cellulos ecovering of the special heat-sensitive paper, thus exposing the black under-surface and producing a black-on-white trace. For the higher paper speeds microswitches are connected to the gearbox of the paper drive so as to automatically increase the power supplied to the stylus. The heating power required to produce a good contrast at 25 mm per second or more would burn a hole in the paper at the low speeds. In order to maintain good contrast tracings over a period of

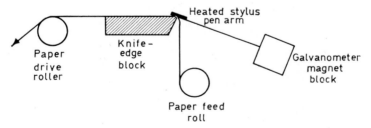

Figure 1.10. The use of a pen arm carrying a heated stylus writing over a knife-edge

27

time, it is necessary periodically to remove deposits of wax from the stylus and check that the stylus pressure is kept at the maker's recommended value. Hot-stylus recording has been generally adopted for portable recorders and electrocardiographs where the need to stock ink and the possibility of its spilling in the recorder rule out the use of ink recording. For an 8-cm writing arm, the frequency response of a hot-stylus pen motor is typically from 0–70 Hz (3 dB down) over a 3-cm deflection. In the case of the same motor fitted to an ink pen, the frequency response would be extended to 3 dB down at 100 Hz. The linearity of the pen motors would be typically 2 per cent of the deflection or 0·3 mm whichever is the greater, over the central $\pm$ 2 cm deflection. Over the outer 5 mm, the linearity becomes 3 per cent of the deflection or 0·3 mm whichever is the greater. For use with such pens, a modern multi-channel recorder such as the Type M4 by Devices Ltd., *Figure 1.11*, provides

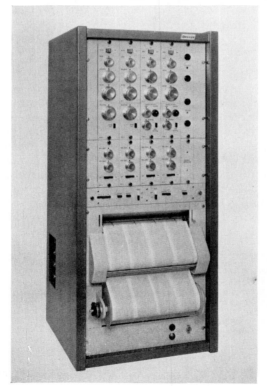

Figure 1.11. Multi-channel pen recorder system. (Reproduced by courtesy of Devices Ltd.)

twelve push-button selected paper speeds to cover the range 2·5 to 100 mm/s, the speeds being controlled by a velodyne servo system to within 1 per cent accuracy. The power requirement for a four-channel Type M.4 recorder including the paper drive is 350 VA at 230 V a.c.

Moving-coil pen motors
In a moving-coil pen motor (galvanometer) a cylindrical soft iron core is placed inside the coil which rotates in the annular gap between the core and the curved pole-pieces of the powerful galvanometer magnet. In this way the moving coil rotates in a radial magnetic field, so that the angular deflection in radians of the coil is proportional to the coil current. The pen motors used in physiological recording systems have their coils suspended by helical or flat strip springs which also serve to carry the current to and from the coil. In a typical case, the natural resonant frequency of the pen motor and pen arm is about 50 Hz and with the damping set to give a 5 per cent overshoot a frequency response from d.c. to 3 dB down at 70 Hz is obtained. A better frequency response, out to 150 Hz, can be obtained with a pen motor designed on the lines of a moving-coil loudspeaker, the coil being totally enclosed within the electro-magnet. This arrangement is used in the Swiss Leichti range of recorders.

Moving-iron pen motors
Some multi-channel physiological recording systems make use of robust moving-iron pen motors. In this form of construction fixed electromagnet coils are employed and the pen arm is attached to a suspended permanent-magnet system. This system is used in the German Schwartzer range of recorders.

Ultra-violet and photographic recorders
In photographic types of recorders, the pattern of the tracing is produced by means of a beam of light moving over a light-sensitive recording paper. The beam of light, being weightless, enables the construction of recorders having the highest frequency response. Multi-channel recorders are easily built up by the use of 'pencil-galvanometers' (*Figure 1.12*). A coil of fine aluminium wire is suspended between two vertical metal strips, and carries a small plane mirror. The complete assembly is mounted in a pencil-shaped housing. Connections to the coil are made via two insulated metal rings at the top of the housing. A number of these galvanometer assemblies can be mounted into a magnet block. On pushing a

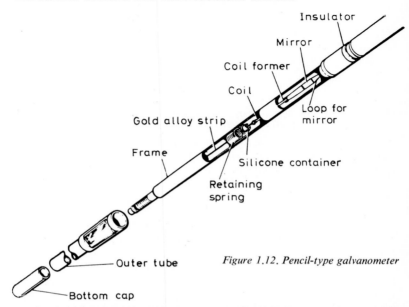

Figure 1.12. Pencil-type galvanometer

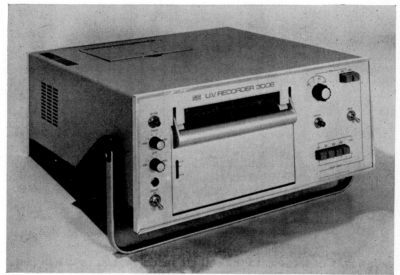

Figure 1.13. Multi-channel ultra-violet recorder. (Reproduced by courtesy of S. E. Laboratories Ltd.)

galvanometer into a mounting hole in the block, spring contacts connect with the metal rings. The galvanometers are insulated from one another in the block so that they can be at different voltage levels if desired. For adjustment of the galvanometer zeros in the horizontal plane, the head of each galvanometer is provided with a slot so that the whole assembly can be turned. For vertical adjustments, each segment of the magnet block containing a galvanometer can be tilted by adjusting a screw placed behind each galvanometer station. For medical work, recorders fitted with 6 or 12 galvanometers are usual. A typical focal length for the lens used with each galvanometer would be 35 cm. The incident light path and the galvanometer focal length are comparable in order to ensure a minimum recording-spot size without loss of sensitivity. Photographic recorders are much used in cardiac catheterization studies where a good frequency response and contrast are essential. The recorder is provided with a rapid developer attachment in order that the tracings can be quickly made available.

When an almost instantly visible trace is required, then the galvanometers are illuminated with ultra-violet light from a high-pressure mercury vapour lamp. This is usually mounted in a self-contained sub-unit having its own cooling system, and is adjustable for the correct focusing. A high-voltage (10 kV) generator is provided to strike the arc of the lamp which is run from a regulated power supply. A typical 6- or 12-channel recorder (without preamplifiers) is the Type S.E. 3006 by S.E. Laboratories Ltd. (*Figure 1.13*). An eight-speed gearbox is provided driven by a hysteresis motor with a non-slip belt drive to the final roller. Three optional gearbox ratios allow a range of paper speeds from 5 mm/minute to 1,250 mm/second. A 60 : 1 jump speed control operates solenoid clutches to give paper speeds in either seconds or minutes. Ultra-violet-sensitive recording paper of any width up to 6 inches can be used. An adjustable iris diaphragm in front of the lamp controls the intensity of the light spots from the galvanometers at the point of writing. Grid lines are projected on to the recording paper by means of a secondary light beam derived from the mercury lamp. A timer unit synchronized with the mains frequency provides a time scale on the recording paper by pulsing a photoflash tube at predetermined intervals, timing lines being produced across the full width of the paper. Either minute or second marks are available. The grid lines are spaced at 2 mm intervals with every fifth line accentuated. The maximum writing speed on the recording paper is 60,000 inches per second.

31

The tracing from an ultra-violet recorder will fade in strong sunlight unless the paper has been fixed by wet processing. The contrast of the trace is not as good as that obtained with a visible-light recorder and photographic recording paper, but is normally quite acceptable. The great disadvantage of photographic recorders lies in the fact that the trace cannot be observed until the reel of recording paper has been developed and fixed. For this reason, a slave cathode-ray tube monitor unit is usually run in parallel with the recorder. In order to enable the operator to judge the amplitude of the traces, the light spots from the galvanometers fall on to a ground glass screen where they can be observed. A similar screen is provided with ultra-violet recorders. It can be a tedious business setting up several tracings and baselines.

CHARACTERISTICS OF GALVANOMETERS

Characteristics of pencil galvanometers

A galvanometer is unable to follow instantaneously the deflection arising from the application to it of a step change in the coil current. The response of the moving coil lags behind the driving signal due to the mechanical inertia of the movement. The effect of inertia will also be to tend to cause the coil to overshoot its final deflection. The response of the coil to a sudden signal change can be altered by adjusting the damping of the system. The degree of damping is assessed by means of a damping factor. This is unity when the galvanometer is 'critically damped'. With critical damping, the coil will deflect smoothly to take up its final position (*Figure 1.14b*). If the damping factor is much less than the critical value, then the coil will overshoot and oscillate about its final rest position, (*Figure 1.14a*). These considerations apply not only to pencil galvanometers but also to pen motors carrying an ink-pen arm or a hot stylus. For

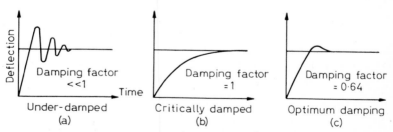

Figure 1.14. The effect of the damping factor upon the response of a pen galvanometer to the application of a step input function

example, the presence of underdamping in the pen motor of an electrocardiograph can give rise to overshoot on the down stroke of the R-wave having the appearance of a clinically significant degree of S–T segment depression. The amount of damping present depends on the resistance in the coil circuit. The value of the external damping resistor which must be placed in parallel with the galvano-meter coil is quoted by the manufacturer. When the output impedance of the driving amplifier is greater than the required damping resistance, then a suitable resistor must be placed in parallel with the amplifier output. On the other hand, when the output impedance of the amplifier is lower than the required damping resistance, a series resistor must be inserted between the amplifier output and the coil. Oil damping alone, or in combination with a damping resistor is used for the lower resistance, high-frequency galvanometers. The damping is normally pre-set by the recorder manufacturer.

The application of the correct amount of damping reduces the overshoot of a galvanometer to a minimum while providing for the best frequency response. The value usually chosen is 65 per cent of critical, that is, a damping factor of 0·65. At this damping, the galvanometer will have a frequency response which is flat to within $\pm$ 5 per cent up to 60 per cent of the natural frequency. The natural frequency is the frequency of oscillation of the under-damped coil, (*Figure 1.14a*). The undamped natural frequency required for a galvanometer can be estimated by multiplying the frequency response needed by a factor of 1·6. The higher the frequency response, the stiffer must be the system and hence the sensitivity is reduced. These considerations are evident in the following table for galvanometers by S.E. Laboratories Ltd. The sensitivities are obtained with (1) An optical path length of 325 mm; (2) a sensitivity tolerance of $\pm$10 per cent; (3) no external damping resistor.

TABLE 1.2.

Type	Natural frequency Hz	Flat frequency response Hz ($\pm$5%)	Nominal galvo. resistance Ω($\pm$10%)	Damping resistor Ω	Max. safe current mA r.m.s.	Galvanometer sensitivity ($\pm$10%)	
						mA/cm	mV/cm
A.35	35	20	47	350	10	0·0008	0·038
A.100	100	60	35	100	10	0·0037	0·130
B.450	450	300	120	250	25	0·05	6
A.1000	1000	600	75	oil+ 250	35	0·34	25
A.8000	8000	5000	42	oil	50	25	1050

The damping factor in each case is 0.65.

33

Frequency response of pen motors

The damping associated with a pen motor carrying a pen arm or hot stylus is greater than that of a pencil galvanometer. Two mechanically resonant systems now exist. These are formed by the compliance of the pen-motor control spring acting in conjunction with the inertia of the coil, and the inertia of the pen arm or stylus. The resonant frequencies of the two systems are adjusted by the manufacturer to give the best frequency response for the complete assembly. A control may be provided to alter the output impedance of the driving amplifier and thus affect the damping of the pen motor. In the case of a push-pull valve driver amplifier where each half of the centre-tapped pen-motor coil forms one anode load, the damping control may be a variable resistor joining the two cathodes.

Referring to *Figure 1.15(a)* and neglecting friction, a second-order differential equation relates the angular deflection of the galvanometer coil to the input current to the coil I:

$$J\mathrm{d}^2\theta/\mathrm{d}t^2 + c\mathrm{d}\theta/\mathrm{d}t + k\theta = K\,I(t)$$

where J is the moment of inertia of the moving-coil assembly including the pen arm or mirror,

$\mathrm{d}\theta/\mathrm{d}t$ is the angular velocity of the coil assembly

$\mathrm{d}^2\theta/\mathrm{d}t^2$ is the angular acceleration of the coil assembly

c is the damping factor

k is the restoring force per unit deflection due to the spring

K is constant of proportionality between the turning force and the coil current.

Thus the force resulting from the flow of current is such as to overcome inertia, the restoring force of the spring and the damping force. The damping factor c includes viscous damping (by air or oil) and electromagnetic damping. The viscous damping is determined by the construction of the galvanometer, but the electromagnetic damping arises from the back e.m.f. which is induced in the moving coil. The back e.m.f. proportional to the angular velocity ($\mathrm{d}\theta/\mathrm{d}t$) generates a current in the coil which opposes the signal current and hence reduces the rate of rotation of the coil. Reducing the resistance R in series with the coil can appreciably increase the value of the damping constant. The interaction of the natural frequency and damping factor on the frequency response of a galvanometer is shown in *Figure 1.15(b)*. The corresponding phase shift variation is shown in *Figure 1.15(c)*.

34

For a moving-coil galvanometer

$$\frac{\theta}{\theta_0} = \frac{1}{\sqrt{\left[1-\left(\frac{f}{f_n}\right)^2\right]^2+\left(\frac{2.f.c}{f_n.c_0}\right)^2}} \; . \; \sin\left(2\pi\, ft - \alpha\right)$$

and $\quad \alpha \quad = \quad$ arc tan $\quad \left\{\dfrac{\left(2\dfrac{f}{f_n}\cdot\dfrac{c}{c_0}\right)}{\left[1-\left(\dfrac{f}{f_n}\right)^2\right]}\right\}$

where $\dfrac{\theta}{\theta_0}$ is the ratio of the deflection θ at frequency f to the static deflection θ_0, f_n is the natural or resonant frequency, $c_0=1$ is the critical damping factor and α is the phase angle. The solution of these equations is shown in *Figures 1.15(b)* and *1.15(c)*.
When the damping is less than critical, the response of the galvanometer to an input step function is given by

$$\frac{\theta}{\theta_\infty} = 1-\exp\left(-2\pi\cdot\frac{c}{c_0}\cdot\frac{T}{T_n}\right)\cdot\cos\left(2\pi\cdot\frac{c}{c_0}\cdot\sqrt{S}\right)$$

where $\quad S = -\left[\left(\dfrac{c}{c_0}\right)^2-1\right]$

and $\quad\theta\quad$ is the deflection at time T after the application of the step function
$\quad\theta_\infty\quad$ is the steady state deflection
$\quad c/c_0\quad$ is the ratio of actual to critical damping
$\quad T/T_n\quad$ is the ratio of the time to the period of the galvanometer's natural frequency.

The solution of this equation gives the damped oscillation executed by the galvanometer (*Figure 1.15d*).

The role of friction
In ink-pen or heated-stylus recorders it is necessary to have a certain pressure existing between the writing element and the paper in order to produce a clear tracing. This means the presence of a considerable amount of friction. Friction indirectly affects the sensitivity of the galvanometer. The final deflection of the galvanometer coil is brought about by a balance arising between the deflecting force due to the current flow on the one hand and the restoring force of the suspension plus the frictional force on the other (*Figure 1.15a*). As a result of friction the pen will tend to stop a little short of its theoretical deflected position. Since the pen can approach a given deflection from either direction the result is a 'dead zone' around the

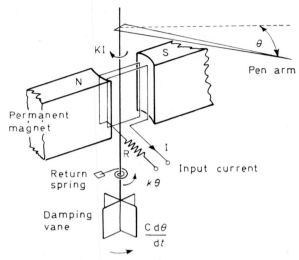

Figure 1.15(a) Forces governing the motion of a moving-coil galvanometer

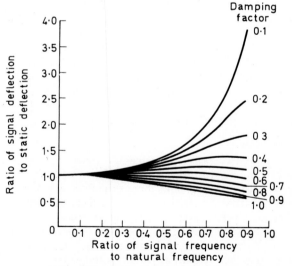

Figure 1.15(b) The ratio of galvanometer deflection at any signal frequency to the static deflection as a function of the ratio of the signal frequency to the natural frequency for various degrees of damping

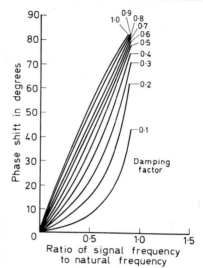

Figure 1.15(c) The phase shift between the sinusoidal driving signal and the resultant coil motion as a function of the ratio of the signal frequency to the natural frequency

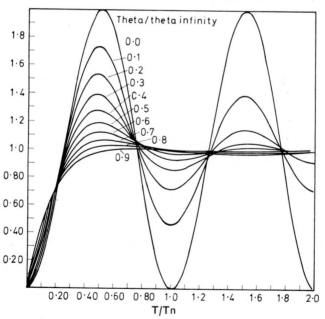

Figure 1.15(d) The effect of applying a step input current to a galvanometer with varying degrees of damping. The ordinate is the ratio of the deflection at a particular time to the steady state deflection. The abscissa is the ratio of time to the periodic time of the galvanometer's natural frequency. The ratio (actual damping/critical damping) increases from 0 to 1 in steps of 0·1 for successive traces

theoretical deflection. The magnitude of the dead zone can be reduced by the use of a stiffer suspension, but this reduces the sensitivity. Increased sensitivity is incompatible with a faster response, for if the number of turns on the coil is now increased to raise the sensitivity, the inertia of the coil will be raised, reducing the frequency response.

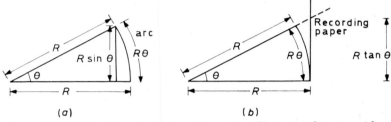

Figure 1.16. (a) Sine distortion with a galvanometer; (b) tangent distortion with an ink-jet or optical recorder

Linearity aspects of galvanometer and pen-motor recorders

For most ink-pen recorders, the tracing is in curvilinear co-ordinates. In a well-designed galvanometer or pen motor, the angle turned through by the moving coil is proportional to the magnitude of the input signal. As in *Figure 1.16*, the pen tip traces out the arc of a circle of radius R where R is the length of the pen arm. If θ is the angle of deflection then the length of the arc will be $R\theta$. However, if the deflection is measured with a rule from the normal time axis, the distance measured will be $R \sin \theta$. For deflections up to 14 degrees the difference between $R\theta$ and $R \sin\theta$ is less than 1 per cent. With an 8-cm pen arm this amounts to a deflection of $\pm$ 2 cm. The distortion is thus less than the ink trace width of 0·5 mm. When a larger deflection amplitude is required with this or a better accuracy, an error-correcting signal system may be employed as has been described for the Beckman Type S–11 Dynograph recorder. An alternative system which has been used by the Cambridge Instrument Company is shown in *Figure 1.17*. Here the recording paper is formed into a suitably shaped trough. The pen motor is now mounted above the paper, the pen making an angle to the paper. This system proves difficult when several traces are used, wide chart paper having to be pulled uniformly through the troughs.

Sine distortion occurs in a recorder having a rigid pen arm, the tip of which traces out an arc on the chart paper. When a hot stylus is used, the stylus rubs along the knife-edge in a direction at right angles to the direction of paper travel, (*see Figure 1.10*). The true deflection, proportional to the applied signal, is again the arc $R\theta$, but the deflection as measured on the chart in rectangular co-ordinates is now the distance $R \tan \theta$. For deflections of plus or

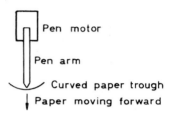

Pen motor

Pen arm

Figure 1.17. The use of a galvanometer mounted vertically above the chart paper

Curved paper trough

Paper moving forward

minus 2 cm with an 8-cm writing arm, the deflection measured in rectilinear coordinates as the tangent will be 3·5 per cent greater than the true arc deflection. On the other hand, the same angle of deflection will give a deflection measured in curvilinear coordinates as the sine which is 1·0 per cent less than the true arc deflection. Tangent error arises appreciably in the case of ultra-violet and ink-jet recorders which can have quite large amplitude deflections. The jet or light beam always falls on the paper at right angles to the paper motion. In the case of the ink-jet recorder using a 52-mm long ink-jet, a deflection of ± 42 mm is possible. The corresponding angle of deflection is ± 46 degrees. Compensation must be introduced for the tangent distortion. This is achieved by the use of straight rather than curved magnet polepieces.

Error-correction system for pen recorders

With an 8-cm pen arm, an angular deflection of $\pm 14\cdot5$ degrees will give a deflection, measured as the sine of the angle, of $\pm$ 2 cm. The distortion between the sine and the true arc deflection will not be more than 1·5%. Using an error-correcting system, as is done in the Beckman Type S–11 Dynograph direct writing recorder, the distortion can be kept down to 0·5 per cent for curvilinear recording over a $\pm2\cdot5$ cm deflection. With this system, the recording pen not only records the input signals on to a graduated chart, but it also serves as a moving contact on to a precision slide-wire voltage divider. The d.c. voltage tapped off from the slide-wire is pro-portional to the position of the pen on the chart. This pen-position signal is then compared with the input signal to the channel amplifier.

Any difference between the two constitutes an error signal. The amplified error signal is used to drive the pen in a direction such as to cancel the error signal. It is necessary to reduce the momentum of the moving pen arm and pen-motor coil before the reduction of the error voltage to zero. If this is not done, the pen will overshoot and possibly oscillate about it deflected position. A signal proportional to the pen velocity is added to the position signal. As the error signal diminishes, the velocity signal predominates retarding the pen motion and preventing or minimizing overshoot and possible oscillation. Referring to *Figure 1.18*, the channel input and position error signals are compared in a differential amplifier using two silicon transistors. All the pens of the multi-channel recorder use a common slide-wire, so that potential differences will exist between the various pens. Means are provided for backing-off these voltage differences in a further differential amplifier. The negative feedback path of the main pen-motor driving amplifier is so arranged that the amount of negative feedback is reduced for rapidly changing position signals. The gain thus increases with increase in the rate of change of the position signal, so that the basic pen position signal now depends on both pen position and velocity. A damping control allows adjustment of the velocity signal. It is arranged to provide a limit to the pen-motor coil current for large deflections in order to prevent damage to the pen. A zero pen control is provided to minimize the deflection force applied to the pen when it is disconnected from the slide-wire for extended periods. The control provides a pseudo pen-position signal.

THE INK-JET RECORDER

Ink-pen and hot-stylus recorders offer the advantages of an instantly visible tracing that is permanent, but are limited by the effects of friction and inertia in their frequency responses. In order to overcome this difficulty, the Swedish Elema–Schonander Company has developed an ink-jet recorder system which is linear up to 500 Hz and usable up to 900 Hz. The writing speed of the ink-jet recorder is given by $V = \omega A = 2\pi f A$, where ω is the angular frequency in radians per second, f is the writing frequency and A is the writing amplitude. For a 6-cm deflection at 500 Hz, the writing speed of the jet is 60 m/s; this compares with approximately 15 m/s for a hot-stylus waxed-paper recorder and optical light-beam recorders which have writing speeds between 1,000 and 10,000 m/s. Earlier models of the ink-jet recorder used moving coil galvanometers having single-turn

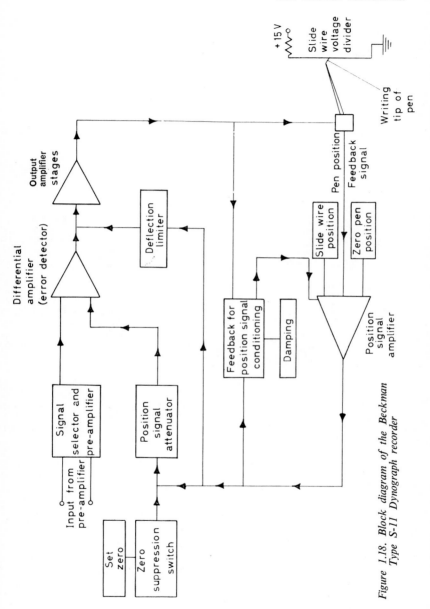

Figure 1.18. Block diagram of the Beckman Type S-11 Dynograph recorder

41

hairpin-type coils, requiring a drive current of 300 mA at 210 mV. Later models use a moving-magnet system. In this arrangement, a glass capillary tube 30 mm long is situated between the poles of an electromagnet, the coils of which are driven from a push-pull transistor amplifier. Glued to this capillary, so that it lies between the polepieces of the electromagnet is a small cylindrical permanent magnet (length 1 mm, diameter 0·7 mm, bore 1·2 mm). The electromagnetic field fluctuates in sympathy with the signal applied to that recording channel amplifier, and the interaction of the

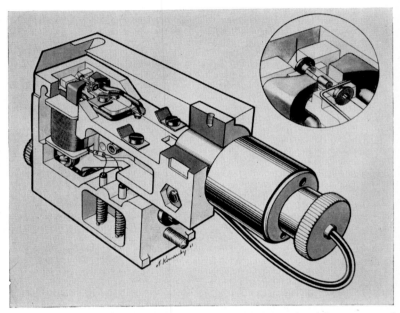

Figure 1.19. Moving-magnet ink-jet galvanometer. (Reproduced by courtesy of Elema-Schonander)

electromagnetic field with the permanent magnet deflects the capillary. The upper end of the capillary is shaped to a nozzle and bent through a right angle (*Figure 1.19*). Carefully filtered ink is pumped through the nozzle and the signal waveform is thus traced out on porous paper. The natural resonant frequency of the hairpin coil type is some 550 Hz and that of the moving magnet type some 600 Hz. In each case the frequency response of the galvanometer alone is flat to about two thirds of the natural resonant frequency.

The gain of the driving amplifier is arranged to fall off in an inverse fashion to the galvanometer resonance peak, so that the frequency response of the combination of galvanometer plus amplifier is linear up to 500 Hz. In both types of jet-recorder, the frequency response is given by:

$$f_0 = \frac{1}{2\pi}\sqrt{\frac{\text{deflection moment}}{\text{restoring force}}}$$

The stream of writing fluid beyond the jet no longer contributes mass to the moving system, so that in this respect it is superior to a purely mechanical system. As a result of air friction and air resistance, the fine stream of writing fluid from the 10 μm-diameter jet orifice breaks up into fine drops and reduces the available jet length.

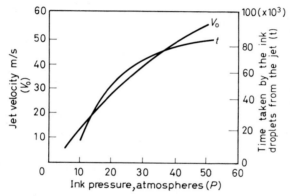

Figure 1.20. Relationship between the time taken by the ink droplets from the jet, the jet velocity and the ink pressure (after Sima, 1966)

Behaviour of the writing mass of fluid

The breaking-up of the jet after a certain distance means that the length of the writing 'arm' must be considerably shorter than that possible with optical galvanometers. In practice, a greater angle of deflection must be used and the deflection limited to 8 cm per channel. The jet stream consists of a large number of flying droplets; the maximum number per second limits the use of the liquid jet and governs the maximum possible writing speed. In *Figure 1.20* is shown the relationship between the time occupied by the droplets forced out of the jet (t), the velocity of the jet stream (V_0) and the fluid pressure (P). For a jet length of 40 mm and a 33·6 mm deflection

43

with a fluid pressure of 30 kp/cm², the transit time of a jet from nozzle to paper is given by $t = b/V_0 = 0.04/35 = 1.12$ ms for the zero line and $t = 0.052/35 = 1.48$ ms for the 40 degree deflection angle. The resulting phase shift when tracing a sine wave between the peak value and crossing point is of the order of 0.36 ms. In the case of the highest possible paper speed (1 m/s) the phase shift produced by the ink velocity is about 0.36 mm. This, for practical purposes is the thickness of the trace.

The ink leaves the orifice with a cross-section of about 0.01 mm and spreads during its travel to a diameter of about 0.03 mm at the correct pressure setting. As a result of the high energy imparted to the ink stream, on impact with the paper the ink is evenly distributed in the form of a circular ring having a diameter some ten times greater than the jet. When the ink pressure and impact velocity are too great, the drops of ink break up into many droplets to give what appears to be a fine mist and a liquid area forms around the recording arc.

The writing fluid is a pure chemical solution, not to be confused with normal inks. The addition of glycerin ensures that the ink will not dry out in the fine jet orifice on standing. In order to force the ink out of the nozzle a pump is required which can produce a maximum pressure of 45 atmospheres. The pressure used varies from 10 atmospheres at the lowest paper speeds to 35 atmospheres at the highest. In the standard model of the ink-jet recorder, an oscillating diaphragm pump is used, but other models use a d.c. motor driving an eccentric. In order to maintain a constant pressure the pump is followed by a pressure-reducing valve. For the model with the oscillating diaphragm pump driven by a solenoid, the pressure regulator alters the pump supply voltage continously to hold the pressure constant. The ink system is fitted with a relief valve, which releases the pressure when the recorder is switched off. This stops the jet when it is not required and reduces the possibility of the formation of air bubbles. After the trace has been formed, the paper drive pulls the paper under a porous ceramic roller. This removes any surplus ink and leaves a dry record. The roller should be washed at the end of each recording session. The recorder is also provided with a low-amplitude 1,000 Hz signal which modulates the trace produced by each channel. This acts to give a controllable width to the trace and reduces the formation of droplets on the paper. Since the writing fluid contains distilled water, the ink jet recorder cannot be used below 0°C. On average, about 5 ml of fluid will be used per hour of recording.

44

Tangent error in the ink-jet recorder

The ink-jet recorder, like the hot-stylus recorder, suffers from a tangent error. This is offset by using straight polepieces in the galvanometer to give a linear field, rather than the conventional curved pole-pieces which would give a radial magnetic field. The effective magnetic field is now proportional to the cosine of the angle of deflection and reduces the sensitivity at the larger deflections. This acts to compensate for the tangent error of the larger deflections. Oil damping is used with the moving-magnet system, together with a constant-current drive. This arrangement gives a frequency response flat up to 500 Hz. With a constant-voltage drive, the frequency response falls off sharply due to the increasing reactance of the coil. A detailed account of factors affecting ink-jet recorders is given by Sima (1966).

Hertz and Simonsson (1969) describe a simple arrangement for the intensity modulation of ink-jet recorders. This facility is useful for the introduction of time and event markers and direction indicators into the traces. It is also possible to adapt an ink-jet recorder to serve as a computer peripheral and to use the jet to write alpha-numeric characters, for example, to annotate the processed analogue output signal from the digital-to-analogue converter of a digital computer system. Lloyd *et al.* (1972) show how this arrangement can be used with the computer analysis of electro-encephalograms.

SLOW-RESPONSE RECORDERS

Strip or roll chart recorders

The most commonly encountered slow-speed recorder, apart from the potentiometric types, is the moving-coil instrument fitted with a pen arm. Essentially the movement is a more robust variation of the moving-coil meter movement, a typical full-scale sensitivity being 5 mA, although types fitted with a powerful magnet are available having a full-scale sensitivity of 1 mA. When the coil is attached directly to the pen arm, the pen writes in curvilinear coordinates. To produce a rectilinear trace a special linkage may be used, or the galvanometer mounted vertically above the chart paper so that the pen arm deflects at right angles to the motion of the chart. Although this type of recorder is widely used in industrial equipment, it is tending, for slow-speed applications, to be replaced in medical equipment by potentiometric recorders. These offer the advantages of a low input current requirement and the availability of a rectilinear tracing with chart widths normally of 6 or 10 inches as compared with a chart width commonly of 4 inches in moving-coil recorders. Small, chopper bar type recorders having a 1 mA moving-coil movement are convenient for use with apparatus such as portable oxygen polarographic electrode systems. At regular intervals the pointer is pressed down on to pressure-sensitive paper to form the tracing.

It is worth mentioning that paper chart dimensions can be affected by changes occurring in the relative humidity of the atmosphere. Lambert (1946) showed that for strip charts the width of the chart changed by 0·42 per cent at 30 per cent relative humidity and by 1·01 per cent at 90 per cent relative humidity. Carnes (1966) reported that the chart width is unlikely to change by more than 1 per cent for a relative humidity change of from 25 to 75 per cent.

Circular-chart recorders

In a circular-chart recorder the chart typically revolves once in 6, 12 or 24 hours. The technique of a circular chart is not easy to use with direct moving-coil movements. One system employs a moving-coil meter having a linkage which tracks the movement of a vane attached to the moving coil, a radiofrequency-coupled capacitance system being used. Circular-chart recorders are particularly useful for recording the baseline stability of an apparatus throughout the period of a working day, the chart, being compact, is easily filed for reference. In practice the time scale becomes very cramped for small deflections towards the centre of the chart making the trace difficult to read.

Recording inks

The cost of a good potentiometric recorder will be several hundred pounds and the weakest part of its performance may well lie in its pen design, particularly in its ink feed mechanism and the choice of ink. Most pens rely upon simple capillary attraction of the ink along the capillary tube feeding the pen tip. The tip may be a stainless steel hypodermic tube, a glass nozzle or a hole in a jewel. The ink reservoir is normally located slightly above the plane of writing to assist the flow of ink. The main requirements for a recorder ink are as follows:

(1) Fluidity. The ink must flow from the pen tip in an even manner so that the production of an intermittent trace is avoided.

(2) Evaporation. The ink must not dry in the pen feed tube and thus stop writing.

(3) Drying. The ink should dry on the chart paper within a few minutes to avoid the possibility of smudging the trace.

(4) Non-corrosion. The ink composition must be such that it does not corrode the ink reservoir, feed tube and pen tip.

Some inks are water based, some spirit based. It is advisable to use the brand of ink recommended by the recorder manufacturer and not to mix inks. The combination of recorder paper surface and ink must be compatible with a good writing action. It may be found that the pressure of the pen on the paper is insufficient to maintain a good contact across the full chart width, and this gives rise to gaps in the tracing. When it is found that ink will not flow freely from the pen, there is, in the author's experience, only one procedure to follow. This is to empty the reservoir of old ink, clean it and refill with fresh ink. Rod through the pen tip and feed tube with a fine wire to clear any deposits of dried ink. Using a tightly fitting narrow plastic tube attach a 2-ml disposable syringe to the pen tip and suck a substantial amount of ink through the pen tip to establish a continous column of ink in the feed tube. As an alternative to ink pens, many potentiometric recorders can be fitted with a ball-point pen.

POTENTIOMETRIC RECORDERS

The principle of a potentiometric recorder is illustrated in *Figure 1.21*. A slide-wire CD, which can be straight or circular, is supplied with a constant current from a battery or power supply B. The unknown d.c. input voltage to be measured is applied between the moving contact F of the slide-wire and one end, C. When the voltage tapped from the portion FC of the slide-wire is equal to the input voltage, a galvanometer placed as shown will indicate zero since there is no potential difference existing across its terminals. The slide wire is carefully constructed from a length of resistance wire of uniform

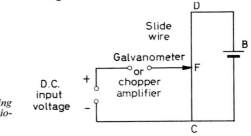

Figure 1.21. Basic operating principles of a potentio-metric recorder

71/72 (1·21)

cross-section so that the resistance per unit length is constant. With the slide wire supplied with a constant current, then, at balance, the distance CF is proportional to the unknown input voltage. The sliding contact F carries a pointer which moves across a linear scale, calibrated in voltage, typical scale spans being 1 mV or 10 mV In a practical potentiometric recorder the galvanometer is replaced by the input terminals of a high-gain chopper/type d.c. amplifier. This is a servo amplifier, the output of the amplifier feeding a servo motor which moves the sliding contact F through a cable linkage. If the input voltage to the recorder is greater than the voltage tapped off at CF then the motor will rotate in one direction, if it is less, then the motor will rotate in the opposite direction. In either case the sliding contact is moved in such a sense as to reduce the voltage applied to the amplifier input to zero. When this occurs the motor stops and the voltage indicated on the recorder scale is equal to the input voltage.

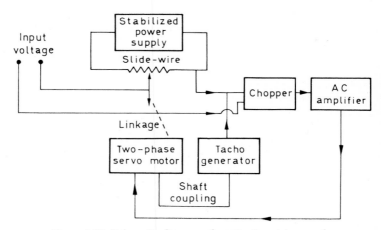

Figure 1.22. Schematic diagram of a potentiometric recorder

The system is illustrated in *Figure 1.22*. The chopper relay contacts are driven at the mains frequency, and their action converts the voltage difference between the input voltage and the slider voltage into a square-wave signal. This is amplified by the servo amplifier and applied to the control winding of a two-phase a.c. servo motor. The other winding is supplied with 50 Hz from a mains transformer and acts as a reference phase winding. When the voltage at the slider is greater than the input signal, the phase of the square wave from the chopper is such that the motor rotates in a direction to reduce the square-wave voltage to zero. If the voltage at the slider is less than the input signal, then the phase of the square wave becomes reversed and the motor rotates in the opposite direction. A typical balancing time for a potentiometric recorder is one second. Mechanical choppers with gold-plated contacts are preferred to transistor switches in order to minimize noise and d.c. offset potentials The shaft of the servo motor is coupled to a tacho-generator in order to minimize overshoot of the balance position. The function of the generator is to produce an output voltage which is proportional to the rotational speed of its shaft. The generator voltage is now applied as a feedback so that the servo motor slows down as it approaches the balance point. When the damping thus introduced is correctly adjusted, the effect is to cause the slider to move smoothly up to the balance position and stop. Were this arrangement not adopted, the slider would move rapidly up to the balance position, overshoot and then execute a damped oscillation.

In some potentiometric recorders, the slide-wire is energized from a 1·5-V Lechlanché cell. This will gradually run down, so that at 15-minute intervals a portion of the slide-wire voltage is automatically compared against that provided from a Weston (cadmium-mercury) standard cell. When the calibration of the recorder was initially established, the voltage from this fixed tap on the slide-wire was arranged to be equal to the standard cell voltage. Any difference found between the two due to the battery ageing is compensated by automatically reducing the resistance of a small rheostat placed in series with the slide-wire so that more current flows through the slide-wire in order to raise the voltage picked off at the tap.

At balance, the input resistance of a potentiometric recorder will be high since it is not drawing any current from the signal source. The actual value depends upon the setting of the input attenuator. Off balance, the input resistance may be quite low, perhaps 400 ohms in the case of a recorder having a transformer-coupled input to the servo amplifier. The resistance of the signal source may have a marked effect on the balancing time of the recorder. A source resistance which is too high for the particular recorder can make the recorder's response very sluggish. As an example, a recorder which has been designed specifically to work from low-resistance sources such as thermocouples may prove to be unsuitable for general-purpose work. Potentiometric recorders are available which will work with source resistances up to 800 ohms or so.

Typical paper speeds are 6, 12 or 20 inches per hour, the chart being driven from a synchronous electric motor via a gear box. When it is necessary to be able to record several slowly varying input signals in sequence, a printing-type potentiometric recorder may conveniently be used. An electrically driven selector switch connects the input signals in turn to the recorder. For each input signal, the recorder comes to a balance and then prints a number or symbol on the chart, the printing serving not only to measure the amplitude of that input signal but also to identify the input channel concerned. Such a recorder is useful for recording a number of temperatures during hypothermia such as rectal, nasopharyngeal and the cooling-bath temperatures. Another example occurs in the recording of renograms where three ratemeters are used connected to three scintillation counter channels, one counter being placed over each kidney and the third over the heart to record the blood background level of radioactive isotope.

A versatile potentiometric recorder is the Servoriter by Texas Instruments. This can have two potentiometric recorders writing on a common chart paper with a wide range of chart speeds ($1\frac{7}{8}$–30 cm, per minute, or per hour). The sensitivity is variable from 1 to 1000 mV full scale, on a 10-inch chart. In a typical application, one recorder-pen displays the dye dilution curve obtained during cardiac output measurements. The second pen shows the output from a special-purpose analogue computer which calculates the area under the dye curve and hence the cardiac output. This is a flat-bed recorder in which the chart is horizontal as opposed to conventional potentiometric recorders in which it is vertical. Thomas (1972) surveys the various types of chart recorder including moving coil, chopper bar, potentiometric and X–Y types.

X – Y RECORDERS

The recorder just mentioned has two separate potentiometric movements, but like most potentiometric recorders it is an Y–T recorder, since the movement of the chart on the X axis is simply a function of time. In an X–Y recorder, the chart sheet is fixed on a flat bed and the movement of the pen carriage is controlled along two mutually perpendicular axes by means of two independent potentiometric recorder systems. In this way the pen trace gives the relationship existing between two variables. In some X–Y recorders the paper sheet is held in place by clips, in others by means of suction developed by a fan, or by the use of magnetic paper. A time-base voltage is normally available for application to the X-input in order to convert the X–Y recorder into a Y–T recorder. In respiratory investigations X–Y recorders are useful to display pressure-volume and pressure-flow loops. They are also much used to display the output waveforms from analogue computers, for example, computer-simulated multi-component exponential curves.

ORDERS OF INSTRUMENTS

For a moving system such as a pressure transducer or pen recorder, the relationship between the forces giving rise to the motion and those tending to oppose it, is a second order differential equation of the form
$$F = M\mathrm{d}^2x/\mathrm{d}t^2 + R\mathrm{d}x/\mathrm{d}t + Sx$$
Where x = displacement, t = time, M = constant due to inertia, R = frictional or damping constant, S = stiffness constant, F = input signal or forcing.
This equation also holds for an electrical circuit if M is replaced by L the inductance, R is now an electrical resistance and S is replaced by the reciprocal of capacitance $1/C$. The velocity $\mathrm{d}x/\mathrm{d}t$ is replaced by the current $I = \mathrm{d}Q/\mathrm{d}t$ where Q is the electrical charge and $\mathrm{d}^2x/\mathrm{d}t^2$ is replaced by $\mathrm{d}I/\mathrm{d}t$.

The zero-order instrument

Here it is assumed that the effects of inertia and friction can be neglected, the result being a zero-order differential equation, that is, $F = Kx$ where K is a constant. The instrument thus responds immediately to the applied signal with no distortion. As an example, one can consider a pointer held in position by a spring.

The first-order instrument

Friction is now present, and the response of the instrument will lag behind the input force or signal. Friction slows down the build-up of the required motion as in the electrical case resistance slows down the current build-up. The first-order differential equation is $F = R\mathrm{d}x/\mathrm{d}t + Sx$. When a step response is presented, the instrument deflection is of the form $x = x_{max}(1 - \exp(-t/T))$ where $x_{max} = F/S$ and $T = R/S$. This is similar to the charging equation of a capacitor. There is no overshoot, the deflection increasing smoothly to a maximum. If a sine wave input is presented, the instrument responds in a sine wave fashion but with a time lag.

The second-order instrument

The response of a second-order instrument resembles that of a

51

first-order instrument in that it tends to lag behind the input signal, but the actual form of the response depends on the degree of damping present. Depending on this, overshoot or oscillation can occur for a step-function input, or resonance for a sinusoidal input. These factors are described in detail in relation to the behaviour of galvanometers.

CRITERIA FOR THE FAITHFUL REPRODUCTION OF A PHYSIOLOGICAL QUANTITY

A system designed to display physiological signals is, in general, composed of three main parts – transducer, processor and display. In order to ensure that the system faithfully reproduces the physiological event of interest, three conditions must be met by the individual parts of the system, or alternatively compensation must be introduced so that the whole system meets those conditions which are as follows.

(1) Linearity over the required range of signal amplitudes, both positive and negative.

(2) An adequate bandwidth for the signal of interest.

(3) Any phase shift introduced must be linearly related to the phase shift.

Amplitude distortion

The recording system should be capable of accepting any amplitude of signal up to the stated maximum, in both positive and negative directions, without causing distortion due to overloading. Doubling the input signal should double the output signal, and so on. This factor should be checked after it has been verified that the frequency and phase responses are adequate.

Frequency response

Any complicated waveform of a periodic nature can, by Fourier analysis, be represented as a constant plus harmonically related sine and cosine waves. Any signal which is a function of time, $F(t)$, can be expressed as:

$$Ft = A_0 + A_1 \cos 2\pi ft + A_2 \cos 4\pi ft + A_3 \cos 6\pi ft \ldots A_n \cos 2n\pi ft$$
$$+ B_1 \sin 2\pi ft + B_2 \sin 4\pi ft + B_3 \sin 6\pi ft \ldots B_n \sin 2n\pi ft.$$

If the waveform does not have a mean d.c. level then $A_0 = 0$, and for other waveforms some of the coefficients may be zero. In order to faithfully reproduce a given waveform it is necessary that all the significant harmonic frequencies be reproduced. For example, in an arterial blood pressure waveform the sixth harmonic has an amplitude of about 10 per cent that of the fundamental. For this type of rounded waveform, a flat frequency response out to at least the tenth harmonic will be adequate. For fine detail it will be necessary to be flat out to the twentieth harmonic or more. In the case of the electrocardiogram it may be necessary to be able to exceed 100 Hz for full accuracy. Hence the extent of the required frequency response is closely related to the degree of fidelity desired. It is the high-frequency end of the response which governs the reproduction of the rapidly changing portions of the wave. The bandwidth needed also extends below the fundamental frequency, by how much depends on the waveform. For example, in ECG recording it should go down to at least 0·2 Hz.

Phase distortion

If the various harmonics are preserved in their proper amplitude relationship, but are displaced in time, a form of distortion known as phase distortion results. Phase advance or retardation (lead or lag) is expressed as a fraction of a cycle by the phase angle θ. If the time displacement between the harmonics is t seconds, then $\theta = t/T \times 360$ degrees since 360 degrees corresponds to the periodic time T for one cycle of the wave. Since $T = 1/f$, $\theta = ft \times 360$ degrees, if each harmonic is to have an equal time displacement, k, then $\theta = kf \times 360$ degrees, that is, the phase angle must be directly proportional to the frequency of the particular harmonic. The harmonic components must be passed through the system in such a way that their phase relationship to the fundamental is preserved. It is possible to have phase distortion present with very little amplitude distortion.

Transient response

When a transient signal, such as a step function is applied to the input of a system, the rise-time of the output signal and the amount of overshoot occurring depend both upon the natural frequency of the system and upon its damping ratio. A linear system having a uniform frequency response and a linear phase shift over a defined frequency band will reproduce the components of a complex input signal with their correct amplitude and phase relationships provided that they lie within the frequency band. This happens even when there is an overshoot on transient signals. It will be remembered that in a second-order system a damping ratio of about 0·7 will produce an overshoot of about 4 per cent. The effect of damping, phase shift and frequency response on the characteristics of a useful low-pass filter is well illustrated by Goodman (1968).

Step function testing

In addition to the sine wave testing of recording systems, the step function test provides a useful additional method. As the name implies, a step function is a waveform which rapidly changes from one level to another.

Poor low-frequency response

In *Figure 1.23* it is shown that if the frequency response does not go down to d.c. the step cannot be maintained at the output, the output being of an exponential form. The time constant T of the

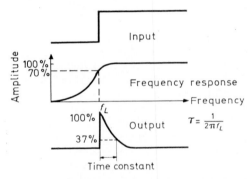

Figure 1.23. The effect of applying a step function input to a system having a poor low-frequency response

system is the time for the output amplitude to fall to 37 per cent of the maximum. The time constant is related to the sine wave frequency response by $T=1/2\pi f_L$ where $f_L=70$ per cent of flat frequency response. When a square wave is passed through an a.c. amplifier the amplifier time constant will introduce some degree of tilt on the flat top and bottom of the wave. For a single, lumped, time constant the sag will be 10 per cent if the duration of the square wave is about one tenth that of the time constant of the circuit, that is, 0·2 seconds for a 2-second time constant ECG recorder. The low frequency time constant of an ECG recorder is conveniently checked by observing the droop introduced on the calibration pulses produced by depressing the 1 mV button.

Poor high-frequency response

The effect of applying a step function to a system having a sine wave frequency response extending to d.c. but limited at the high frequency end is to slow down the rise time of the output signal, *Figure 1.24.*

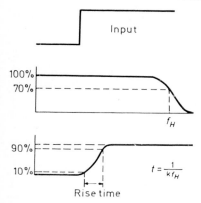

Figure 1.24. The effect of applying a step function input to a system having a poor high-frequency response

If the rise time, t is taken from 10 per cent to 90 per cent of the maximum amplitude, then $t = 1/kf_H$ where f_H is the frequency at which the response has fallen to 70 per cent and k depends on the high-frequency roll-off of the circuit. In practice k is often about 2 to 3.

STIMULATORS FOR NERVE AND MUSCLE

Stimulator circuits of various kinds are widely used to provide test signals in order to estimate the response of both nerve and muscle. Basically, the stimulator generates either a single pulse or trains of pulses having known characteristics of amplitude and width.

The simplest types of stimulator can consist only of a battery-powered blocking oscillator circuit which can be held in one hand. A typical application would arise in the testing of peripheral nerve response during anaesthesia. A suitable pulse width would be 1 ms with a pulse repetition rate of one per second, the output voltage being 90 V maximum. The circuit is provided with a high-impedance constant current output stage so that the current delivered to the patient is independent of normal variations in the electrode contact impedance. The stimulus current is variable between 0–15 mA.

More versatile stimulators use a variable-rate multivibrator to set the basic stimulus frequency. The output from the astable multivibrator triggers a monostable multivibrator circuit which sets the pulse width. Finally, the output pulse from the monostable is fed either to an emitter-follower stage in order to provide a low-output impedance constant-voltage output, or to a high-output impedance constant-current stage. A trigger pulse is usually available for triggering the timebase of a cathode-ray tube oscilloscope in order that the leading edge of the stimulus pulse can be observed on the screen. Typically, the pulse interval would be in the range 10 ms to 10 seconds in three switched ranges, with pulse widths from 0·1 ms to 100 ms covered in four switched ranges. For inducing tetanus, trains of pulses from 0·1 ms to one second are available. The stimulus amplitude can be varied from 0 to 1, 0 to 10 and 0 to 100 V. The constant-voltage output impedance would be less than 100 Ω, the constant-current output impedance being greater than 100,000 Ω.

It is necessary to guard against stimulus break-through. That is to say, the swamping of the evoked potential on the recorder by the much larger stimulus pulse. The stimulus is usually fed to the preparation via a balanced output transformer, the windings of which have sufficient inductance so that no significant droop is introduced into the pulse shape. The transformer provides a bipolar output which is isolated from earth, and is fitted with an electrostatic screen to reduce capacitive coupling. The response evoked by the stimulus is often detected by means of a low-noise parametric amplifier. This would have a floating input, an input impedance of (10 MΩ shunted by 1 pF) from each input terminal to earth and a broad-band noise level of less than 5 μV peak-to-peak. The capacity to earth of both the stimulating and pick-up electrodes to earth is thus low and the resistance to earth is high. This arrangement practically eliminates the stimulus artefact which arises from leakage current to earth through the preparation. If these precautions are not taken, stimulus break-through can completely mask the evoked potential.

For many purposes feeding the stimulus from a screened, balanced, transformer will reduce the stimulus artefact to a sufficient degree. However, other more sophisticated methods of isolating the stimulus from earth are available. One approach is to provide the stimulator circuit with a radio-frequency output stage. A radio link of a centimetre or two path is used to transfer energy into a tuned circuit coupled to the stimulator electrodes, thus removing any direct contact with the stimulator. Tomaszewski and Kadziela (1968) describe the use of a d.c. amplifier fitted with a radio-frequency output stage feeding into a cathode-ray tube oscilloscope as a stimulus current monitor. Barry and Davies (1968) employ a pair of field-effect transistors followed by two silicon transistors to form a simple stimulus isolation unit. It is suitable for use with a mains-powered stimulator for class studies of nerve *in vitro*. A new device

56

of interest for this application is a semiconductor device which functions as a light-activated coupler. The output of the stimulus pulse generator is fed to a gallium arsenide diode which emits pulses of infra-red radiation at about $0 \cdot 9$ μm. The intensity of the emitted radiation is controlled by the forward input current. The radiation descends upon a silicon photodiode which responds well at this wavelength. The d.c. current transfer ratio from input diode to output diode is approximately $0 \cdot 002$. In order to provide a current gain close to unity, the isolator is normally used in conjunction with a transistor current amplifier. The stray coupling impedance consists of 2 pF in parallel with 10^{11} Ω (Rose and Bassett 1967).

Constant-current stimulators are employed for muscle stimulation particularly for obtaining strength-duration curves. A high-current stimulator for the massive stimulation of isolated skeletal muscles is described by Ross and Brust (1968). The design of a constant-current stimulator for general use is that of Meyer (1967), while details of a constant-voltage stimulator are given by Bakema and Koopmans (1968). The latter circuit can supply pulses from 20 mV to 24 V in amplitude with a duration variable from $0 \cdot 5$ to 120 ms and a pulse repetition rate variable from $0 \cdot 25$ to 100 pulses per second.

THE USE OF COMPUTERS IN PATIENT MONITORING

Digital computers are being used increasingly in patient monitoring applications, not only to control data logging activities, but also to detect statistically significant trends in the patient's condition. Less frequently, they may also be used on-line to control the replacement of blood loss or the infusion of diuretic agents (Sheppard *et al.* 1968). A central processor with a core cycle time of the order of 1 micro-second and a size of at least 8 K and preferably 16 or 32 K is required for work with perhaps four patients. Since a digital computer operates upon a series of discrete numerical values, it is necessary to sample on a pre-determined basis the various physiological variables involved such as arterial blood pressure, body temperature, ECG, EEG and respiratory pattern. The sampling rate of the analogue-to-digital converter involved is chosen to suit the particular variable. It might be 100 per second for the arterial blood pressure, 60 for the EEG, and 10 for a dye dilution cardiac output curve. In order to identify the waves of each ECG complex, a sampling rate of 300 per second would be required. When only details of each R–R interval and R-wave width are needed for an arrhythmia analysis, the use of an analogue pre-processor in front of the digital machine can reduce

57

the number of samples needed to 2 per ECG complex (Sandman *et al.* 1972). *Figure 1.25* illustrates the effect of the intravenous injection of propranolol on the heart rate of a patient with a tachycardia. It is basically a plot of 128 successive R–R intervals in milliseconds, with each beat categorized by the computer. An average R–R interval and an R–Wave width is found for each group of 8 beats and each beat compared with the average for its group. A beat is called premature if its R–R interval is less than 80 per cent of the

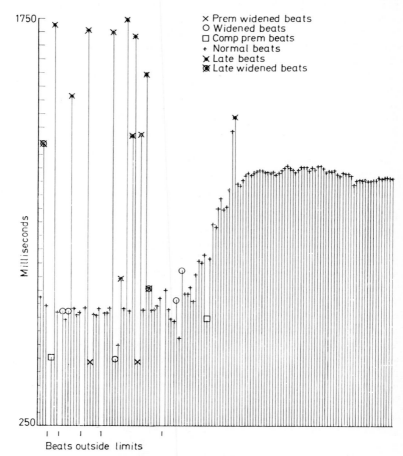

Figure 1.25. A computer plot of 128 successive R-R intervals illustrating the effect of the drug propanolol in terminating cardiac arrhythmias.

average, and wide if its R–wave width is more than 20 per cent greater than the average. The effect of the propranolol in slowing the heart and stopping the arrhythmias is clearly seen. Propranolol is a beta blocking agent. Another obvious application for an analogue pre-processor lies in the analysis of an arterial blood pressure waveform to yield the systolic, diastolic, pulse and mean pressures. If an analogue pre-processor is not suitable, then a reduction of stored ECG data by a factor of about 20 can be obtained if the turning points of the ECG are stored. That is to say, the time at which each turning point occurs, the amplitude of the ECG at that point and a symbol characterizing the nature of the turning point, e.g. whether it is from a plateau to positive or positive to negative, etc. This information is stored on-line on magnetic tape or on a disk and interrogated later to give details of P–R interval changes, for example.

The speed of a digital computer makes results available much more quickly than would be possible with manual calculation. A good example occurs in the calculation of cardiac outputs from dye dilution curves (Shubin, Weil and Rockwell, 1967). Within about one minute from the end of the description of the curve, the cardiac output is available, together with the appearance time, area under the curve, cardiac index, left ventricular work, and total systemic resistance (Gil-Rodriguez *et al.*, 1971). The use of the Fast Fourier Transform has made it possible to perform on-line frequency analyses of the EEG during surgery.

Most commercial patient monitoring modules provide a 1 V output which can be selected by the input multiplexer high level switches of the computer system (*Figure 1.2b*). Any additional analogue amplification or filtering (low-pass or mains frequency notch) can be supplied by an analogue conditioning amplifier provided for each channel prior to the high level channel selector multiplexer. Complicated programs such as those for EEG and ECG arrhythmia analysis may require more than 8 K of store. When several programs have to be run interleaved, it is necessary to have available a disk on the computer system. For storing data from three patients over periods of 10 hours, a 1 mega word fixed head disk would be suitable. The worst case time to *access* a given area of the disk is only 75 ms. In the case of digital magnetic tapes, blocks of data are stored serially, and the access time may be several hundred milliseconds or more.

Whilst it is convenient to print-up data from patient monitoring on a teleprinter or line printer in the computer˙room, the noise of

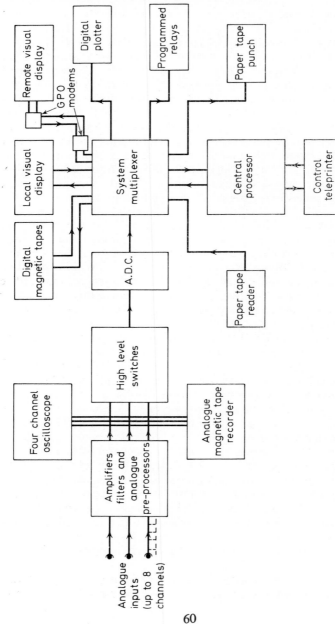

Figure 1.26. Block diagram of a digital computer system used for patient monitoring

these devices is too great for use in a surgical or intensive care environment. Here it is preferable to use some form of visual display unit. Alphanumeric information is displayed on the cathode ray tube or television screen of the visual display. A keyboard is usually provided for the entry into the computer system of numerical data concerning the patient. A digital graph plotter is a most useful off-line device for the production of trend curves and plots showing the effects of drugs.

The great advance brought by computers lies in the ability to take logical decisions. Hence more subtle warning and alarm systems are possible than the simple upper and lower limit conditions normally provided on patient monitors. Various tracking functions have been adapted from industrial stock control procedures to give warning of statistically significant trends in a patient's condition.

Although small, dedicated, bedside computers are available for patient monitoring purposes; the larger disk-based configurations need to be located at a distance from the patients concerned. Multi-way cabling is often used, but three-channel (0–100 Hz) analogue telephone data links make it possible to operate from distances of many miles if required (Hill and Payne, 1972). Standard digital telephone links operating at 1200 bauds can be used to return data from the computer to visual displays in the hospital.

Systems which are wholly core-based tend to be limited in their versatility and the relatively slow transfer rates for programs from magnetic tapes is also a severe limitation. In the case of a fixed head disk, the longest access time is of the order of 75 milliseconds so that the chaining together of programs drawn from the disk is very much faster than is possible with magnetic tapes.

A number of successful multi-bed patient monitoring systems have been reported from the U.S.A. Sheppard *et al.* (1968) have been particularly interested in monitoring patients following cardiac bypass. Using a visual display they monitored the values of the systolic and diastolic arterial pressures, the heart rate, central body temperature and right and left atrial pressures, the volume of fluid removed from the chest drains, the urine output and the volume of blood infused. The attending doctor enters into the computer system a value for the systolic arterial pressure for that patient. When the actual pressure is above the pre-set value, no blood is infused no matter how low the atrial pressures may be. It is assumed that above this level further increase in blood volume does not result in increased cardiac output. The physician also enters a value for atrial pressure, usually the left, which is considered the maximum level that can be attained without deleterious effect. The limit set for the left atrial pressure is generally between 12 and 25 mm Hg. When neither the systolic arterial nor atrial pressure limits are being exceeded, an increment of 20 ml of blood is automatically infused by the computer, using a roller pump actuated by a stepper motor.

Osborne *et al.* (1969) and Raison *et al.* (1970) have also developed a comprehensive computer-based monitoring system for patients requiring intensive care. An integrating pneumotachograph was used in conjunction with a fast response oxygen fuel cell to measure respiratory volumes and oxygen consumption. Airway pressure was also monitored, and this led to a monitoring of the patient's compliance and respiratory work. These parameters have proved valuable in the management of patients on a ventilator.

Jensen *et al.* (1966) have used a computer monitoring system in a unit dealing with patients in shock. In this connection it is important to monitor not only rectal temperature, but temperatures at the periphery such as the finger and big toe temperatures. Systolic, diastolic, pulse and mean arterial pressures were also logged, and the heart rate together with any deficit found between the pulse and ECG values for heart rate. The central venous pressure was measured and, using a low-pass filter, the respiratory swings were extracted from the signal and used to actuate a respiratory rate recording. The computer was also programmed to measure cardiac outputs by means of the dye dilution technique. A number of other computer applications to the monitoring of patients have been reported (Boam *et al.*, 1972; Cox *et al.*, 1968; Hilberman *et al.*, 1972; Neely *et al.*, 1971a, b; Rosi *et al.*, 1969; Siegal *et al.*, 1968; Hill, 1969; Weil *et al.* (1966); Wixson (1972).

Whereas conventional patient monitors are fitted merely with upper and lower limit alarm facilities—for example, bradycardia and tachycardia alarms—it is possible to point out trends which are statistically significant within defined limits by making use of the computer's power to take logical decisions. One approach to this problem is to make use of a tracking signal which will take on a positive or negative critical level when the quantity being tracked changes its value by a pre-determined amount based on an exponentially weighted-average value. This places more weight on recent data points than on points which occurred further back in the past. A good account of the use of Trigg's tracking signal (Trigg, 1964) is that of Lewis (1971). Yet another approach to detecting trends in a patient's condition using a digital computer is that of Taylor (1971).

Digital computers also have wide application to the sorting of patient's records of various kinds. Thompson and Moore (1971) describe the use of a computerized study to compare the action of three intravenous anaesthetic agents, whilst Hill and Bodman (1968) describe the computer sorting of the anaesthesia records of two groups of prostatectomy patients. Kolstad and Nordbye (1971) report on the use of a computer based medical record at the Norwegian Radium Hospital. The patients concerned had gynaecological cancer, the forms for computer input forming an integral part of the record. A simple and relatively inexpensive form reader was developed for the transfer of numerical data and written text into the computer. Thatcher (1971) discusses the changes which must come about in hospital medical record systems in order for full advantage to be taken of computer facilities. Vahl *et al.* (1971) have designed an editing system using a light pen for enhancing interesting features and removing artefacts from physiological data before automatic analysis.

Data logging systems are being used to record a large number of relatively slowly changing variables such as patients' pulse rates, body temperature and blood pressure. The output data from the logger can be stored on magnetic tape and subsequently analysed by a digital computer (Campbell *et al.*, 1970).

Computer systems of any complexity are expensive and require air-conditioned accommodation in order to achieve their best reliability. The effort required to produce a comprehensive set of applications programs is considerable and highly trained programmers are expensive. Thus a medical computer project should not be embarked upon without considerable planning and careful consideration of what is to be attempted and the time scale envisaged in relation to the currently available resources. With proper precautions, computers can provide invaluable assistance in the processing and statistical analysis of large amounts of data or of data which is generated in a short space of time.

TERMS COMMONLY ENCOUNTERED IN COMPUTING

Access time—The time required to locate a particular store address and either read the data in it or write data into it.

Absolute address—A number identifying a location in store.

Accumulator—A register or specific location in the central processing unit is which arithmetic or logical results can be formed.

Analogue signal—A representation of a variable by a physical quantity such as a voltage whose amplitude continuously represents the magnitude of the variable.

Alphanumeric—Letters of the alphabet; special symbols and numerals.

Application program—A set of program instructions for dealing with one aspect of the task to which the computer is being applied.

Arithmetic unit—That part of the computer which performs arithmetic operations.

Assembly language—Program instructions in the form of symbols or mnemonics. It is converted into machine code by the computer to enable the instructions to be used for controlling the computer's operation.

Background programming—Some executive programs support the use of computing time on a low priority basis concurrently with the running of on-line programs.

Backing store—Magnetic tape units, disks or drums.

Batch processing—A technique by which items are collected into groups for processing.

Bit—Binary digit (0 or 1).

Block—A group of data on paper tape or magnetic tape of convenient size for input-output operations to be performed.

Byte—A group of 8 bits.

Character—A digit, letter or special symbol.

Compiler—A program which converts high level language statements into machine code.

Control programs—Systems software—programs which govern the transfer of data to and from peripheral equiment and ensure its coordinated operation.

Control unit—That part of the computer which controls the execution of program instructions.

Core store—Date storage contained within the computer's central processor with an access time usually of the order of one microsecond. It is usually constructed from rows of ferrite cores and is almost always in slabs of 4096 (4 K) locations.

CPU central processing unit—Contains the arithmetic unit and core store. It directs the operation of the other equipment and performs computations. It usually has a control panel and on-line teleprinter.

Cycle time—The minimum time which must elapse between two successive references to a store location to insert or extract a word or character.

Data base—A file of data which fulfils a general rather than a specific information use.

Data link—A communications system used for transmitting and receiving data between remote terminals.

Dedicated—Devoted to one particular application.

Digit—A decimal digit (0 to 9).

Direct access store—A store in which data are not accessed in a serial manner and in which the time taken to access a location does not depend on the position of that location in store.

Disk store—A backing store in which data are stored on a number of concentric circular tracks on magnetic disks which rotate at a high speed giving direct access. Disks may be either fixed or exchangeable.

Duplex—Applies to communication channels providing transmission in two directions simultaneously. In half duplex operation, transmission is possible in both directions but not simultaneously.

Executive—A set of complicated routines mainly resident in the core store which control and monitor the computer's basic operations.

Fail soft—A computer or peripheral failure occurring without loss of data.

File—A collection of records.

Flagging—A method for tagging or identifying certain items in a file.

Hardware—The electromechanical and electronic portions of a computer system.

High level language—A programming language orientated to the natural language of the programmer (e.g. English). Each instruction generates several machine code instructions. A compiler is required to perform the conversion.

Instruction—The basic step in a program.

Jump—To transfer control of the computer to an instruction which is not necessarily the next in sequence; the jump may be conditional upon the result of a test, or unconditional.

Location—Part of a store; for example, an address.

Loop—A repetition of a sequence of instructions.

Low level language—See machine language.

Machine language (code)—The basic computer language consisting of instructions, each having a numerical code to describe the particular operation and one or more absolute addresses specifying the location of data.

Magnetic tape—A method for storing data on reels of magnetizable tape in computer accessible form. Records must be organized sequentially.

Mnemonic language—See assembly language.

Modem—MOdulator/DEModulator: a device used to transmit information by a frequency modulation system over telephone lines.

Multi-access—A system allowing several terminals to have access to one central computer.

Multi-programming—A computer system capable of storing more than one program at a time. Each program is obeyed for a short time in an appropriate sequence in order to achieve an optimum utilization of the computer and its peripherals.

Multi-processing—A computer system in which two or more processors are under the control of a single operating system and share memory, input-output control units and peripherals.

Object language—Machine language.

Off-line—A computer system in which the output from other off-line equipment is transported to an on-line input device directly connected to the computer.

On-line—Applies to any equipment or function in the system connected directly to the computer.

Operation—The action required to be performed by the computer and specified in an instruction.

Operating system—A set of routines for supervizing the operations of a computer system.

Overlay—A section of a program, held in a backing store, which is transferred to the core store only when it is actually required for immediate execution.

Pack—To store several small items in the area normally provided for one word or record.

Packing density—The amount of information which can be recorded in a given space, e.g. the density in bits per inch on magnetic tape.

Random—A sequence in which it is impossible to predict, from a knowledge only of the preceding numbers of the sequence, what the next number will be.

Real time—Processing of data by a computer sufficiently rapidly for events to be detected or influenced as they occur.

Record—A related group of data comprising a number of items.

Register—A unit of internal storage in the computer normally associated with the arithmetic and control units.

Routine—Part of a program.

Source language—The programming language used by the programmer.

Subroutine (procedure)—A routine arranged so that control can be passed between it and the main program in order to avoid duplicating similar sequences of instructions and to provide for the inclusion of previously proven sections of program.

Time-sharing system—A computer system which uses one device for two or more concurrent operations, e.g. a computer system in which several users share direct on-line access to separate programs and data files.

Word—A unit of storage comprising a number of bits, e.g. a 16 bit word length.

REFERENCES

Carnes, F. C. (1966). 'Selecting paper for recorder charts.' *J. Instrum. Soc. Am.*, (Dec.) 55

Ertel, P. Y., Lawrence, M., Brown, R. K., and Stern, A. M. (1966). 'Stethoscope acoustics, I, II. *Circulation*, **34**, 889

Gibson, J. M., Gibson, M. M., and Hirsch, H. R. (1970). 'Distortion of neural data by "notch" filters.' *Med. biol. Engng.*, **8**, 95

Goodman, A. H. (1968). 'Low-pass filters for electromagnetic flow meters.' *Med. Electron. biol. Engng.*, **6**, 477

Hertz, C. H., and Simonsson, S. I. (1969). 'Intensity modulation of ink-jet oscillographs.' *Med. biol. Engng.*, **7**, 337

Holdack, K., Luisada, A. A., and Lieda, H. (1965). 'Standardization of phonocardiography.' *Am. J. Cardiol.*, **15**, 419

Lambert, L. B. (1946). 'The production of recorder charts.' *Instrum. Pract.*, **1**, 24

Lloyd, D. S. L., Binnie, C. D., Stenfors, S. G. B., and Roberts, J. R. (1972). 'Character generation on a moving chart recorder.' *Bio-Med. Engng.*, **7**, 274

Mable, S. E. R., and Stone, R. N. (1965). 'An oscilloscope for clinical display.' *Wld. med. Electron. Instrum. (Lond.)*, **3**, 256

Prior, Pamela, F., Maynard, D. E., Sheaff, P. C., Simpson, B. R., Strunin, L., Weaver, E. J. M., and Scott, D. F. (1971). 'Monitoring cerebral function: clinical experience with new device for continuous recording of electrical activity of brain.' *Br. med. J.*, **2**, 736

Shackel, B. (1967). 'Eye movement recording by electro-oculography.' In *Manual of Psycho-physiological Methods*, p. 310, Amsterdam; North Holland Pbl.

Sima, H. (1966). 'Flussigkeitsstrahl-Oszillografen.' *Elektronik*, **6**, 179 and **7**, 213

Smale, A. J. (1967). 'Recording medical signals.' *Electron. Pwr.*, **13**, 452

Thomas, J. A. (1972). 'Chart recorders.' *Electronic Pwr.*, **18**, 244

Van Vollenhoven, E., Van Rotterdam, A., Dorebos, T., and Schlesinger, F. (1969). 'Frequency analysis of heart murmurs.' *Med. biol. Engng.*, **7**, 227

— and Wallenburg, J. (1970). 'Calibration of air microphones for phonocardiography.' *Med. biol. Engng.*, **8**, 309

Stimulators

Bakema, H, and Koopmans, J. J. C. (1968). 'A transistorized constant voltage stimulator for use in combination with mechanical recording.' *Med. Electron. Biol. Engng.*, **6,** 199

Barry, W., and Davies, H. E. F. (1968). 'F.E.T. isolation unit for a nerve stimulator.' *Electron. Engng.*, **40,** 143

Meyer, A. A. (1967). 'A transistorized stimulator for student's use, with constant-current output, for use in physiology.' *Med. Electron. Biol. Engng.*, **5,** 61

Ross, S. M., and Bassett, A. L. (1967). 'Stimulus isolation employing a light-activated coupler.' *J. Appl. Physiol.*, **22,** 820

— and Brust, M. (1968). 'A transistorized high-current, long-pulse amplifier for massive stimulation of isolated skeletal muscle.' *J. Appl. Physiol.*, **24,** 583

Tomaszewski, R., and Kadziela, W., (1968). 'A d.c. Amplifier with Radio-frequency output used as a stimulus current monitor.' *Acta physiol.pol.* **19,** 127

Computers

Boam, B., Ostlund, J., Stauffer, W., and Reed, J. (1972). 'Use of the digital computer in monitoring paediatric intensive care patients.' *J. Advancem. med. instrum.* **6,** 70

Campbell, D. E. S., Ekstedt, J., Hedberg, A., and Oldberg, B. (1970). 'Automatic data collection for computer calculation of instrument measurements in research laboratories.' *Comput. Prog. Biomed. (Amst.)*, **1,** 171

Cox, J. R., Jnr., Nolle, F. M., Fozzard, H. A., and Oliver, G. C. (1968). 'Aztec, a pre-processing program for real-time ECG rhythm analysis.' *I.E.E.E. Trans Bio-med. Engng.*, BME. **15,** 128

Gil-Rodriguez, J. A., Hill, D. W., Horny, J. T., Lundberg, S., and Wilcock, A. H. (1970). 'A comparison of some methods for estimating the area under a dye dilution curve.' *Br. J. Anaesth.*, **42,** 981

Hilbermand, M., Patitucci, P. J., and Peters, R. M. (1972). 'On-line assessment of cardiac and pulmonary patho-physiology in the acutely ill.' *J. Advancem. Med. Instrum.*, **6,** 65

Hill, D. W. (1969). 'Computers in the management of shock.' In *Physiological and Practical Aspects of Shock*, Ed. by J. Freeman (Int. Anesthesiology Clin., Vol. 9, p. 1035). Boston; Little, Brown.

— and Bodman, R. I. (1968). 'The application of a computer sorting program to prostatectomy patients.' *Br. J. Anaesth.*, **40,** 785

— and Payne, J. P., (1972). 'The use of analogue telephone data links for the transmission of physiological signals.' *Br. J. Anaesth.*, **44,** 562

Jensen, R. E., Shubin, H., Meagher, P. F., and Weil, M. H. (1966). 'On-line computer monitoring of the seriously ill patient.' *Med. biol. Engng.*, **4,** 265

Kolstad, P., and Nordbye, K. (1971). 'A computer based medical record.' *Acta obstet. gynec. scand.*, **50,** supp. (57).

Lewis, C. D. (1971). 'Statistical monitoring techniques,' *Med. biol. Engng.*, **9,** 315

Neely, W. A., Robinson, W. T., Holloman, G. H., and McMullan, E. H. (1971a). 'An inexpensive bedside analogue computer for measuring respiratory work and certain other parameters.' *Surgery*, **69**, 309

—, — Hardy, J. D., and Bubo, W. O. (1971b). 'A computer analysis of pulmonary function in surgical patients.' *Ann. thorac. Surg.*, **11**, 565

Osborn, J. J., Beaumont, J. O., Raison, J. C. A., Russell, J., and Gerbode, F. (1969). 'Measurement and monitoring of acutely ill patients by digital computer.' *Surgery*, **64**, 1057.

Raison, J. C. A., Osborn, J. J., Beaumont, J. O., and Gerbode, F. (1970). 'Oxygen consumption after open heart surgery measured by a digital computer system.' *Ann. Surg.*, **171**, 471

Rosi, P. S., Yokochi, H., Deller, S., Quinn, M., Greenberg, A. G., Rabib, S., Blatt, S., Lewis, J., and Jacobs, J. E. (1969). 'Non-invasive patient monitoring.' *Surg. Forum.*, **20**, 234

Sandman, A., Hill, D. W., and Wilcock, H. A. (1973). 'An analogue pre-processor for the measurement, by a digital computer of R–R intervals and R–wave widths. *Med. biol. Engng.* (In Press)

Sheppard, L. C., Kouchoukos, N. T., Kurtts, M. A., and Kirklin, J. W. (1968). 'Automated treatment of critically ill patients following operation.' *Ann. Surg.*, **168**, 596

Shubin, H., Weil, M. H., and Rockwell, M. A. (1967). 'Automated measurement of arterial blood pressure in patients by use of a digital computer.' *Med. biol. Engng.*, **5**, 353

Siegal, J. H., Greenspan, M., Cohen, J. D., and DelGuercio, L. R. M. (1968). 'A bedside computer and physiologic nomograms.' *Arch. Surg.*, **97**, 480

Taylor, D. E. M. (1971). 'Computer-assisted patient monitor systems.' *Bio-med. Engng.*, **6**, 560

Thatcher, R. A. (1971). 'New concepts in design of medical records in the computer era.' *Med. J. Aust.*, **1**, 1080

Thompson, G. E., and Moore, D. C. (1971). 'Ketamine, Diazepam, and Innovar: A computerized comparative study.' *Anesth. Analg. Curr. Res.*, **50**, 458

Trigg, D. W. (1964). 'Monitoring a forecasting system.' *Opl. Res. Q.*, **15**, 271

Vahl, S. P., Vickery, J. C., Monro, D. M., and Tinker, J. (1971). 'An interactive computer-based editing system for physiological data.' *Comput. biol. Med.*, **1**, 317

Weil, M. H., Shubin, H., and Rand, W. M. (1966). 'Experience with a digital computer for study and improved management of the critically ill.' *J. Am. med. Ass.*, **198**, 147

Wixson, S. E. (1972). 'Acute myocardial infarction computer applications.' *J. Advancem. Med. Instrum.*, **6**, 55

2 –Pressure Transducers and Myographs

PRESSURE TRANSDUCERS

Quantitative information concerning a patient's condition can be obtained by applying to him various sensing devices. Those physical properties such as temperature, pressure, sound intensity and force to name but a few examples, have to be changed into a corresponding electrical signal. Devices which convert one physical property into another are called transducers. While mechanical transducers are encountered, for example, the aneroid pressure manometer, or mercury-in-glass thermometer, there is a particular interest in those transducers which give an electrical output signal. This type of transducer can be made very versatile and offers a number of advantages in practice. These include the following.

(1) The transducer can be placed in a relatively inaccessible recording site. For instance, in the recording of heart sounds or blood pressure from the tip of a cardiac catheter; or pressures in the gut by means of an endoradiosonde.

(2) The sensitivity of the transducer is often very high and the gain of the associated amplifier can be varied over a wide range.

(3) The frequency response of the transducer and its amplifier can often be very high, so that high fidelity recording of dynamic phenomena is possible.

(4) It is axiomatic that the taking of measurements should not interfere significantly with the quantity being measured. The high sensitivity of modern transducers means that they impose a negligible loading upon the system under test. In some cases there need be no physical contact between the transducer and the subject. This occurs in arrangements which measure heat or gamma radiation emitted by the subject, or which sense changes in the direction or intensity of light or ultrasound reflected from the subject.

(5) Modern practice is to arrange to normalize the electrical signals produced by each transducer used in a particular investigation. That is to say, that a transducer is followed by a 'signal conditioner' which adjusts its output to a common signal level, typically one volt. The signal conditioner will provide any necessary gain or frequency response adjustment. In this way the signal from any transducer is made compatible with the input signal required for the driver amplifiers of the channels of a multi-channel display unit. This is normally either a cathode-ray tube display or pen recorder. By this means it is easily possible to interchange recording channels and to observe the time relationships of a number of physical quantities. Provision is normally made to be able to feed the signals from each recording channel into a magnetic tape recording system or into some additional data processing system such as a frequency analyser or an analogue or digital computer.

In order that it can be recorded electrically, a physiological pressure must first be transformed or transduced into a corresponding electrical signal which can be subsequently amplified and displayed on a recorder. In medical applications, probably the most widely encountered transducers are the various forms of pressure transducer. The range of pressures to be measured extends from a few millimetres of water in pneumotachograph work, through millimetres of mercury in venous pressure measurements, centimetres of water in respiratory pressure studies, to centimetres of mercury in arterial blood pressure measurements. Transducers are also available for recording gas pressures up to hundreds of atmospheres. Lower pressure versions can be used to monitor pressure fluctuations in hospital pipeline systems.

Pressure is defined as 'force per unit area'. Pressure transducers normally operate upon the principle of applying the pressure to be measured to a stiff diaphragm and sensing the movement of the diaphragm. In its simplest form a diaphragm is a thin flat plate of circular shape, attached firmly by its edge to the wall of a containing vessel. On applying a higher pressure to one side than the other, the diaphragm deflects away from the high pressure, the movement being greatest at the centre (*Figure 2.1.*) Only for small deflections is there a linear relationship between the diaphragm deflection and the applied pressure, non-linearity becoming noticeable when the deflection approaches half the diaphragm thickness. A larger, and more linear deflection than could be obtained from a flat diaphragm is given by a circular diaphragm having concentric corrugations. The linear range of the diaphragm depends on a number of factors including the number of corrugations, the depth of each corrugation, the thickness of the diaphragm material, the radius of each corrugation from the centre and the physical properties of the material. In order to achieve a high-frequency response and a low-volume sensitivity in physiological pressure transducers it follows that the diaphragm movement must be small, and that a sensitive system is required to detect the diaphragm motion. Typical diaphragm materials are phosphor bronze, stainless steel and beryllium copper.

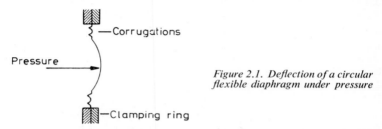

Figure 2.1. Deflection of a circular flexible diaphragm under pressure

The three most common arrangements for use with diaphragms are; (1) to make the diaphragm one plate of a capacitor; (2) to connect the diaphragm to the core of a differential transformer; and (3) to attach to the diaphragm a strain gauge bridge.

Variable capacitance transducers

Capacitance transducers operate upon the principle that the electrical capacitance existing between a pair of metal plates alters with the separation of the plates. The closer the plates, the greater the capacitance existing between them. One plate is normally stationary, the other forming the diaphragm to which the pressure is applied. Provided that care is taken to exclude dirt, the plate separation can be made very small, so that small movements of the diaphragm can give rise to appreciable capacity changes. Capacitance manometers are suitable for use when a high sensitivity and natural frequency are required, the high natural frequency arising from the use of a stiff diaphragm. Particular care must be taken in the construction of capacitance manometers to ensure that their temperature stability is comparable with strain gauge and differential transformer types. A differential contraction or expansion of the manometer component parts will produce a capacitance change which is recorded as an artefact. Pressey (1953) discusses the reduction of temperature effects in capacitance transducers in relation to the choice of materials and method of construction.

72

The capacitance of the gauge is used as part of the tuning element in a radiofrequency modulation system. In some cases it may be possible to have the capacitance manometer and its associated oscillator mounted together on a chassis as, for example, in manometers designed to measure down to fractions of a millimetre of water pressure (Hill, 1959). If the capacitance manometer is connected directly to its modulation circuit via a cable, the capacity of the cable in parallel with the manometer will tend to reduce the sensitivity of the arrangement. In addition, the temperature coefficient of the cable capacitance may give rise to a significant shift in the baseline of the recording. Haines (1960) has described a very useful circuit which can be used with the capacitance transducer situated at the end of up to 300 feet of coaxial cable. With the advent

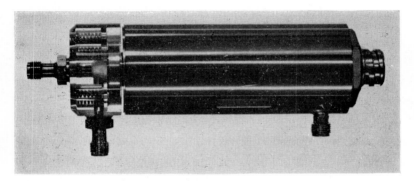

Figure 2.2. Capacitance blood pressure manometer with housing holding the oscillator and demodulator. (Reproduced by courtesy of Elema-Schonander)

of compact transistorized circuitry, an alternative approach is now possible. In *Figure 2.2* is shown a capacitance manometer designed for physiological measurements. The housing includes the oscillator and demodulator for the frequency modulation system, the cable connecting to the main recorder supplying power and carrying the output signal from the gauge. The arrangement provides a d.c. signal which can be used with any driver amplifier in a multi-channel recorder. The classical papers on the use of capacitance manometers in blood pressure measurement are those of Lilly, Legallais and Cherry (1947) and Hansen (1949). One disadvantage of capacitance manometers is the need for a special radiofrequency energizing system, and they cannot always be directly interchanged for strain gauge manometers in multi-channel recording systems.

73

Variable inductance transducers

The effective inductance of a coil can be altered by changing the position of a core of magnetic material lying within the magnetic field of the coil. The coil forms part of an audiofrequency a.c. bridge, or it can act as the tuning inductance of a radiotelemetry transmitter, as in an endoradiosonde or 'radio pill' (Mackay, 1968; Gleason and Lattimer, 1962). The principle of this type of gauge is shown in *Figure 2.3*. Movement of the core due to a pressure increase on the diaphragm will increase the frequency of the transistor oscillator if the diaphragm is made from a ferromagnetic material and decrease it if the diaphragm is of aluminium. The restoring force on the diaphragm comes mainly from the compressibility of the air trapped behind the diaphragm, rather than from the elasticity of the diaphragm. This might change due to contact with body fluids if the

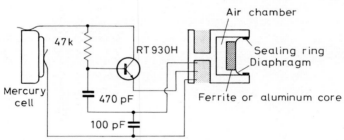

Figure 2.3. Schematic diagram of a radio pill designed to monitor pressure fluctuations in the gastrointestinal tract (after Mackay, 1968)

endoradiosonde is placed in the gut. If there are no leaks present, the action of the air behind the diaphragm will stay constant, giving a constant pressure calibration before ingestion and after passage from the body. The battery life with continuous operation is about 3 days. The radiated signal is received on an f.m. receiver which has a d.c. output from its discriminator circuit. This output is fed to a pen recorder, the pen deflection being related to the pressure applied to the diaphragm. Juhasz and Harris (1965) mention a miniature inductive pressure transducer 2 mm in diameter and 8 mm long. Its sensitivity was 0·15 mV/mmHg pressure per volt excitation, and the transducer was produced for intracardiac pressure measurements. Juhasz and Harris state that the main difficulties encountered in the construction of this type of transducer lie in non-linearity associated with the magnetic materials and problems of magnetic screening.

The optical de-focusing pressure manometer

In a de-focusing pressure manometer, the pressure to be measured is applied to a capsule which consists of two chambers from a flexible optically-reflecting diaphragm (Greer, 1964). Light from a low-voltage lamp is divided by mirrors into two beams which fall one on to each face of the thin polyester diaphragm which is aluminized on both sides to provide mirror surfaces (*Figure 2.4a*). When there is no pressure differential across the diaphragm, both faces act as plane mirrors so that the intensities of the light reflected from each side will be approximately equal. If a positive pressure is applied to the left side of the chamber with respect to the right, then the diaphragm will tend to bow inward towards the right-hand side. This forms a concave or converging mirror on the left-hand side and a convex or

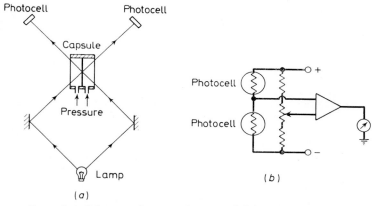

Figure 2.4. Schematic diagram of an optical defocusing manometer

diverging mirror on the right-hand side. As a result, the intensity of light falling on the left-hand photocell is increased whilst that falling on the right-hand photocell is decreased. The pair of photocells is connected in a bridge arrangement with an operational amplifier, as shown in *Figure 2.4b*. The unbalance of the bridge is linearly related to the pressure difference across the capsule. This is used to deflect a meter scaled in terms of pressure and to provide a 1 V FSD output signal. Pressure ranges of 1, 3, 10, 30, 100, 300, 1,000 and 3,000 mm of water are available, and the capsule is said to be able to withstand an overload equal to 10 times the full-scale pressure for 5 minutes. The response time is quoted as 100 ms. Whelpton (1968) finds that silicon solar cells are able to provide a more stable baseline than do cadmium sulphide photocells. This is important when the de-focussing manometer is to be followed by an integrator as in an integrating pneumotachograph. The manometer can be run from a battery or d.c. power supply in the range 12–18 V at about 60 mA, so that it is suitable for portable applications.

Linear variable-differential transformer pressure transducers

The principle of the linear variable-differential transformer is illustrated in *Figure 2.5*. When the ferromagnetic core is symmetrically disposed between the primary winding and the two secondary windings, the construction is such that the a.c. voltage induced in each of the secondaries is of equal magnitude but opposite phase.

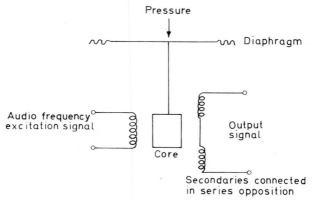

Figure 2.5. Principle of the linear variable differential transformer

When this occurs there will be no output from the combined secondary windings which are connected in series opposition. The effect of applying a pressure to the diaphragm is to move the core and produce an electrical imbalance. This results in the production of a net output voltage from the combined secondaries. The phase of the output voltage will reverse as the core moves through the central position. By using a phase-sensitive rectifier, the sign of the resulting d.c. output voltage will depend upon whether a positive or negative pressure difference exists across the transducer diaphragm. In practice there is not a complete absence of output at the null position of the core, since any harmonics of the excitation frequency (usually a few kilocycles per second) are still present. These are backed-off electrically by means of the circuit zero control.

Differential transformer pressure transducers are supplied in the well known Sanborn range of physiological recording equipment. The audiofrequency carrier pre-amplifier with which they are used can also operate with strain gauge transducers. The transducer is excited with 6 V at 2,000 Hz.

An example of a differential transformer pressure transducer is shown in *Figure 2.6*.

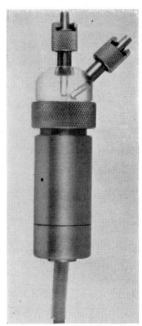

Figure 2.6. Differential transformer pressure transducer. (Reproduced by courtesy of Hewlett Packard)

Juhasz and McPherson (1963) describe the construction of a differential transformer pressure transducer for use in biological experiments.

STRAIN GAUGES

The development of strain gauges arose from the need in engineering practice to be able to measure the effects of tension and compression in beams. The applied force per unit area is known as the *stress,* and the resulting increase in length per unit length is known as the *strain*. In a rigid structure the strain will be small, and sensitive gauges capable of measuring it had to be developed. The

77

basic operation of the original wire strain gauge lies in the fact that if a wire is stretched, its electrical resistance will increase. Conversely, if the wire is caused to contract, its resistance will decrease. An increase in the wire resistance will arise from an increase in its length, a decrease in its cross-sectional area, and possibly a small change in the resistive properties of the material. The 'gauge factor' of a wire wire strain gauge is defined as

$$F=\frac{r/R}{l/L}$$

where R is the original resistance of the gauge, r is the change produced in its resistance, L is the original length of wire used, and l is the change produced in its length. Typically, a gauge made from Nichrome wire might have a resistance of 220 Ω and a gauge factor of 2·25, while a similar gauge in stainless steel wire might have a

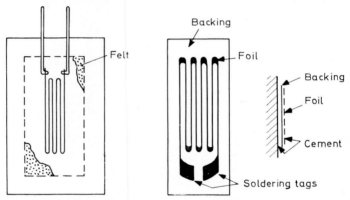

Figure 2.7. Wire strain gauge   Figure 2.8. Etched foil strain gauge

resistance of 200 Ω and a gauge factor of 3·1. The gauge factor of the wire material mainly determines the sensitivity of the gauge. The wire used should be chosen to possess a low temperature coefficient of resistance. In a practical wire strain gauge (*Figure 2.7,*) the wire is formed into a zig-zag pattern and is firmly bonded on to an impregnated paper. The dimensions of the 200 Ω Nichrome wire gauge are 25 mm long by 4 mm wide. Etched metal foil gauges are also available, *Figure 2.8.* In use, these gauges are firmly bonded with an adhesive to the member or diaphragm whose movement is to be recorded. Hence this type of strain gauge is known as a 'bonded strain gauge'.

78

Consider a cantilever beam as shown in *Figure 2.9*, having one strain gauge bonded to the upper surface, and a second gauge bonded to the lower surface. The two gauges are placed in opposite

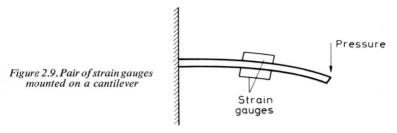

Figure 2.9. Pair of strain gauges mounted on a cantilever

arms of a Wheatstone bridge network as shown in *Figure 2.10*. As a result, changes in the resistances of the two gauges arising from changes in the ambient temperature are cancelled. The effect of strain in the cantilever, however, is to increase the resistance of the upper gauge and decrease the resistance of the lower gauge, thus unbalancing the bridge. This type of bridge arrangement is known

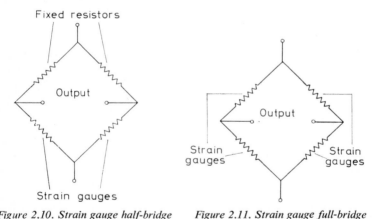

Figure 2.10. Strain gauge half-bridge   *Figure 2.11. Strain gauge full-bridge*

as a 'half-bridge'. Double the sensitivity is obtained by the use of a 'full-bridge'. Two gauges are now placed on top of the cantilever and two on the under-surface. The positions of the gauges in the bridge are shown in *Figure 2.11*. In some recording systems, the strain gauge bridge is energized with a stabilized d.c. voltage and the bridge output amplified with a chopper-type d.c. amplifier

(Offner Dynograph). In other systems (Sanborn), the bridge is energized with a stabilized audiofrequency supply and the output fed into a carrier amplifier. Both full and half bridge input positions are provided. For the half bridge position, a pair of matched reference resistors is built into the strain gauge pre-amplifier to complete the bridge circuit.

A stiff metal cantilever fitted with strain gauges makes a convenient isometric myograph for recording contractions of muscle; the tip of the cantilever is joined to the muscle via a length of thread, for example, in an organ bath study of a smooth muscle strip.

Silicon bonded strain gauges

In recent years attention has transferred from bonded wire and foil strain gauges to bonded gauges made from silicon semiconductor material and making use of the piezo-electric effect. Whereas a Nichrome wire strain gauge might have a gauge factor of 2·4, that of a semiconductor gauge might be 120, or 50 times greater than that of the wire gauge. A disadvantage of semiconductor strain gauges lies in their greater temperature sensitivity, and to a lesser extent, in their non-linearity. Both of these effects can be minimized by using a full bridge configuration. A description of semiconductor strain gauges is given by Thorp and Jones (1968). The conventional wire or foil element is now replaced by a single crystal filament of silicon. The thin strip of silicon is cut from a single crystal and processed to a finished size of less than 0·0005 inch thick by 0·01 inch wide. The silicon element is mounted on a substrate of epoxy resin and glass fibre, with nickel strips for the electrical connections. The interconnection between the silicon and the nickel strips is made by gold wires, bonded to the silicon and welded to the nickel. The complete assembly is coated with epoxy resin to give protection from abrasion and environmental condition. The high output from silicon gauges means that they can often be worked into a simple battery and meter circuit, no chopper amplifier being necessary.

A useful feature of silicon strain gauges lies in the fact that by suitably doping the material, the gauge can be made to have either a positive or a negative gauge factor. In this way, for a strain which is only tensile (or compressive), both positive and negative resistance changes can be produced. With two gauges of each type, a full bridge can be made to respond to strains of the same sign in each of the four arms.

The gauge factor of a silicon gauge is markedly temperature dependent. Typically for a gauge made from p-type silicon, the gauge factor increases by some 2·5 per cent for a 20°C increase in temperature. Thermistors can be incorporated in the bridge for temperature compensation, or a combination of suitably chosen p-type and n-type gauges used.

Forse (1965) gives a full account of the manufacture and mounting of semiconductor strain gauges. The doping of single crystal silicon with phosphorus produces gauges with negative resistance/strain characteristics, while boron doping gives gauges having positive resistance/strain characteristics. The strain measured by a bonded strain gauge is given by $S=l/L$ where l is the change in length arising from the application of the applied stress, and L is the unstressed length. S is commonly expressed as a percentage, typical values encountered in metal structures lying in the range 0·05–0·5 per cent. For numerical convenience, the strain value is usually multiplied by 10^6 to give values of microstrain. For temperatures in the range —20°C to +80°C and for strains up to 3,000 microstrain, standard epoxy strain gauge cements are satisfactory. Forse (1965) discusses the curing schedule for epoxy cements and the subsequent mounting of the gauge. A general account of strain gauges is that of Neubert (1968).

Silicon-diaphragm pressure transducers

The availability of integrated circuit techniques has led to the development of silicon-diaphragm pressure transducers in which a number of silicon strain gauges have been laid down on the back of the diaphragm. The circular diaphragm of single crystal silicon material first has a layer of silicon dioxide grown over its surface by heating in a furnace at about 1,000°C in a suitable atmosphere. It is necessary to control the thickness of this oxide film. Insufficient thickness will give poor insulation to the aluminium tracks which are later deposited upon it for bringing out the electrical connections. Too great a thickness may spoil the definition of the etching process used to produce the silicon strain gauge elements. The silicon dioxide is next etched free in those positions on the diaphragm where the gauges are to be laid down. The etched diaphragm is replaced in the furnace through which is passed the dopant atmosphere such as boron or phosphorus. Diffusion takes place through the windows etched in the oxide film forming a number of p-n isolated junction resistors. During this process a thin oxide layer will have grown over the diffused area, and contact holes must be then etched out at the ends of the gauges. Contacts are now laid down to the gauges by vacuum depositing a film of aluminium and subsequently etching away the excess. In practice, eight gauge elements might be laid down, four near the centre of the diaphragm and four towards its periphery. As shown in *Figure 2.12*, when the diaphragm is deflected, the resistance of the centre gauges increases while that of the peripheral gauges decreases. The most closely matched pairs at the centre and periphery are connected as a Wheatstone bridge. The diaphragm is held at the edge only by alloying the silicon to a ring of metal having a similar coefficient of expansion. An output of 25 mV per 100 mmHg pressure applied to the diaphragm is possible with a 10 V excitation (a.c. or d.c.). The diaphragm diameter is of

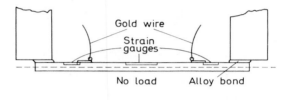

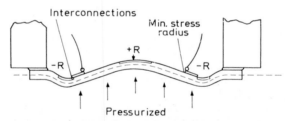

Figure 2.12. Deflection diagram for a silicon diaphragm (after Thorp and Jones, 1968)

the order of 0·2 inch. The natural frequency of such a transducer is approximately 20 kHz. An advantage of silicon gauges lies in their mechanical ruggedness. An applied pressure of 5,000 mmHg did not produce any change in the calibration of such a gauge. The type SE4–81 gauge by S. E. Laboratories Ltd. recommended for blood pressure recording has a full-scale sensitivity of ±300 mmHg and can withstand 5,000 mmHg requiring a 10 V excitation. The input and output impedance of the SE4–81 transducer is 1,000 Ω. Silicon has a Young's modulus close to that of steel and is elastic to the breaking point.

The use of a stiff silicon diaphragm produces a high natural frequency and also makes the gauge proof against a considerable degree of overpressurization. With unbonded strain gauge transducers it is more easily possible to damage the gauge by applying pressure from a flushing syringe when the exit tap from the system is inadvertently closed. These facts, together with the high sensitivity possible are illustrated by the following specification of a typical silicon diaphragm blood pressure transducer (Type 462 by the Birtcher Corporation).

Volume of transducer chamber	0·2 cm³
Diaphragm diameter	6·5 mm
Undamped natural resonant frequency	5 kHz
Excitation	11·4 mA d.c.
Pressure range	−100 to +300 mmHg
Over pressure	Not greater than 10 times full scale
Linearity and hysteresis	±1 per cent full scale (±3 mmHg)
Temperature coefficient	±2 mmHg/°C maximum at 25 mV output
Output voltage	15 mV d.c. ±5 per cent at 300 mmHg at operating temperature

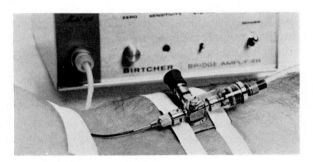

Figure 2.13. Silicon-diaphragm blood pressure transducer.
(Reproduced by courtesy of Birtcher Corporation)

In *Figure 2.13* is illustrated the Type 462 gauge mounted on a small metal plate for positioning on the body surface. The calibration stability is such that for most purposes an electrical rather than a pressure calibration can be used. For this the bridge is unbalanced by means of a push-button control to give an output signal equivalent to that produced by a pressure of 100 mmHg. The three-way stopcock enables zero pressure to be set or the system flushed. When the rubber septum is fitted to the side-arm, an anticoagulant or drugs can be injected through it. The solid-state d.c. amplifier used with the gauges provides zero-setting, sensitivity controls and a calibration facility.

The high sensitivity of silicon-diaphragm gauges is well illustrated by the S.E. Laboratories Type SE4–81 arterial blood pressure gauge which requires a volume displacement of only 0.01 mm^3/100 mmHg. A flat frequency response out to 100 Hz is obtainable with this gauge plus a 1 metre-long No. 7F catheter.

Mercury strain gauges

Thin, flexible, rubber tubes filled with mercury are commonly used to estimate changes produced in the diameter of a limb during use of the technique of venous plethysmography to investigate the magnitude of the peripheral circulation. The venous return to the limb is occluded when an observation is to be made. The resultant swelling of the limb gives rise to an output from the strain gauge bridge which is related to the inflow of blood to the limb. The method is normally used to observe relative blood flow changes, and care must be taken to minimize artefacts due to temperature changes. Mercury strain gauges have a low impedance of the order of an ohm or two, and are usually worked into an a.c. bridge via a step-down matching transformer. Some relevant papers are those of Elsner, Eagan and Anderson (1959), Whitney (1953) and Greenfield, Witney and Mowbray (1963).

Unbonded strain gauge transducers

Unbonded wire strain gauges have been, perhaps, the most well known of the popular pressure transducers for direct blood pressure recording. The American Statham and CEC gauges are of this type. The arrangement is shown schematically in *Figure 2.14a*. Four strain-sensitive wires are connected as shown, to the two supporting frames. One frame fits loosely inside the other. The inner, movable, frame is connected to the diaphragm upon which the applied pressure acts. The outer frame is fixed. Enough initial tension is applied to the wires to keep them under some residual tension when the moving frame is at either end of its travel. Mechanical stops prevent overload of the wires. A positive pressure applied to the diaphragm stretches wires B and C, and relaxes wires A and D. The wires form a four-arm active (full) bridge. The inner frame is mounted on springs which act to return the moving frame to a central position in the absence of pressure applied to the diaphragm. Referring to *Figure 2.14(b)*, extra resistors are placed inside the gauge housing to adjust the performance to a standard specification. The unbonded strain gauge transducer is preferred for the measurement of low pressures, since hysteresis errors are less than would be the case if wire gauges were bonded to the diaphragm. Typically, an unbonded strain gauge transducer might be energized with a 10 V d.c. supply. The bridge output is of the order of microvolts, so that a high-gain d.c. amplifier is required to follow the bridge.

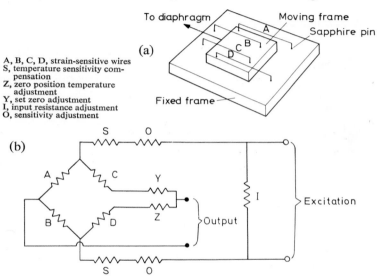

A, B, C, D, strain-sensitive wires
S, temperature sensitivity compensation
Z, zero position temperature adjustment
Y, set zero adjustment
I, input resistance adjustment
O, sensitivity adjustment

Figure 2.14. (a) Schematic diagram of an unbonded strain gauge pressure transducer; (b) compensation resistors mounted in the pressure gauge housing

The characteristics of a well-known unbonded strain gauge pressure transducer are:

Statham Type P 23 D pressure transducer

Pressure range	0–750 mmHg
Excitation	10 V maximum (a.c. or d.c.)
Output resistance	300 Ω
Output voltage	50 μV/mmHg at 10 V excitation (d.c.)
Volume displacement	0·04 mm³/100 mmHg

Unbonded strain gauge pressure transducers, such as the Statham Type SF 1 are small enough to be mounted at the tip of a cardiac catheter. The catheter has a union which can be used for flushing or the withdrawal of blood samples.

Ayling (1968) gives a design for an accurate transistorized control unit for use with strain-gauge pressure transducers. Corbett and Macmillan (1967) give details of a simple control box for use with two strain-gauge pressure transducers. The box has outputs giving the sum or the difference of the two pressures, or the individual pressures.

Ardill, Fentem and Wellard (1967) describe a modification to the dome-shaped cuvette normally supplied with the Consolidated Electrodynamics Corporation strain-gauge arterial blood pressure transducer. The volume of the original cuvette plus two conventional three-way taps was 1·15 ml and the new design reduces this to 0·15 ml, and makes it possible to flush out all small bubbles. All junctions where bubbles might lurk are visible through the Perspex. For the measurement of human arterial blood pressure the transducer is connected by 20 cm of flexible transparent tubing (Portex No. 3, 1 mm bore) to a 21 S.W.G. needle. The CEC cuvette with this system had a natural frequency response to 80 Hz and a response flat to within ±5 per cent up to 30 Hz. The redesigned cuvette had a natural frequency of 159 Hz. A degree of mechanical damping was made possible in the new head by incorporating a stainless steel plug which could be rotated in order to partially occlude the pressure-transmitting channel. When this was correctly adjusted the frequency response was flat to within ±5 per cent out to 70 Hz. Bacteriological tests confirmed that the cuvette could be effectively sterilized by leaving it full of a 2 per cent formalin solution for 12 hours. Macmillan and Stott (1968) describe a helical stenosis for providing hydraulic damping.

Catheter-tip pressure transducers

The problems associated with the inertia of the metre long fluid column contained in a cardiac catheter connected to an external pressure transducer can be eliminated by placing a miniature pressure transducer at the tip of the catheter. Millar and Baker (1972) describe a catheter-tip transducer which is 12 mm long by 1·65 mm in diameter and is mounted at the end of a 1·5 metre long No. 5 French cardiac catheter. In addition to the electrical connection wires, the catheter also contains a tube which is used to connect the rear of the transducer's diaphragm to atmospheric pressure. The transducer employs discrete semi-conductor strain gauge elements bonded to a miniature silicon diaphragm. The measurement pressure range is plus and minus 300 mm Hg and an overpressure of up to 1500 mm Hg will not damage the gauge. The volume displacement is 2×10^{-3} mm³ per 100 mm Hg and the nominal sensitivity is 0·1 V per 300 mm Hg for a 3·5 V excitation. This can be either a.c. or d.c. The natural frequency of the transducer is 15 kHz, so that it may also be used to record heart sounds. The linearity and hysteresis are within plus or minus 0·5 per cent of full scale from 0 to 300 mm Hg. Using temperature compensation gauges on the diaphragm a temperature stability of plus or minus 0·15 mm Hg per °C is obtainable.

In view of the difficulty and risk associated with the placing of a cardiac catheter, it is highly desirable that its base line and calibration should drift as little as possible during the recording period and that means should be provided for checking these. Millar and Baker (1972) state that because of the good physical and thermal stability of their transducer, they can switch in a separate reference half of the associated Wheatstone bridge. One setting simulates the zero pressure situation; others provide known amounts of unbalance corresponding to different pressure steps. A high-pass filter is switched in when it is required to record heart sounds. With an excitation of 5·4 V d.c., the leakage current into the patient from the catheter was only 22×10^{-9} A.

An alternative approach is to make use of fibre optic bundles to transmit white light from an external source up and down the catheter. A small mirror at the distal end of the catheter also acts as a diaphragm and is distorted by the pulsatile blood pressure acting on it. The light reflected from the mirror is thus modulated by the blood pressure and, falling on a photocell, gives an electrical output. Lekholm and Lindstrom (1969) describe such a transducer and state that its frequency response extends out to 15 kHz.

MANOMETER CALIBRATION SYSTEMS

Henry, Wilner and Harrison (1967) describe a calibrator for catheter-manometer systems. It is capable of applying simultaneously a static pressure (0–200 mmHg) and a sinusoidal pressure (0–70 mmHg) at a continuously variable frequency (5–2 kHz). Bubbles in the system are detected by significant changes occurring in the resonance frequency with changing static pressure. Another form of pressure generator for calibrating catheter-manometer systems is that of

Stegall (1967). It uses an oscillograph's power amplifier to drive an underwater loudspeaker.

A four-tap arrangement for use with arterial pressure transducers is proposed by Hepburn (1967) based upon a functional analysis of the requirements for recording, flushing, calibrating and setting the zero.

RESONANCE EFFECTS WITH NEEDLES AND CATHETERS

The purpose of a complete pressure transducer system is to reproduce a varying pressure with minimal amplitude and phase distortion and with a maximal frequency response. Wiggers (1928) states that a frequency response linear out to the tenth harmonic of the pressure signal is adequate, while Macdonald (1960) suggests an upper limit of about 100 Hz. To this end the damping factor of manometer plus cannula or catheter should be adjusted to be about 0·7. The un-damped natural frequency of the manometer alone must be considerably above that of the complete system. With modern silicon gauges the resonant frequency of the gauge alone can be greater than 5 kHz. By fitting an adjustable damping segment between the transducer and the catheter or cannula it is possible to select the optimal damping to give a flat frequency response. For a 78-cm, 19-gauge polyvinyl catheter the frequency response could be flat out to 70 Hz (*Figure 2.15*).

Hansen (1949) discusses the effects of damping on cardiac catheter systems in detail, and illustrates how resonant vibrations in the system, if not damped out, can distort the tracings. Damping adjustment is also discussed by Ardill, Fentem and Wellard (1967).

An interesting paper is that by Latimer and Latimer (1969). By the use of transmission line theory it is shown how it is possible to determine the properties of a catheter-manometer system with a view to establishing the optimum frequency response.

The use of small diameter catheters

The small volume displacement required by modern electronic blood pressure transducers makes possible the use of small-lumen arterial catheters having an external diameter of only 0·8 mm. These can be left in position for up to 8 days without risk of a thrombotic occlusion of the vessel. The small calibre prevents haematoma formation after withdrawal. Care must be taken to see that the cutting tip of the needle used to puncture the artery does not sever

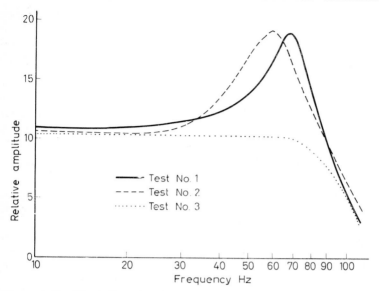

Figure 2.15. Effect of varying the damping on the frequency response of a capacitance pressure transducer and catheter system

the catheter as it is introduced. In use, a steady flow of 4·5 ml of sterile saline per hour is passed through the catheter to prevent blood clotting in it. The saline, in a disposable plastic bag, is pressurized by surrounding the bag with a cuff inflated to about 300 mmHg. The flow rate is set by a stainless steel capillary leak. A wider tube can be switched in parallel with the leak to give a higher rate of flow for rapid flushing. Venous catheters of 0·8 mm external diameter are also available for right heart catheterization. The narrow, flexible tube is floated by the venous blood stream into the right heart and on into the pulmonary artery. The frequency of such a catheter extends out to 40 Hz. No hydraulic damping control is required.

The use of miniature cardiac catheters has been described by Bradley (1964) and by Etsten *et al.* (1955). Scheinman *et al.* (1969) showed the value of miniature catheters for the investigation of cardiovascular function in patients who might be considered to be too ill for the use of conventional catheter techniques. Mostert *et al.* (1970) used 90 cm long catheters of 1·65 mm outside diameter radiopaque polyethylene tubing to catheterise the right ventricle and pulmonary artery of patients in chronic renal failure. In their paper they show a dramatic photograph of a catheter which has formed into a series of knots. The movement of the heart spontaneously initiated the formation of the knots after the catheter was allowed to curl up in the right atrium. Following this, the distance from the site of venepuncture to the right atrium was always ascertained by holding the catheter first over the patient along the route it was to follow and then over a measuring stick. Care was taken not to float the catheter further than about 1 cm distal to the tricuspid valve so as to avoid its coiling up inside a dilated cardiac chamber or its tributaries.

THE DISPLAY OF SYSTOLIC, DIASTOLIC AND MEAN ARTERIAL PRESSURE FROM A PRESSURE TRANSDUCER

Although the systolic, diastolic and mean blood pressures can be estimated from the tracing of a pen recorder connected to the output from a suitable pressure transducer, this becomes tedious when the readings have to be made known to an operator at regular intervals, perhaps while the transducer needle is being inserted into a chamber of a patient's heart. McGough and McDonald (1968) describe a battery-powered display unit for use with the carrier amplifier supplying an unbonded strain gauge pressure transducer. A pair of capacitors are charged via silicon diodes to store a voltage proportional to the positive (systolic) and negative (diastolic) peaks of the arterial pressure waveform. The reading circuit for each capacitor consists of a balanced pair of metal-oxide-silicon transistors with a 50-μA full-scale deflection meter connected with a series resistor across their sources. The gate of one M.O.S.T. is connected to the capacitor, the gate of the other M.O.S.T. serving as a 'set zero' control. The circuit is given a 5·5-second time constant so that the meters will follow changes in the systolic and diastolic levels. When required, a smoothing circuit can be switched in to show the mean arterial pressure.

The site of pressure measurement

Conventionally, blood pressure is referred to atmospheric pressure at the height of the heart. A correction of $-7·8$ mmHg must be applied for every 10 cm the site of measurement is below the height of the heart. This is obviously particularly important in the measurement of venous pressure (Borrow and Escaro, 1968).

The recording of central venous pressure

The use of a central venous catheter is an important aid to the management of patients who are seriously ill with, for example, cardiac failure, and those with low blood volumes. It can provide a valuable guide to the replenishment of blood volume and the fact that this has not overloaded the circulation. The catheter is commonly made from polytetrafluoroethylene (TEFLON) and its tip is usually located in the superior vena cava to avoid complications associated with placing it in the right atrium. Sykes (1963) reports a wide range of central venous pressures (0–12 cm H_2O with a mean of 5 cm H_2O) in normal patients. No correlation has been found between central venous pressure, and age, race, arterial pressure, heart rate, height or weight (Latimer, 1971). Latimer suggests a reference level for central venous pressure measurement of 10 cm above the table with the patient supine. Central venous pressure is commonly measured with a saline manometer or an aneroid capsule pressure gauge. Latimer connects the gauge by an air-filled tube to a small plastic coil taped to the patient's chest at the reference level. The coil is filled with saline and is connected to the central venous catheter by a saline-filled tube. The saline-air interface within the coil is free to move with the pressure but is localized within the coil. The air-filled tube allows the manometer to be positioned anywhere as convenient. The coil localizes the interface at the reference level so that levelling of the gauge is not required even if the patient moves from lying to sitting.

Because a frequency response of a few Hz is adequate for venous pressure recording, special venous pressure transducers have been developed with a high sensitivity and which can be taped to the patient at the reference level. A typical bonded strain gauge semiconductor pressure transducer for this application would have a sensitivity of 200 micro-volts per mm Hg at 10 V d.c. excitation and a pressure range of -10 to $+100$ mm Hg. The transducer is excited from a small mains powered unit carrying a meter scaled -5 to 30 mm Hg and -5 to 40 cm H_2O. The unit's supply isolation transformer has a screened primary winding to minimize leakage currents, and one side of the transducer's excitation is earthed so that any residual leakage current flows directly to earth.

PHYSICAL ASPECTS OF ELECTROMANOMETRY

As has been previously mentioned, in order to obtain accurate dynamic recordings of rapidly changing pressures, such as the arterial blood pressure, particular attention must be paid to the design of the hydraulic system as a whole. This includes not only the pressure transducer but the associated tubing, adapters and taps. In order that the recording is not distorted, the recording hydraulic system must be capable of performing simple harmonic oscillations at frequencies in excess of the highest harmonic component of the pressure signal. That is to say, a high undamped natural frequency is required. Noble (1953) shows that the behaviour of the pressure transducer system can be considered in terms of a simple mechanical analogue consisting of an oscillating spring, fixed at one end and carrying a mass at the other (*Figure 2.16*.) The behaviour of the transducer system is governed by three main factors:

(1) The mass of the liquid column which oscillates in the catheter or needle attached to the manometer.

(2) The stiffness of the transducer diaphragm. This provides the spring factor.

(3) The viscous resistance providing damping in the catheter or needle. This arises from the motion of the liquid as the diaphragm moves.

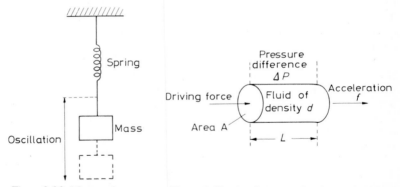

Figure 2.16. Mass-spring analogue for a hydraulic pressure transducer-catheter system

Figure 2.17. Acceleration of a segment of fluid in a catheter

The action of the system is controlled by the simultaneous influence of three physical laws. Newton's Law of Motion directly relates the acceleration of the mass to the force acting upon it. Hooke's Law relates the movement of the elastic diaphragm to the

92

force it experiences and Stoke's Law relates the resistance offered by the fluid column to the force acting upon it. These proportionalities can be expressed as:

M = mass = force/acceleration
R = resistance = force/velocity
S = stiffness = force/displacement

For this type of mass-spring analogue, Noble (1953) shows that the undamped natural frequency, $f_0 = \dfrac{1}{2\pi}(S/M)^{\frac{1}{2}}$. In the practical case when damping is present, let the damped frequency be f_d. Then $f_d/f_0 = (1 - R^2/4MS)^{\frac{1}{2}}$. Clearly, damping lowers the oscillation frequency. When the damping is two-thirds of critical then

$$f_d/f_0 = \sqrt{[1 - (\tfrac{2}{3})^2]} = \sqrt{5/3} = 74 \cdot 5 \text{ per cent}$$

of the undamped natural frequency.

Further comparison of the electromanometer with the mass-spring analogue

In purely mechanical systems such as recording pens there exists a relationship between the applied force, the resulting displacement and acceleration and the mass of the system. The hydraulic system differs in that it has a distributed volume of fluid rather than a discrete mass. It is desirable to work in terms of volume and pressure rather than displacement and force. It is then possible to obtain an equivalent mass for the fluid.

In *Figure 2.17*, let ΔP be the pressure differential existing across an element of fluid of cross-sectional area A, length L and density d. Applying Newton's Law of Motion, force = mass × acceleration, that is, $A\Delta P = (dLA) \times f$ where f is the acceleration. If the volume acceleration is defined as $F = Af$, then $\Delta P = dLF/A$. This is similar to force = mass × acceleration where dLA is the equivalent mass of fluid. The volume of the pressure transducer chamber is normally small, typically $0 \cdot 2$ ml. Suppose that a transducer has a silicon diaphragm 5 mm in diameter. For a chamber volume of $0 \cdot 2$ ml, the chamber length will be 10 mm. Let this be connected to a metre-long catheter of internal diameter 1 mm. The equivalent mass of fluid in each case is $dL\pi r^2$. The ratio of the effective masses is 2,700 : 1. Hence the fluid inertia (effective mass) of the catheter is much greater than that of the chamber. This result is to be expected since the velocity of the fluid will be greater in the narrow-bore catheter than in the wider chamber.

In the spring-mass analogue, the spring possesses a stiffness. The stiffness of the diaphragm in a pressure transducer is defined in terms of the pressure which must be applied in order to give rise to a unit increase in volume. Thus $S=\Delta P/\Delta V$. The reciprocal of the stiffness is the compliance (slackness). This is generally known as the volume displacement ($\Delta V/\Delta P$). It is usually quoted in terms of mm³/100 mmHg pressure. For the SE 4–81 silicon diaphragm blood pressure transducer made by S.E. Laboratories it is less than 0·01 mm³/100 mmHg.

Damping of the motion of the fluid in the catheter arises from the viscous resistance of the catheter. Assuming streamline flow conditions, Poiseuille's equation gives $V=\pi P.r^4/8\eta L$ where V is the volume flow per second, P is the pressure differential across the catheter, r is the radius and L the length of the catheter. The resistance to flow is $P/V=8L\eta/\pi r^4$, where η is the viscosity of the fluid.

Frequency response of the transducer-catheter system

The undamped natural frequency of the mass-spring system was given by $f_0=1/2\pi.(S/M)^{\frac{1}{2}}$. For the system of transducer plus catheter or needle this expression becomes $f_0=(r/2).(\Delta P/\pi L.\Delta V)^{\frac{1}{2}}$ where r is the catheter or needle radius in cm, L is the catheter or needle length in cm, ΔP is the pressure increment in dynes/cm² and ΔV is the volume increment in cm³; f_0 is in Hz.

In order to obtain a high undamped natural frequency, the bore of the needle or catheter should be as large as possible and its length as short as possible. The diameter is far more important than the length in determining f_0 which also varies as the square root of the pressure/volume ratio. This means that the stiffness of the diaphragm must be made very much greater in order to significantly increase f_0.

The damping factor for the system is $D=R/2(MS)^{\frac{1}{2}}$. On substituting for M, R and S this becomes $D=(4\eta/R^3).(L\Delta V\pi)^{\frac{1}{2}}$ assuming that the density $= 1$. It can be seen that the radius of the catheter or needle is an all-important factor in determining the damping. Since D is proportional to $1/R^3$ and to $L^{\frac{1}{2}}$ the effect of length will be less important. The damping can be varied by introducing an adjustable constriction into the line. As in the case of recorders for optimum frequency response D should be set at 0·7. The use of narrow catheters demands a pressure transducer which has a very low volume displacement. Clearly, the stiffer the diaphragm the smaller will be the sensitivity so that a compromise has to be reached. Great care must be taken, by boiling the system if possible, to remove any air

94

bubbles which may be present. The compressibility of the gas in the bubble will greatly reduce the frequency response of the system.

Adjustment of the damping

As with recorders, the frequency response of the hydraulic system can be determined either by observing the sine-wave frequency response with a manometer-calibration pressure generator as has been previously described, or by applying a step function input, and setting the damping to give about a 6 per cent overshoot. The fluid-filled catheter is connected to a syringe having a metal plunger, the last few inches of catheter proximal to the syringe being filled with air. The syringe plunger has a hole along its axis which can be occluded by placing a finger on top of the plunger. With the hole open the plunger is placed in the barrel, the hole is then closed and the plunger rapidly withdrawn to give a negative-going pressure step. Hydraulic damping is the best. Adjustment of the electrical damping control on the transducer amplifier may not give the same results.

ISOMETRIC MYOGRAPHS

An isometric myograph measures the contractile force of a muscle or muscle fibre under such conditions that the muscle undergoes a negligible change in length. One end of the muscle might be fixed to a stiff cantilever carrying strain gauges. If only sharp contractions are to be sensed, the movement of the cantilever can be detected with the aid of the stylus and crystal from a gramophone pick-up. Biro, Rusnakova and Rusnak (1966) use the RCA Type 5734 triode valve as a mechanoelectric transducer. The output voltage developed by this triode is very sensitive to small displacements of its anode. Biro, Rusnakova and Rusnak mention that muscle fibres are extended by a constant tension 10–100 times greater than the changes arising from contraction of the muscle. The signal due to the residual tension can be backed off and the full sensitivity preserved.

A myograph featuring an electrical-to-mechanical transducer for loading the preparation is discussed by Noyes (1967). This system employs a thermoelectric heat pump to achieve a close temperature regulation of the muscle. Bassett, Ross and Hoffman (1967) have studied the contractile force of isolated cardiac muscle. Their apparatus enabled the length and force of the contracting muscle to be controlled and monitored.

Cardiac force and blood vessel stress transducers

A requirement exists to measure the contractile force of the beating heart. Feigl, Simon and Fry (1967) describe force transducers which are coupled to the heart by a set of pins thrust through the myocardium. The transducers can be used to measure tensile stress (force per unit area) in the beating myocardium under isometric or auxotonic conditions. Boniface, Brodie and Walton (1953) used a strain gauge arch sutured to the wall of the left or right ventricle. Brown (1960) used strain gauges to investigate the effect of anaesthesia upon the contractile force of the heart.

Janicki and Patel (1968) have designed a force gauge for the measurement of the longitudinal stresses developed in a blood vessel *in situ*. It consists of two parallel beams joined at the ends by means of brass flexure plates. A fixed extension (leg) is attached to the lower beam and a movable leg to the upper beam. The distance between the two legs can be varied from 9 to 11 cm. The bottoms of the legs can be attached to cylindrical plugs which are inserted inside the blood vessel. Each flexure plate carries a pair of strain gauges, the whole forming a full bridge.

INDIRECT METHODS FOR MEASURING AND RECORDING ARTERIAL BLOOD PRESSURE

Electrical pressure transducers offer the advantage that they can be used to measure and record both venous and arterial blood pressures, even in cases of shock when the pressure is low. It is, however, necessary to perform an arterial puncture to connect the transducer to the artery of choice unless the patient already has such a connection available. For the routine monitoring of blood pressure in comparatively fit patients there is often no justification for performing an arterial puncture and arrangements based upon the traditional Korotkoff sounds principle must be employed.

The sphygmomanometer

The most commonly encountered arrangement for measuring the systolic and diastolic blood pressure is the sphygmomanometer. A mercury-column or aneroid pressure gauge is connected to an inflatable cuff which is usually placed around an upper arm. The cuff is pumped up to a pressure in excess of the systolic and the cuff pressure is then gradually released. Pulsations can be detected when the intra-arterial pressure just exceeds the cuff pressure, using a stethoscope placed over an artery distal to the cuff. The diastolic pressure point is identified by the changing character of the Korotkoff sounds. Geddes and Moore (1968) show that by mounting a sound transducer wholly within the conventional arm-encircling cuff, high-intensity sounds can be detected with the cuff placed in any location on the upper arm.

Automated sphygmomanometer

A number of commercial patient monitoring systems make use of some form of sphygmomanometer for the monitoring of systolic and diastolic pressures. In the simplest arrangement a tube runs from each patient to a central nursing station where pressure can be applied. A microphone is placed under the cuff usually over the brachial artery and the Korotkoff sounds can be heard via the amplifier and microphone which are normally switched to act as a cardiophone. In more sophisticated versions a pump is started on command or at multiples of five minutes to inflate the cuff. Once the pre-set pressure has been attained, the cuff is deflated via a linear leak, As soon as Korotkoff sounds are detected by the microphone, a moving arm which was being driven downwards by the pointer of the pressure gauge is locked in position to indicate the systolic pressure. The cessation of the Korotkoff sounds when the artery is fully open causes a second arm to be locked in position to indicate the diastolic pressure. The readings from such a system compare well in quiet, normotensive patients with those obtained using a stethoscope. Difficulties may be experienced in patients who are obese, hypotensive or restless. If an ECG is being simultaneously recorded this can be utilized to operate a gating circuit to activate the microphone only when the Korotkoff sounds occur. In this way artefacts arising from extraneous noises or brushing of the cuff can be greatly reduced.

A greater reproducibility in the determination of the diastolic point is when the microphone output is amplified and fed to one possible channel of a fast-response pen recorder. The change in character of the Korotkoff sounds at the true diastolic point can then be seen from the recording. A convenient transducer for this arrangement can be made from a crystal gramophone pick-up. The stylus is adapted to carry a small diaphragm which is placed under the cuff over the artery. Smith (1962) described this type of system which he used for monitoring the blood pressures of dental patients. A mercury-column pressure gauge was used fitted with platinum contacts which made contact with a chain of resistances fed with a constant d.c. supply voltage. As the mercury column descended, it shorted-out fewer of the resistances. In this way a voltage related to the cuff pressure was available for feeding to a second channel of the pen recorder. It was actually the out-of-balance voltage from a bridge circuit. A somewhat similar system is that of Geddes, Spencer and Hoff (1959) where the piezo-electric crystal is fitted to the inside distal third of the cuff surface. A Bourdon gauge type of electrical pressure transducer recorded the cuff pressure. A full description of an automatic blood pressure system using a crystal pick-up and superimposing the Korotkoff sound tracing upon the cuff pressure tracing is that of Lywood (1967). Groedel and Miller (1943) state that the Korotkoff sounds have prominent frequencies in the range 45—60 Hz for normo-tensive subjects, and in the range 45—125 Hz for hypertensive subjects. Lywood (1967) found that the bandwidth 25—125 Hz gave a good signal-to-noise ratio when recording Korotkoff sounds from the brachial artery beneath the lower edge of the cuff. It is important that the amplifier for the Korotkoff sounds should have the maximum gain possible with a tolerable noise level otherwise false readings may be obtained for the systolic and diastolic pressures. Lywood mentions that the rate of fall of cuff pressure should be such as to allow about 20 beats to be recorded between the systolic and diastolic points. With a heart rate of 60 beats per minute and a blood pressure of 120/80 mmHg this is equivalent to a fall of 2 mmHg per second. It is feasible to stop deflation at a pressure of 20 mmHg since this is sufficient to hold the cuff in position but will offer little restriction to blood flow.

DOUBLE-CUFF METHODS FOR INDIRECT BLOOD PRESSURE RECORDING

The oscillotonometer

The methods described so far have used only a single cuff. However, a greater sensitivity and thus accuracy is attainable by the use of a double cuff system. A simple, non-automatic version, known as an oscillotonometer has been in use by anaesthetists for many years. Referring to *Figure 2.18*, both cuffs are connected to an airtight cylindrical box which carries on its top face a pointer and pressure scale. The case contains two pressure-sensitive capsules A and B. Capsule A is relatively stiff and its interior is open to the atmosphere. Capsule B is more sensitive so that for a given pressure difference it will be more compressed than will A. The two capsules are connected by means of an arm pivoted at C, and connected by a linkage to the pointer P. In use both of the cuffs and the interior of the case are inflated to a pressure above the patient's systolic pressure. As a result, capsule A is compressed, the pointer indicating the cuff pressure. Capsule B is unaltered since its internal and external pressures remain the same. The cuff pressure is then released in small steps and after each fall in pressure a lever is operated in order to determine whether the systolic point has been reached. Movement of the lever allows the box still to be at the upper cuff

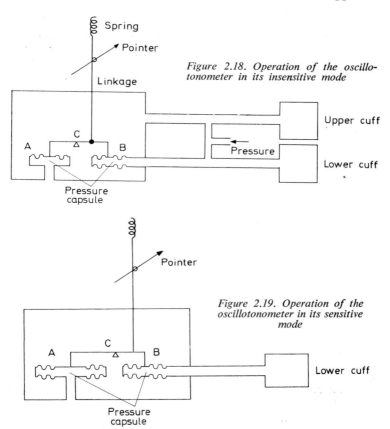

Figure 2.18. Operation of the oscillo-tonometer in its insensitive mode

Figure 2.19. Operation of the oscillotonometer in its sensitive mode

pressure but connects only the lower cuff to the sensitive capsule B, (*Figure 2.19*). When blood can pass under the upper cuff it gives rise to pressure pulsations in the lower cuff which are transmitted via B to the pointer. Thus systole is shown by a sudden increase in the amplitude of the pointer oscillations. When the systolic point is detected, the lever is returned to its original position and capsule A registers the systolic pressure. The diastolic pressure is determined in a similar fashion, except that it is taken to be the pressure at which the oscillations of the pointer suddenly decrease in amplitude. In each case the sensitive capsule B magnifies the phenomena at the systolic and diastolic points.

Automatic double-cuff methods

De Dobbeleer (1965) describes a form of automated tonometer which he developed especially for recording the blood pressure of patients suffering from Parkinson's disease and whose limbs had a marked tremor. The instrument detects the variation in phase difference

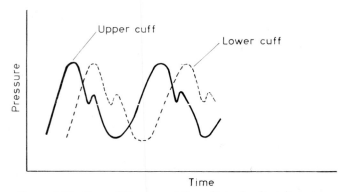

Figure 2.20. Phase difference existing above the diastolic pressure between the pressure fluctuations from the upper and lower cuffs

between the pressure pulsations in the upper and lower cuffs as the pressure changes from systolic to diastolic. The inflating pressure is connected to both cuffs in parallel. Let both cuffs be at a pressure above systolic. Then pressure pulsations will reach the upper cuff but not the lower cuff. As the cuff pressure falls below systolic, pulsations will get to the lower cuff but will be delayed in time (*Figure 2.20*). This delay arises from the inertia of the blood, and the arterial wall. When diastolic pressure is reached, the artery is not completely occluded at any phase of the cardiac cycle and so the phase difference between the pulsations in the cuffs falls to zero. The arrangement for detecting this fact is shown in *Figure 2.21*. The cuffs are cross-connected to chambers S for systolic pressure detection and D for diastolic pressure detection. In each chamber is a bead thermistor mounted in the air stream from the appropriate tube connecting to a cuff. The thermistor in chamber S responds only to pressure fluctuations from the lower cuff, while in chamber D the pulsations from the lower cuff are directed straight at the thermistor and pulsations from the upper cuff are directed to cross the jet from the lower cuff at right angles.

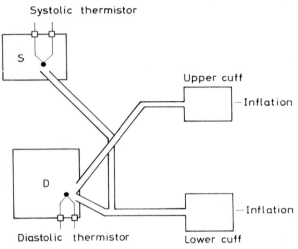

Figure 2.21. Arrangement of the thermistors in De Dobbeleer's double cuff system

In use the cuffs are inflated above the systolic pressure and no pressure pulsations reach thermistor S. When the systolic pressure is reached pressure pulses from the lower cuff puff air past the thermistor in S. These pulses affect the temperature of the thermistor which has taken up an equilibrium temperature as a result of the electric current which is passed through it. The associated pulsatile changes in the thermistor resistance suddenly increase in amplitude at the systolic point. This is a similar action to that produced in the oscillotonometer. The pulses are fed to a circuit which locks the systolic pointer of a panel meter. The cuff is then released slowly, the pressure in the lower cuff being indicated by a second pointer on the meter. Between systolic and diastolic pressures in the cuff, the puffs of air from the upper cuff arrive at the diastolic thermistor in D before the corresponding puffs of air from the lower cuff. Thus the thermistor resistance varies in a pulsatile fashion; again the action is similar to that of the oscillotonometer. When the diastolic pressure is reached the phase difference between the puffs from the upper and lower cuffs falls to zero, and they arrive simultaneously in chamber D. The jet from the upper cuff is now blown away from the thermistor by that from the lower cuff. Hence the resistance of the thermistor in D suddenly becomes steady, and this is arranged to lock the meter pointer at the diastolic pressure. The inflation and deflation of the cuffs can be arranged to occur on demand or automatically at pre-determined intervals as required, and the maintenance of an accurate cuff position is not so important as with some systems employing microphone detectors.

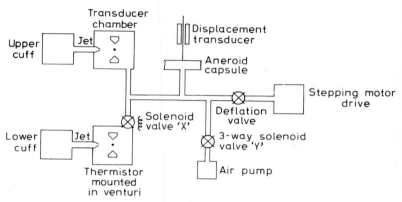

Figure 2.22. Pneumatic circuit of Flanagan and Hull's double cuff system

Another detailed account of a two-cuff system is that of Flanagan and Hull (1968). Their instrument consists of (1) a pneumatic circuit including a double brachial cuff with transducers and an inflation/deflation mechanism; (2) a servo mechanism for controlling the deflation of the cuffs; (3) transducer amplifiers, with their associated pulse circuitry for systolic pressure identification; (4) an electronic logic system for controlling the operating sequence with an automatic alarm facility; (5) an integral chart recorder. The system only measures the systolic pressure. In *Figure 2.22* is shown the pneumatic circuit of the system, and in *Figure 2.23* the electronic control system. Each transducer chamber contains a thermistor mounted in a venturi tube, the jet from each cuff being directed towards the appropriate transducer. The design of the chambers is such that the backflow of air into the cuff following an arterial pulse wave does not flow past the thermistor. By this means only one

102

voltage pulse is obtained from the thermistor for each pulse from its jet. A servo mechanism is used to ensure that the cuff pressure diminishes at a linear rate. The cuff pressure is sensed by means of an aneroid capsule which is connected to a displacement transducer in order to provide an analogue electrical signal. A motor-driven helical potentiometer provides a decreasing reference voltage for

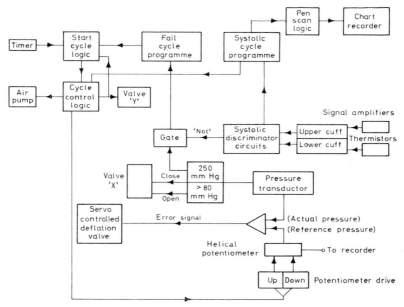

Figure 2.23. Electronic control system of Flanagan and Hull's double cuff system

the servo. A comparator circuit senses any voltage difference existing between the reference voltage and the transducer output and controls a fine needle valve so as to keep the voltage difference zero. Thus the cuff pressure is forced to follow the helical potentiometer voltage in a linear fashion. If the deflation rate is not truly linear any changes in it may result in artefact signals from the thermistors. The pulses from the thermistors actuate integrated circuit logic elements to stop the helical potentiometer turning when the systolic point is reached. The cuffs are then vented for fifteen seconds and the potentiometer voltage fed to a chart recorder. The inflation cycle is restarted after a pre-determined time interval.

103

Steinberg and London (1966) describe a single-cuff system with a digital read-out of both systolic and diastolic pressures, which could be of interest when applied to the more accurate double-cuff systems.

The accuracy of indirect blood pressure recording methods

The phenomenon of the Korotkoff sounds was described by Korotkoff (1905), an English translation of his paper being given by Lewis (1943). Roberts, Smiley and Manning (1953) found that the systolic values recorded by indirect methods are usually lower than those obtained by direct measurement with an arterial puncture by at least 10 mmHg. Van Bergen et al (1954) also found that the indirect method underestimated, and that the greatest error occurred in the 'young hypertensive' group of subjects. Holland and Humerfelt (1964) found that the error was not related to arm diameter or skin fold thickness, but to the directly measured blood pressure itself. Karvonen, Telivuo and Jarvinen (1964) found that errors apparently related to arm size in obese subjects arose from the use of a brachial cuff which was too short. The error was greatly reduced with a 40-cm cuff. Trout, Bertrand and Williams (1956) also reduced the error by applying the cuff to the forearm of obese patients.

Finger-cuff systems for recording systolic pressure only

Finger cuffs usually consist of an outer rigid tube having an inner wall of rubber which transmits pressure to the finger when inflated. Ball, Pallett and Shillingford (1961) used a sensitive volume-displacement transducer to detect the systolic point. Green (1955) devised a finger-cuff blood pressure follower, the cuff pressure being made to automatically cycle within a range of 2–4 mmHg around the systolic pressure.

A useful review of both direct and indirect methods for the measurement of blood pressure in animals and man is the book by Geddes (1970).

REFERENCES

Ardill, B. L., Fentem, P. H., and Wellard, M. J. (1967). 'An electro-magnetic pressure generator for testing the frequency response of transducers and catheter systems.' J. Physiol., Lond. **192**, 19P

Ayling, A. B. (1968). 'A transistorized control unit for accurate gas-pressure measurement with strain gauge pressure transducers.' J. sci. Inst. **1**, 86

Bassett, A. L., Ross, S. M., and Hoffman, B. F. (1967). 'An apparatus for varying the length of isolated heart muscle.' J. appl. Physiol. **22**, 813

Biro, E., Rusnakova, M., and Rusnak, J. (1966). 'A device for measuring isometric contractions mechanoelectrically.' *Physiol. bohemoslov.* **15**, 391

Boniface, K. J., Brodie, D. O., and Walton, R. P. (1953). 'Resistance strain gauge arches for direct measurement of heart contractile force in animals.' *Proc. Soc. exp. Biol. Med.* **84**, 263

Borrow, M., and Escaro, R. (1968). 'The reliability of control versus pressure monitoring and errors in its interpretation.' *Surgery Gynec. Obstet.* **127**, 1288

Bradley, R. D. (1964). 'Diagnostic right-heart catheterization with miniature catheters in severely ill patients.' *Lancet.*, **2**, 941

Brown, J. M. (1960). 'Anaesthesia and the contractile force of the heart.' *Curr. Res. Anesth. Analg.* **39**, 487

Corbett, J. L., and Macmillan, A. L. (1967). 'Differential pressure measurement.' *J. appl. Physiol.* **22**, 843

Elsner, R. W., Eagan, C. J., and Andersen, S. (1959). 'Impedance matching circuit for the mercury strain gauge.' *J. appl. Physiol.* **14**, 871

Etsten, B., Reynolds, R. N., and Li, T. H. (1955). 'The effects of controlled respiration on circulation during cyclopropane anaesthesia.' *Anesthesiology*, **16**, 365

Feigl, E. O., Simon, G. A., and Fry, D. L. (1967). 'Auxotonic and isometric cardiac force transducers.' *J. appl. Physiol.* **23**, 597

Forse, M. S. (1965). 'Semi-conductor strain gauges.' *Wld. med. Electron. Instrum. Lond.* **3**, 20

Gleason, D. M., and Lattimer, J. K. (1962). 'A miniature radio transmitter which is inserted into the bladder and which records voiding pressures.' *J. Urol.* **87**, 507

Greenfield, A. D. M., Witney, R. J., and Mowbray, J. F. (1963). 'Methods for the Investigation of peripheral blood flow.' *Br. med. Bull.* **19**, 101

Greer, J. R. (1964). 'Greer micromanometer.' *Wld. med. Electron. Instrum. Lond.* **2**, 141

Hansen, A. T. (1949). *Pressure Measurement in the Human Organism.* Copenhagen; Technisk Forlag

Henry, W. L., Wilner, L. B., and Harrison, D. C. (1967). 'A calibrator for detecting bubbles in cardiac catheter-manometer systems.' *J. appl. Physiol.* **23**, 1007

Hepburn, F. (1967). 'Foolproof tap systems for manometry.' *Lancet* **1**, 481

Hill, D. W. (1959). 'The rapid measurement of respiratory pressures and volumes.' *Br. J. Anaesth.* **31**, 352

Janicki, J. S., and Patel, D. J. (1968) 'A force gauge for measurement of longitudinal stresses in a blood vessel in situ.' *J. Biomechan.*, **1**, 19

Juhasz, L., and McPherson, A. (1963). 'Inductive-type pressure transducer.' *J. Phys., Lond.* **165**, 60P

— and Harris, G. F. (1965), 'Electromedical transducers.' *Wld. med. Electron. Instrum. Lond.* **4**, 186

Latimer, R. D. (1971). 'Central venous catheterization.' *Br. J. hosp. Med.*, **5**, 369

Lekholm, A., and Lindström, L. (1969). 'Optoelectronic transducer for intravascular measurements of pressure variations.' *Med. biol. Engng.*, **7**, 333

Lilly, J. C., Legallais, V., and Cherry, R. (1963). 'A variable capacitor for the measurement of pressure and mechanical displacement.' *J. appl. Phys.* **18,** 513

Macdonald, D. A. (1960). *Blood flow in Arteries.* London; Edward Arnold

Mackay, R. S. (1968). *Bio-medical Telemetry.* New York; Wiley

MacMillan, A. L., and Stott, F. D. (1968). 'Continuous intra-arterial blood pressure measurement.' *Bio-Med. Engng,* **3,** 20

McGough, A. R., and McDonald, R. D. (1968). 'Systolic-diastolic Heart pressure monitor.' *Electron. Engng,* **40,** 673

Millar, H. D., and Baker, L. E. (1972). 'A stable ultra-miniature catheter-tip pressure transducer.' *Med. biol. Engng.,* **11,** 86

Mostert, J. W., Evers, J. L., Hobika, G. H., Moore, R. H., Kenny, G. M., and Murphy, G. P. (1970). 'The haemodynamic response to chronic renal failure as studied in the azotaemic state.' *Br. J. Anaesth.,* **42,** 397

Neubert, H. K. P. (1968). *Strain Gauges, Kinds and Uses.* London; MacMillan.

Noble, F. W. (1953). *Electrical Methods of Blood Pressure Recording.* Springfield; Thomas

Noyes, D. H. (1967). 'Muscle balance with electrical-to-mechanical loading transducer.' *J. appl. Physiol.* **22,** 177

Pressey, D. C. (1953). 'Temperature-stable capacitance pressure gauges.' *J. scient. Instrum.* **30,** 20

Scheinman, M. M., Abbott, J. A., and Rapaport, E. (1969). 'Clinical uses of a flow-directed right heart catheter.' *Archs intern. Med.,* **124,** 19

Stegall, H. F. (1967). 'A simple, inexpensive, sinusoidal pressure generator.' *J. appl. Physiol.* **22,** 591

Sykes, M. K. (1963). 'Venous pressure as a clinical indication of adequacy of transfusion.' *Ann. R. Coll. Surg.,* **33,** 185

Thorp, W. and Jones, T. (1968). 'Silicon microcircuit piezo resistive transducers for medical applications.' In *Proc. 2nd European Conf. Med. Electron.,* 33. London; Hanover Press

Whelpton, D. (1968). 'A modified respiratory integrator system.' *Br. J. Anaesth.* **40,** 392

Whitney, R. J. (1953). 'The measurement of volume changes in human limbs.' *J. Physiol., Lond.* **121,** 1

Wiggers, C. J. (1928). *The Pulse Pressure in the Cardiovascular System.* London; Longmans, Green

Indirect measurement of blood pressure

Ball, G. R., Pallett, J., and Shillingford, J. P. (1961). 'An automatic finger blood-pressure recorder.' *Lancet* **2,** 1178

De Dobbeleer, G. D. P. (1965). 'Measurement of systolic and diastolic blood pressure by means of phase shift.' *Wld. med. Electron. Instrum. Lond.* **3,** 122

Flanagan, G. J. and Hull, C. J. (1968). 'A blood pressure recorder.' *Br. J. Anaesth.* **40,** 292

Geddes, L. A. and Moore, A. G. (1968). 'The efficient detection of Korotkoff sounds.' *Med. electron. bio. Engng,* **6,** 603

— Spencer, W. A.. and Hoff, H. E. (1959). 'Graphic recording of Korotkoff sounds.' *Am. Heart J.* **57,** 361

— (1970). *The Direct and Indirect Measurement of Blood Pressure.* Chicago; Year Book Medical Publishers.

Green, J. H. (1955). 'Blood-pressure follower for continuous blood pressure recording in man.' *J. Physiol., Lond.* **130**, 37P

Groedel, F., and Miller, M. (1943). 'Graphic study of auscultatory blood pressure measurement.' *Expl. Med. Surg.* **1**, 148

Haines, J. (1960). 'A versatile mechano-electrical transducer system.' *Proc. 3rd Int. Conf. Med. Electron.* London; Inst. Electrical Engineers.

Holland, W. W., and Humerfelt, S. (1964). 'Measurement of blood pressure: Comparison of intra-arterial and cuff values.' *Br. med. J.* **2**, 1241

Karvonen, M. J., Telivuo, L. J., and Jarvinen, E. J. K. (1964). 'Sphygmo-manometer cuff size and the accuracy of indirect measurement of blood pressure.' *Am. J. Cardiol.* **13**, 688

Korotkoff, N. S. (1905). 'On methods of studying blood pressure.' *Izv. imp. voenno-med. Akad.* **11**, 365

Lewis, W. H. (1943). 'The evolution of clinical sphygmomanometry.' *Bull. N.Y. Acad. Med.* **17**, 871

Lywood, D. W. (1967). 'Blood pressure.' In *Manual of Psychophysiological Methods*, Eds. P. H. Venables and Irene Martin. Amsterdam; North-Holland

Roberts, L. N., Smiley, J. R., and Manning, G. W. (1953). 'A comparison of direct and indirect blood pressure determinations.' *Circulation* **8**, 232

Smith, W. D. A. (1962). 'A method of recording systolic blood pressure.' *Br. J. Anaesth.* **34**, 136

Steinberg, B. L., and London, S. B. (1966). 'Automatic blood pressure monitoring during surgical anaesthesia.' *Anesthesiology* **27**, 861

Trout, K. W., Bertrand, C. A., and Williams, M. H. (1956). 'Measurement of blood pressure in obese persons.' *J. Am. med. Assoc.* **162**, 970

Van Bergen, F. H., Weatherhead, D. S., Treloar, A. B., Dobkin, A. B. and Buckley, J. J. (1954). 'Comparison of direct and indirect methods of measuring arterial blood pressure.' *Circulation* **10**, 481

3 – Measurement of Gas Flow, Volume and Respiratory Rate

THE PNEUMOTACHOGRAPH

A pneumotachograph head is essentially a small resistance to gas flow which is placed in series with the flow to be measured. The design of the head is such that the flow through it is laminar, that is the pressure drop appearing across the head is linearly related to the gas velocity up to a specified maximum flow. A sensitive manometer connected across the head can now be calibrated in terms of gas velocity, or more usually in terms of volume flow rate since the cross-sectional area of the head can be considered to be constant. The fact that the resistance to flow of the head is small (a few mm of water) means that it can be inserted into a breathing circuit with minimal interruption to the respiration of the patient.

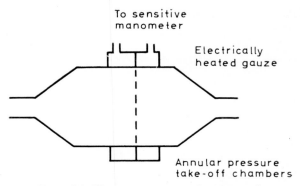

Figure 3.1. Wire gauze pneumotachograph head

One common design of pneumotachograph head, often called a flow-can, is that of Fry *et al* (1957). Referring to *Figure 3.1*, the head is seen to consist of a sheet of fine mesh wire gauge, typically 400 mesh, fastened between a conical inlet and outlet tube. The gauze can be electrically heated, using a low-voltage supply, to prevent the condensation of expired water vapour. Immediately on either side of the gauze is a series of small holes situated around the periphery of the conical tubes, each set of holes communicating with an annular chamber which leads to a metal side-arm. These are connected one to each side of a sensitive differential manometer. The use of the pressure take-off chambers minimizes any negative pressure effect which may arise at a single orifice due to interaction with the flowing gas stream.

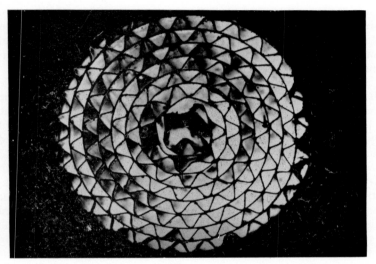

Figure 3.2. Fleisch-type concentric tube pneumotachograph head (from 'Physics Applied to Anaesthesia', Butterworths)

Another popular form of pneumotachograph head is that due to Fleisch. In effect the Fleisch head consists of a large number of small, parallel, metal tubes. It is made as can be seen from *Figure 3.2* by rolling a sheet of thin corrugated metal with a plane strip of metal, and inserting the resulting coil within an outer protective metal cover. This construction helps to maintain a laminar flow at higher flow rates than would be possible for a gauze of similar area. The Fleisch head also contains a low-voltage heating element with the object of preventing condensation of water vapour upon the interior during expiration. Four standard Fleisch heads are available covering the range from 60 litres per minute up to approximately 1,000 litres per minute. In each case the pressure drop developed for the maximum flow rate is of the order of 7 mm water. Unbonded strain gauges, differential transformers, capacitance and defocusing manometers have all been used successfully with pneumatachograph heads.

For a given flow rate, the pressure drop developed across the head is dependent upon the viscosity of the gas mixture. For accurate work during anaesthesia, a calibration curve must be constructed for the head concerned, using various mixtures of oxygen and nitrous oxide. Hobbes (1967) gives such a graph and shows that the pressure drop increases linearly with increasing nitrous oxide concentration. Smith (1964) also discusses the use of a pneumotachograph (in studies on the uptake of nitrous oxide during dental anaesthesia) under conditions of a wide range of nitrous oxide-oxygen concentrations.

The head cannot be heated very strongly because of possible discomfort to the patient when the metal head is placed close to the mouth of the patient. Hobbes (1967) raised the temperature of the Fleisch head from ambient to 37°C and noted that the output increased by 1 per cent for each degree C rise. Hobbes also showed that the effect of saturating air at 37°C with water vapour was to reduce the output from the head by 1·2 per cent as compared with dry air at the same temperature. Smith (1964) describes the construction of a low-resistance multi-gauze passive humidifier for holding both the temperature and water vapour content of expired air constant for use with a pneumotachograph head. During expiration, some of the water vapour passes into the relatively cool gauzes and condenses upon them. As a result the gauzes become warmed. During inspiration, a proportion of the condensed water is re-evaporated. Mapleson, Morgan and Hillard (1963) discuss the performance of a ten-gauze passive humidifier and show that it should give an inspired humidity which is 58 per cent of the expired humidity. Noe (1963) gives an account of a system in which a computer is used to determine the flow rate from a pneumotachograph head, the computer being fed with gas composition data from a mass spectrometer, and temperature data from a temperature sensor placed in the head. Problems associated with the calibration of pneumotachographs are also dealt with by Grenvik, Hedstrand and Sjogren (1966).

The calibration of a pneumotachograph head in terms of volume flow rate can be accomplished by passing known gas flows through it. The flows can be conveniently produced from a multi-bladed compressor (a good quality vacuum cleaner) and a large rotameter-type gas flow meter. Alternately, if the output from the pressure manometer connected to the head can be taken to a pen recorder, then a sine wave pump, Cooper (1961), Hill, Hook and Bell (1961), may be used. For a sine wave-flow pattern, the peak volume flow rate is equal to π times the minute volume (Fry *et al* 1957). Thus for a minute volume of 20 litres the peak flow rate is 63 litres per minute.

While the use of a pneumotachograph with spontaneously breathing patients is relatively simple, it is much harder in the case of patients connected to an automatic lung ventilator or who are having intermittent positive pressure respiration administered by squeezing a rubber bag. Unless great care is taken, there is a high probability that a pressure wave from the ventilator will reach one side of the pneumotachograph head before it reaches the other. This will give rise to a transient high pressure drop appearing across the head, and thus to an artefact of high flow. Clearly the pneumatic capacities must be accurately balanced on either side of the head. Thick-walled rubber tubes should connect the head to its manometer, and these should be tied together. A head consisting of a rigid bundle of metal tubes should be preferred for this application to a gauze-type head. The cross-sectional area of the gauze may not be the same in the forward and reverse flow directions, and the gauze is likely to be deflected by a pressure pulse.

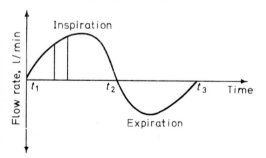

Figure 3.3. The integration of a pneumotachograph signal to yield the inspiratory and expiratory tidal volumes (from 'Physics Applied to Anaesthesia', Butterworths)

The integrating pneumotachograph

Pneumotachographs are of considerable interest in their own right for recording gas flow patterns, as for example in obstetric practice, or when evaluating the performance of a ventilator. Clinically, the requirement is more usually to record tidal, and hence, minute volume. This can easily be done by electrically integrating, with respect to time, the output from the pneumotachograph pressure transducer. A typical respiratory flow pattern over one breathing cycle is illustrated in *Figure 3.3*. By dividing the curve into a number of strips each of width dt seconds it can be seen that the inspiratory and expiratory tidal volumes are given by:

$$\int_{t=t_1}^{t=t_2} f.dt \quad \text{and} \quad \int_{t=t_2}^{t=t_3} f.dt$$

where f is the instantaneous flow rate in litres per minute. The integral gives the area under the curve and clearly the product (litres/minute $\times$ minutes) is equal to a volume in litres. In *Figure 3.4* is shown a pneumotachogram and its integral. The height of the lower tracing is proportional to the tidal volume. If the inspired and expired tidal volumes are equal (respiratory quotient $=1$) the vertical height from A to B would be the same as from B to C so that the level of the trace would not drift. The curves of *Figure 3.4* were obtained by connecting the integrating pneumotachograph to a sine waveform respiratory pump (Hill, Hook and Bell, 1961). It is seen that the tidal volume tracing is 90 degrees out of phase with the flow tracing. Mathematically this follows since the integral of a sine wave is a cosine wave.

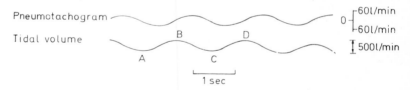

Figure 3.4. The upper tracing shows a pneumotachogram and the lower shows its integral (from 'Physics Applied to Anaesthesia', Butterworths)

In order to be able to record the minute volume, the output signal from the pneumotachograph pressure transducer is passed through a half-wave rectifier. The appropriate polarity of the rectifier can be selected by a switch to pass either the inspiratory or the expiratory signals. Under these conditions, the output from the integrating circuit consists of a staircase-like tracing, each 'step' indicating the magnitude of a tidal volume. The integrator can be re-set at the end of a pre-set volume or a pre-set time. This may be done automatically, for example whenever a volume of 10 litres has

112

been accumulated. Whelpton and Watson (1966) describe a convenient integrating circuit for use with a pneumotachograph, the integration being performed by means of a transistor operational amplifier. Clinically, trouble is often experienced with the use of integrating pneumotachographs due to the baseline of the integrator output continually drifting. This may arise from a drift in the balanced condition of the integrating amplifier. A check can be made by shorting out the input to the amplifier and observing whether the output still drifts. It should be remembered that the integrator adds up the product with time of any voltage difference applied to its input terminals. Thus the drift may be due to a drift in the balance condition of the pressure transducer used with the pneumotachograph head. Finally, the drift may arise from genuine physiological conditions. For example, if the pattern of respiration of an experimental animal changes markedly, then its respiratory quotient may well alter and this will cause a drift in the integrator output. If a respirator with a markedly peaked waveform is used for inflation, and expiration is passive, then the pneumotachograph may not respond uniformly to the peaks and this will give rise to a drift.

If the degree of drift present is moderate, it can be a great convenience to have the integrating capacitor shorted out automatically at the changeover from each inspiration and expiration and vice versa. This ensures that the integrator output is re-set to zero at regular intervals so that the tracing is always kept in the vicinity of the baseline. The integrator of Whelpton and Watson (1966) employs a second operational amplifier to sense the zero flow points of the pneumotachogram. The output of this second amplifier is connected to a sensitive relay. At the crossing points the input voltage to the amplifier falls to zero and the relay is de-energized. As a result, its contacts close and short out the integrating capacitor. When the pneumotachograph tracing is away from the zero flow line an input signal is fed to the re-set amplifier energizing the relay removing the short circuit from the capacitor so that integration re-commences. This automatic zeroing facility is particularly useful when the respiratory pattern is changing. If a steady drift is present, perhaps due to a change in the zero setting of the pneumotachograph pressure transducer, this can be compensated by applying a suitable offset voltage to the input of the integrating amplifier.

For lung function studies, pneumotachographs can be provided with a number of auxiliary electronic circuits in addition to an integrator. For example a 'catching' circuit can be incorporated to

113

store the peak value of the inspiratory or expiratory flow rate. A timing circuit may be used with the integrator to record the 'F.E.T.1' that is, the forced expiratory tidal volume after one second.

Other applications of integrators

The action of an integrator effectively is to smooth out the input waveform, and hence the integral shows much less fine detail than does the original pneumotachogram. Integrating circuits are also used to derive a mean blood pressure reading from the output of a blood pressure transducer, and also to measure the area under a dye dilution cardiac output curve, or the areas under the peaks of a gas chromatogram. For the latter application it is usual to use a digital integrator. The electrical signal corresponding to the chromatogram is fed into a voltage-controlled oscillator. The frequency of the oscillator is proportional to the input voltage. The sine-wave output from the oscillator is converted into standard pulses and these are then counted for the time of duration of each peak. The number of counts is proportional to the area of the appropriate peak in each case.

THE MEASUREMENT OF RESPIRATORY RATE

Triggering signals for a respiratory ratemeter can be obtained from the output of a pneumotachograph but for the purposes of patient monitoring a simpler arrangement is usual. Several possibilities exist, none of which is perfect, and it is as well to have more than one technique available.

The use of a thermistor probe

If a sensitive thermistor is placed just below the nostril and maintained in a bridge circuit at a temperature above ambient, it will be cooled once each respiratory cycle by the passage of the cooler inspired air. The thermistor resistance will increase significantly during this phase giving rise to an output voltage from the bridge. This can be used to trigger an integrating ratemeter circuit having a long time constant. The method is simple and works well except in the case of some patients who object to having anything attached to the face. In the case of intubated, anaesthetized patients, the thermistor can be mounted so that its tip protrudes into the airway.

For patients who are having oxygen administered via a face mask it is convenient to mount the thermistor in the disposable mask so that it is in the stream of tidal air.

The use of a spring-loaded switch

The thermistor probe has the advantage that it does respond to the movement of tidal air. If it is not feasible to use this method, then an indirect approach must be adopted. A light strap can be placed around the thorax and attached to a sensitive spring-loaded switch. Expansion of the chest during inspiration causes the switch contacts to close and actuate a trigger circuit producing a pulse which is fed to a ratemeter. This method can work well, but finding the correct tension for the strap may require care. Should it happen that the patient's mode of respiration changes significantly so that the main respiratory movement changes from the thorax to the belly, then triggering may fail.

The use of an impedance pneumograph

Provided that the patient is not making a great deal of movement with his thorax, the signals from a two-terminal impedance pneumograph should provide satisfactory signals for triggering a respiratory ratemeter. This method has the advantage of enabling an ECG signal to be obtained from the same pair of electrodes for use in triggering a cardiac ratemeter.

In designing the respiratory ratemaker, it may be arranged that if the rate indicated falls far below 10 breaths per minute for 10 seconds then an alarm will sound.

DRY DISPLACEMENT GAS METERS

When it is required to measure gas volumes of 10 litres and more a large spirometer may not be available. For this reason, if a written record is not required it may be convenient to use a dry displacement gas meter. For example, several expired tidal volumes may be collected in a Douglas bag and the minute volume found from the respiratory rate and the total volume measured by passing the contents of the bag through a gas meter. Cooper (1959) describes the use of dry gas meters in common anaesthetic circuits.

A detailed account of the operation and testing of dry displacement gas meters is that of Adams *et al* (1967). Basically, a dry gas meter is a motor which is driven by the pressure of the gas being measured. The required energy comes from the difference in pressure between the inlet and outlet, and the design aims to keep this small and constant. Referring to *Figure 3.5* the horizontal valve plate divides the case of the meter into two compartments, the upper of which (the valve chamber) receives the incoming stream of gas. The space below the valve plate is divided by a vertical division into identical chambers. To each side of this plate is attached a bellows formed from a metal disc and a diaphragm. The diaphragms are usually made from East Indian sheepskin treated with special oils.

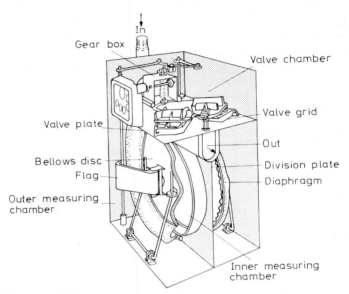

Figure 3.5. Schematic diagram of a dry displacement gas meter. (1) valve chamber; (2) valve grid; (3) diaphragm; (4) inner measuring chamber; (5) division plate; (6) outer measuring chamber; (7) flag; (8) bellows disc; (9) valve plate; (10) gear box (after Adams and colleagues, 1967)

Each bellows together with the space between it and the meter casing on that side forms two separate measuring chambers. The chambers communicate with the valve chamber via two sets of ports in the valve plate. Each set of ports has three openings. The inner port on each side leads to a bellows, the outer port to the corresponding outer measuring chamber and the middle (or outlet) port on each side connects to a common outlet pipe. Each valve cover has a central dome and two flat lateral wings. The dimensions are such that in the dead-centre position the dome exactly covers the outlet port while the wings cover the inner and outer measuring ports. By sliding to and fro over its seating each valve alternately connects the outlet port with one of the two measuring ports via the dome, and simultaneously exposes the other measuring port to the incoming gas. Thus fresh gas must pass through one or other of the measuring ports on each side to a measuring chamber before it can return later on to the outlet tube. The gas is ducted alternatively to the interior and exterior of the bellows causing them to expand and contract. Each bellows is attached by a hinge (the flag) to flag rods that pass up through grease seals to the valve chamber. The rotation of the vertical flag rods is transmitted through a linkage consisting of the flag arms to the tangent (a lever fixed to a vertical crankshaft). The two flag arms are joined together and are connected to the tangent by an adjustable tangent pin. Pivoted on the crank are swivel-jointed arms connecting the crank to each valve cover. The movement of the bellows is thus converted to a circular motion of the crankshaft which results in a push-pull action of the valve arms and a reciprocating radial action of the valve covers over their seatings. It is arranged that the movements of the two sides of the gas meter are a quarter of a cycle out of phase. Thus, whenever one bellows is moving at its maximum rate, the other is stationary. This ensures an uninterrupted flow of gas through the meter. The bellows are never both full or both empty at the same time. The radius of the circle described by the tangent pin is proportional to the movement of the diaphragms. By shifting the tangent pin along the tangent, the stroke of the diaphragms can be altered thus altering the volume of gas displaced per stroke. A worm on the crankshaft meshes with a toothed wheel to which is attached the pointer spindle. The calibration in England of dry gas meters is normally aimed at ensuring that they read within ± 2 per cent of the true volume at maximum capacity and at 10 per cent of this flow. However, to achieve this accuracy, the meter should be well maintained and checked at regular intervals. The accuracy figures refer to the accuracy that is achieved after several cycles of the mechanism. The error within one cycle should not exceed 5 per cent of the true volume in a good meter.

Correction factors for dry gas meters

If a dry gas meter has been tested over the full range of flow rates with which it will be used and found to have a constant calibration error, then a correction factor may be applied to obtain the true reading. Adams *et al* (1967) mention that at normal atmospheric pressure, an increase in pressure of 10 cm water will cause a reduction in volume of approximately 1 per cent. Hence a meter should be used which has a rated maximum capacity in excess of the maximum flow likely to be encountered. At room temperature (65°F, 18·3°C) a temperature change of 5 degF (2·8degC) will also alter the volume by about 1 per cent. The presence of water vapour does not affect the accuracy of the meter, but care must be taken to minimize the condensation of water within the meter. Water in the outer casing measuring chambers will not affect the meter calibration until there is enough to diminish the space swept by the bellows, but water inside the bellows will diminish their effective volume and hence cause over-reading. A dry gas meter is often used to calibrate electrical methods of measuring gas volume.

ELECTRICAL IMPEDANCE PNEUMOGRAPHS

A useful method for obtaining a written record of the respiratory pattern in terms of tidal volumes is that of measuring the electrical impedance between a pair of electrodes placed bilaterally along the mid-axillary lines.

Goldensohn and Zablow (1959) were able to quantify the relationship existing between respiratory volume and the corresponding transthoracic impedance change. Subsequent studies of the relationship have been performed by Geddes *et al* (1962), McCally *et al* (1963), Kubicek, Kinnen and Edin (1963, 1964), Hamilton *et al* (1965), Allison, Holmes and Nyboer (1964), and Baker *et al* (1965, 1966, 1967). A detailed survey of the various instrumental systems available for use with impedance pneumography has been given by Pacela (1966).

Baker, Geddes and Hoff (1965) have shown that in the frequency range 50–100 kHz, the changes observed in the transthoracic impedance accompanying respiration are essentially due to changes in the resistive component only, the magnitude of these changes being independent of frequency over this range.

The block diagram of a two-terminal impedance pneumograph is given in *Figure 3.6*. The impedance existing across the thorax is denoted by $(Z_0 + \Delta Z)$ where Z_0 is the standing impedance and ΔZ is the impedance change accompanying respiration. The output resistances $(\frac{1}{2}R_k)$ are made large in comparison with the value of $(Z_0 + \Delta Z)$ to ensure that the electrodes are in an essentially constant current circuit. By Ohm's law, the input voltage presented to the amplifier is $V_0 + V_1 = iZ_0 + i\Delta Z$. The resting impedance Z_0 may be of the

118

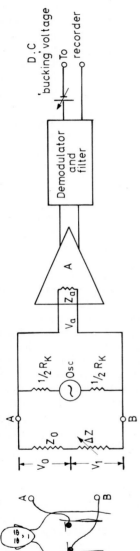

Figure 3.6. Two-terminal constant current impedance pneumograph. (Reproduced by courtesy of Dr. L. E. Baker)

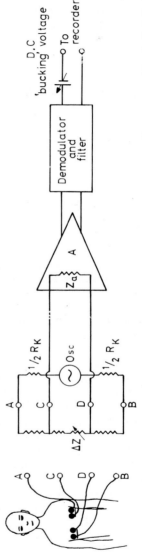

Figure 3.7. Four-terminal (tetrapolar) constant current impedance pneumograph. (Reproduced by courtesy of Dr. L. E. Baker)

119

order of 200 Ω, while ΔZ will be of the order of a few ohms per litre. After amplification with a gain A, the output voltage $AV_0 + AV_1$ is rectified and smoothed to produce d.c. components V_0 d.c. and V_1 d.c. The pneumograph may be calibrated in terms of impedance in ohms by connecting a decade resistance box in place of the thorax. When the standing impedance has been measured, the signal arising from it (V_0 d.c.) can be backed-off by an opposing voltage to establish a baseline on the recorder. Variations from this baseline are then produced by the action of V_1 d.c.

By using an a.c. amplifier, the impedance pneumograph will only respond to the impedance changes accompanying respiration and will ignore the standing impedance. For routine clinical work this arrangement is preferable since the complication of a backing-off voltage is avoided. The impedance electrodes will also pick up an electrocardiogram signal. This can be displayed on an electro-cardiograph by connecting the lead 1 input terminals to the output of the pneumograph. The result is, of course, a non-standard lead, but it is useful for monitoring the heart rate and the presence of arrhythmias. The input circuit to the pneumograph is connected across the transthoracic impedance of a few hundred ohms. Because of this low value of impedance it is not prone to pick up interference signals from the mains wiring. Thus it has proved possible to record clean respiration and ECG signals using the impedance pneumo-graph situated in the anaesthetic room connected to the patient in the operating room via twenty feet of cable. The time constant of the electrocardiograph (1·5 to 2 seconds) will pass the ECG signal, but not the respiration signal. Working with frequencies of either 20 or 50 kHz, does not give rise to cardiac effects of any kind or stimulation of cutaneous receptors under the electrodes with a current of 1 mA r.m.s. With silver disc electrodes 1 cm in diameter, the contact impedance for each electrode (with the skin cleaned and electrode jelly employed) is of the order of 250 Ω. The potential drop at each electrode is 250 mV and the total power dissipation is about 0·5 mW at the electrodes and a further 0·25 mW in the thorax.

The two-terminal impedance pneumograph is convenient for use with a quiet subject such as a resting volunteer or an anaesthetized patient. Since the contact impedance of the electrodes is likely to be greater than the resting transthoracic impedance, significant artefact signals can be expected if movement of the subject gives rise to changes in the electrode-contact impedance. Movement artefacts can be significantly reduced by the use of a four-terminal impedance pneumograph (*Figure 3.7*). The output from the oscillator is applied to the two outer electrodes A and B. The impedance signal is applied to the two inner electrodes C and D. By this means the main oscillator current does not flow through the contact impedances of electrodes C and D, all that flows through these is the small input current of the amplifier. This system is clinically useful for monitoring the respiration of restless subjects such as babies. It is not possible, as with the two-terminal system, to measure the full value of the resting transthoracic impedance but for monitoring purposes this is not usually required.

Calibration of impedance pneumographs

The electrical calibration of an impedance pneumograph can be effected by means of connecting the electrodes (the voltage electrodes in the case of a four-terminal system) to a non-inductive decade resistance box which can provide one-ohm increments. The respired volume calibration will differ for each subject and must be determined individually. With spontaneously breathing subjects it is convenient to have them breathe into an electrically recording fast-response spirometer. The pneumograph and spirometer signals are then displayed on adjacent channels of a multi-channel recorder, and the pneumograph calibration factor (ohms impedance change per litre) determined. With anaesthetized patients who have been given a muscle relaxant drug, the volume calibration can be found by inflating the patient with a known tidal volume from an automatic lung ventilator, or by inflating him with a large volume (400 ml) syringe.

Applications of impedance pneumographs

Berry *et al* (1962) and Catterson *et al* (1963) have used the impedance technique to monitor the respirations of astronauts during space flights. Geddes *et al* (1962, 1964) have used it with conscious patients, and Pallett and Scopes (1965) have monitored the respiration of newborn infants. Baker and Hill (1969) have found the method convenient to use with patients who had been paralysed and anaesthetized. Farman and Juett (1967) found the method of value in the monitoring of post-operative patients. It should be pointed out that the method effectively monitors thoracic movements and not the movement of tidal air directly. Thus if a respiratory obstruction occurs chest movements are likely to occur and will be picked up by the impedance pneumograph. Their pattern will soon become markedly different from that of normal respiration and the fact that something is wrong will be evident to an observer. It would not be wise to rely only upon an alarm signal triggered from a respiratory ratemeter actuated from an impedance pneumograph.

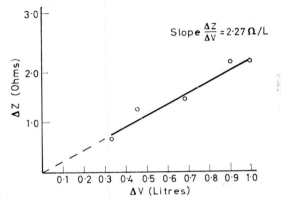

Figure 3.8. Linear relationship existing between peak values of impedance change and tidal volume (after Baker and Hill, 1969)

In *Figure 3.8*, from Baker and Hill (1969), is shown the straight-line calibration obtained for impedance change versus tidal volume in the case of a woman aged 54 years undergoing surgery for the removal of a bladder stone. The slope of the line was $2 \cdot 27$ Ω per litre.

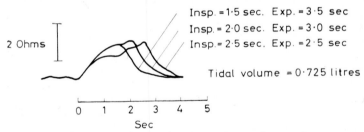

Figure 3.9. Superimposed records of impedance changes for various respiratory patterns (after Baker and Hill, 1969)

Superimposed records are shown in *Figure 3.9* of ΔZ obtained when this patient was ventilated with various respiratory cycles in which the time periods of inspiration and expiration were varied, but the sum of the two periods was maintained at 5 seconds. The tidal volume was kept constant at $0 \cdot 725$ litres. The records show that the peak amplitude of ΔZ is independent of the inspiratory-expiratory ratio and that the system faithfully follows the ventilatory pattern.

Using a two-electrode system, Baker *et al* (1966) examined the impedance-ventilation calibration of 7 normal male subjects and found that the best accuracy was obtained with the pair of electrodes placed approximately 6 cm above the xiphoid level. In general, obese subjects will give smaller signals than patients of a lighter build and it may be necessary to experiment with the placing of the

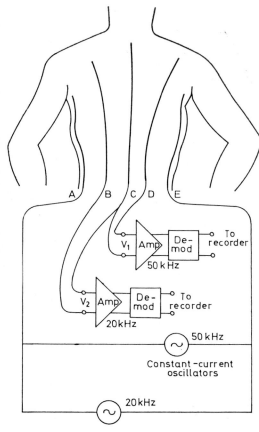

Figure 3.10. The use of two different frequency imped-ance pneumographs to compare the ventilation of the left and right lungs

electrodes in order to obtain the best possible signal. Valentinuzzi *et al* (1971) have shown that the impedance coefficient in ohms per litre obtained by bipolar impedance pneumography exhibits an inverse relationship with the body weight in kilogrammes. This relationship appears to be valid on an inter-species basis and is also probably true from an intra-species viewpoint. The relationship found was; impedance change in ohms per litre of air breathed= log 490—20·8 log W, where W is the body weight in kg.

By means of using 2 four-terminal impedance pneumographs operating respectively at 20 kHz and 50 kHz, Baker (1970) has been able to compare the ventilation of the right and left lungs

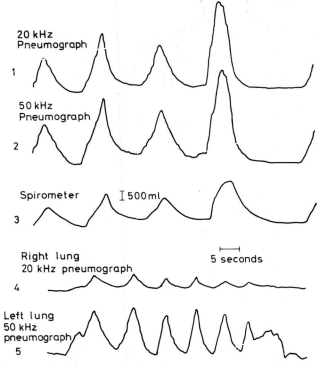

Figure 3.11. A comparison of ventilation of the left and right lungs of an asthmatic boy aged 12 years. Records 1 and 2 were taken simultaneously with the pneumographs connected in parallel to electrodes B and D (Figure 3.10) recording the same signal from both lungs. Records 4 and 5 were taken with the pneumographs connected as in Figure 3.10, recording the impedance changes from each lung. (Reproduced by courtesy of Dr. L. E. Baker)

in patients having a previously diagnosed pulmonary pathology. The results confirmed those of Nyboer (1964) which showed that an unequal distribution of tidal air between the lungs can be detected.

124

Nyboer used a single frequency in conjunction with two pairs of pick-up electrodes. Baker's arrangement is shown in *Figure 3.10*. The electrodes consist of aluminium strips approximately ½-inch wide attached to the centre of 1-inch wide adhesive strips which serve to hold the electrodes in place. The two lateral electrodes are usually placed along the midaxillary lines and the central electrode over the spinal column. The remaining two electrodes are spaced from the outer electrodes by approximately one third of the distance between the lateral and vertebral electrodes. The current sources of the two generators are connected across the two outer electrodes each providing a current of 1 mA r.m.s. The amplifiers use sharply tuned filters to ensure that the two pneumographs are non-interacting. The results obtained by Baker from a boy aged 12 years, are shown in *Figure 3.11*. Channels 1 and 2 record the similar signals recorded from both lungs by connecting the inputs of both pneumograph amplifiers in parallel to electrodes B and D of *Figure 3.10*, the gains of both amplifiers were set to be approximately equal. The tracing on channel 3 is the total uncorrected ventilation measured with a standard water-seal recording spirometer. Channels 4 and 5 display the impedance changes associated with the right and left lungs respectively. A subsequent X-ray examination revealed the right diaphragmatic excursion to be less than the left, thus accounting for the reduced ventilation of the right lung as indicated by the impedance recordings.

Cooley and Longini (1968) used a two-terminal pneumograph in which one electrode is earthed. The active electrode is surrounded by a guard-ring electrode driven from the out-of-balance voltage of an automatically balanced 100 kHz bridge via a separate amplifier. The guard-ring largely suppresses artefact signals arising from motion.

SPIROMETRY

The most common types of spirometer consist of a cylindrical metal bell open at one end and suspended from a pulley via a chain having a counterweight at its other end. The bell, which has a capacity of the order of 6 litres for most purposes, has its open end immersed in an outer container of water. The water acts as a seal on the principle of a 'gasometer'. With a suitable volume of gas in the cylinder or bell, the tidal air of a subject may be led in and out of the bell via pipes passing through the water and the excursion of the bell will be proportional to the tidal volume. The chain can carry an ink pen which marks on a motor-driven drum of paper. Unless a special lightweight bell is provided the normal spirometer is only capable of responding fully to slow respiratory rates, and not to the shallow, rapid, breathing sometimes encountered after anaesthesia. Thus care must be exercised when a spirometer is used to calibrate an impedance pneumograph attached to a spontaneously breathing subject. For the best results, one of the new dry, servo-assisted electronic spirometers should be used. These are fitted with linear transducers to record the displacement of the plastic-sheet spirometer chamber.

Provided that the speed of response of the spirometer is adequate, modern practice is to fit a low-inertia, linear potentiometer to the

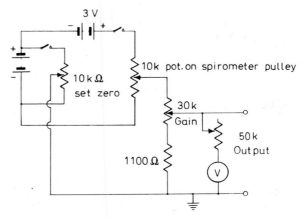

Figure 3.12. Energizing circuit for use with a potentiometer attached to the pulley wheel of a spirometer

pulley-shaft of a water spirometer and to use this to produce a d.c. signal proportional to gas volume. This can be then taken down on a frequency modulation tape recorder and fed into the analogue-to-digital converter of a digital computer system (Rosner and Caceres, 1967). Caceres used a 10 kΩ potentiometer having a $\frac{1}{2}$ per cent linear tolerance and a 5 per cent resistance tolerance. The circuit is shown in *Figure 3.12*. Provision must be made to set the output voltage to zero at any setting of the potentiometer slider. Thus the baseline of the recorder can be set for any resting level of the spirometer bell. The f.m. tape recorder ran at $3\frac{3}{4}$ inches per second with a 1200 Hz carrier. The tape was played into the computer's analogue-to-digital converter which operated for this application at a sampling rate of 200 per second. For this application the sampling rate limits the frequency bandwidth of the spirometer curve to about 80 Hz, which is more than adequate. The same computer system can also be used to break down ECGs into their time intervals and amplitudes, the sampling frequency of the converter now being set to 500 per second. The addition of a potentiometer to a 200-litre Tissot spirometer is discussed by Gillet and Lemarchands (1967).

Good indices of respiratory function are the Forced Vital Capacity (F.V.C.) and the Forced Expiratory Volume (F.E.V.) The F.E.V. is the volume of air a subject can expire from full inspiration with maximum effort in a given time period, most commonly one second. The F.V.C. is the total volume of air a subject can expire from full

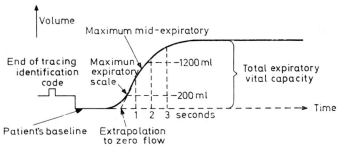

Figure 3.13. Breakdown of a typical F.V.C. spirometer tracing (after Caceres, 1965)

inspiration with maximum effort irrespective of time. The computer is first fed with the clinic location number, the patient's number and data so that it can calculate the spirometer constant, that is a calibration factor allowing for the room temperature. The F.V.C. is computed together with the time taken for the F.V.C., that is the time from the onset of the curve (extrapolated to zero to correct for slow starting (*Figure 3.13*) until maximum expiration is achieved. The F.E.V. is found at 1, 2 and 3 seconds and each is expressed as a percentage of the F.V.C. The Maximum Expiratory Flow Rate is determined as the flow rate existing between the expiration of 200 and 1200 ml and the Maximum Mid-Expiratory Flow Rate found is the flow rate during the middle 50 per cent of the F.V.C. Clearly the use of a computer can relieve the staff of a great deal of tedious calculation from spirometer traces.

McDermott, McDermott and Collins (1968) describe a lightweight

portable instrument consisting of a polythene bellows spirometer
and transistorized timing unit which   dial reading of the
F.E.V and F.V.C   neter and electronic
                                              cribed by Gaensler
                                              1960).

                                              xecutes an angular
                                              in its water-filled
                                              e sensed by means

Fig 3.15   nfortably carried
                                              '). It is fitted with
                                              each respiratory

                                              neter having an
u   counterweights
o

                                              ained in spiro-
m   pe, it may be
ne

Th

Th   ∴ a spirometer must be adequate both for
the measurement of the forced expiratory volume and of rapid
breathing. Any water-sealed spirometer includes moving masses
in the form of the bell and counterweights. This leads to the usual
problems of inertia and possible oscillation of the bell. With conventional spirometers a high rate of gas flow impinging upon the
water surface displaces a volume of water and hence displaces the
bell by an amount which is not related to the ventilatory volume. On
the other hand, at the end of expiration the bell may continue to
rise, drawing air across the valves into the spirometer. This leads
to an over-estimation of the expiratory volume. A partial compensation can be achieved by the use of a spirometer bell having a large
diameter (20 cm for F.E.V. work) and which fits closely over the
central core of the spirometer so that the area of water covered by
the bell is small in relation to that of the water tank. The bell must be
of a constant cross-section and well balanced so that it does not
drag on the core. Nunn (1956) describes a lightweight spirometer
having a frequency response which was within 2 per cent of the
static response up to 35 breaths per minute, the resonant frequency
being 96 breaths per minute with the bell immersed to a depth of
5 cm. The bell was made from anodized aluminium, having a mass

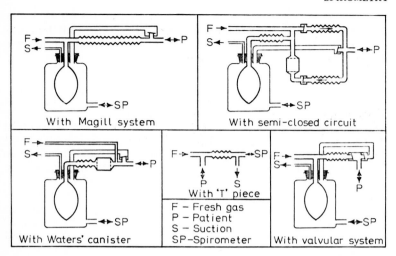

Figure 3.14. The application of continuous flow spirometry to various anaesthetic systems (after Nunn, 1956)

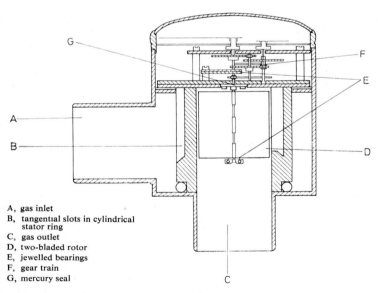

A, gas inlet
B, tangential slots in cylindrical
    stator ring
C, gas outlet
D, two-bladed rotor
E, jewelled bearings
F, gear train
G, mercury seal

Figure 3.15. Longitudinal section through the Wright respirometer. (Reproduced by courtesy of the British Oxygen Co.)

129

of 89·5g, and was suspended by two pulleys. The bell capacity was 2 l, its length was 30 cm, internal diameter 9·2 cm and thickness 0·314 mm. The core diameter was 7·9 cm external and the distance of the core to the sides of the tank was 6·8 cm.

The application of spirometry to anaesthesia

The use of spirometry is complicated in anaesthesia by the variety of the gas circuit configurations in use. It is usual for the circuit to contain a rubber reservoir bag from which the patient breathes during his periods of peak flow. As shown in *Figure 3.14*, the bag is placed inside a rigid box to which is connected the spirometer. The anaesthetic circuit receives a flow of fresh gas from the anaesthetic machine and this, after leaving the anaesthetic circuit, is sucked through the box by means of a suction pump whose flow rate is continuously adjusted to match that of the fresh gas. Nunn and Pouliot (1962) used a 40-litre bag in a box to measure with a spirometer the inspired and expired minute volumes of a patient during nitrous oxide anaesthesia.

THE WRIGHT RESPIROMETER

The Wright Respirometer (Wright, 1955) is shown in section in *Figure 3.15*. It is basically a miniature air turbine with moving parts which have a very low inertia. The revolutions of the two-bladed rotor are recorded by means of a gear train and dial similar to that used in watches. The dial indicates directly the number of litres of gas which have passed through the instrument between two successive readings. The device responds to gas flow in one direction only and hence does not need valves. The response of the respirometer (indicated volume/actual volume) is flow-rate dependent, since slip occurs to a greater degree at the higher rates. At very low flows the rotor will not turn. At high rates the response tends towards a fixed value. Nunn and Ezi-Ashi (1962) investigated the performance of the Wright respirometer and found that it under-read at low flow rates and over-read at high flow rates. However, during anaesthesia, the respiratory waveform and the nature of the respired gas mixture combined to minimize the small error which would otherwise result from hypoventilation. They report that over-reading is always to be expected from hyperventilation, the error will always exaggerate a departure from normality. The Wright respirometer is mechanically fragile and may read incorrectly if it has been dropped. The speed of rotation of the vanes can be counted by means of optical or magnetic coupling to an external counting circuit.

REFERENCES

Flow meters

Adams, A. P., Vickers, M. D. A., Munroe, J. P. and Parker, C. W. (1967). 'Dry displacement gas meters.' *Br. J. Anaesth.* **39,** 174

Cooper, E. A. (1959). 'The estimation of minute volume.' *Anaesthesia* **14,** 373

Cooper, E. A. (1961). 'Behaviour of respiratory apparatus.' *Medical Research Memorandum* **2,** 11 London: National Coal Board.

Fry, D. L., Hyatt, R. E., McCall, C. B. and Mallos, A. S. (1957). 'Evaluation of three types of respiratory flow meters.' *J. appl. Physiol.* **10,** 210

Grenvik, A., Hedstrand, U. and Sjogren, H. (1966). 'Problems in pneumotachography.' *Acta anaesth. scand.* **10,** 147

Hill, D. W. (1959). 'The rapid measurement of respiratory pressures and volumes.' *Br. J. Anaesth.* **31,** 352

— Hook, J. R. and Bell, E. G. (1961). 'Servo-operated respiratory waveform simulator.' *J. scient. Instrum.* **38,** 100

Hobbes, A. F. T. (1967). 'A comparison of methods of calibrating the pneumotachograph.' *Br. J. Anaesth.* **39,** 899

Mapleson, W. W., Morgan, J. G. and Hillard, E. K. (1963). 'Assessment of condenser humidifiers with special reference to a multiple-gauze model.' *Br. med. J.* **1,** 300

Noe, F. E. (1963). 'Computer analysis of curves from an infra-red CO_2 analyser and screen-type airflow meter.' *J. appl. Physiol.* **18,** 149

Smith, W. D. A. (1964). 'The measurement of uptake of nitrous oxide by pneumotachography.' *Br. J. Anaesth.* **36,** 363

Whelpton, D. J. and Watson, B. W. (1966). 'A respiration integrator.' *Br. J. Anaesth.* **38,** 233

Impedance spirometry

Allison, R. D., Holmes, E. L. and Nyboer, J. (1964). 'Volumetric dynamics of respiration as measured by electrical impedance plethysmography'. *J. appl. Physiol.* **19,** 166

Baker, L. E. (1970). 'Biomedical applications of electrical impedance measurements.' In *Progress in Medical Electronics.* Ed. by D. W. Hill and B. Watson. Cambridge; University Press.

— and Hill, D. W. (1969). 'The use of electrical impedance techniques for the monitoring of respiratory pattern during anaesthesia.' *Br. J. Anaesth.* **41,** 2

— and Geddes, L. A. (1967). 'Transthoracic electrical impedance changes with pneumothorax.' Digest of the 7th Int. Conf. Med. and Biol. Engng., Stockholm

— — and Hoff, H. E. (1965). 'Quantitative evaluation of impedance spirometry in man.' *Am. J. med. Electron.* **4,** 73

— — — and Chaput, C. J. (1966). 'Physiological factors underlying transthoracic impedance variations in respiration.' *J. appl. Physiol.* **21,** 1491

Berry, C. A., Minners, H. A., McCutcheon, E. P. and Pollard, R. A. (1962). 'Results of the 3rd United States Manned Orbital Space Flight. October 3rd, 1962.' NASA SP-12. p.27 Washington, D. C.; Office of Scientific and Technical Information, National Aeronautics and Space Administration.

Catterson, A. D., McCutcheon, E. P., Minners, H. A. and Pollard, R. A. (1963). 'Mercury project summary including results of the 4th manned orbital flight, 15 and 16 May.' 1963 NASA SP-45, p. 299. Washington, D.C.; Office of Scientific and Technical Information, National Aeronautics and Space Administration.

Cooley, W. L. and Longini, R. L. (1968). 'A new design for an impedance pneumograph.' *J. appl. Physiol.* **25,** 429

Farman, J. V. and Juett, D. A. (1967). 'Impedance spirometry in clinical monitoring.' *Br. med. J.* **4,** 27

Geddes, L. A., Hoff, H. E. and Spencer, W. A. (1964). 'Monitoring patients in hospitals—an exercise in automation.' *The Slide Rule* **24,** 4

— — — and Valbona, C. (1962). 'Acquisition of physiological data at the bedside.' *Am. J. med. Electron.* **1,** 62

Goldensohn, E. S. and Zablow, L. (1959). 'An electrical impedance spirometer.' *J. appl. Physiol.* **14,** 463

Hamilton, L. H., Beard, J. D. and Kory, R. C. (1965). 'Impedance measurement of tidal volume and ventilation.' *J. appl. Physiol.* **20,** 565

Kubicek, G., Kinnen, E. and Edin, A. (1963). 'Thoracic cage impedance measurements. Calibration of an impedance pneumograph.' *Tech. Documentary Report No. SAM-7 DR-63-41;* U.S.A.F. School of Aerospace, Brooks Air Force Base, Texas.

— — — (1964). 'Calibration of an impedance pneumograph.' *J. appl. Physiol.* **19,** 557

McCally, M., Barnard, G. W., Robins, K. E. and Marko, A. R. (1963). 'Observations with an electric impedance respirator.' *Am. J. med. Electron.* **2,** 322

Nyboer, J. (1964). 'Bilateral pulmonary function by tetrapolar electrical impedance spirometry.' *Harper Hosp. Bull.* **22,** 232

Pacela, A. F. (1966). 'Impedance pneumography—a survey of instrumentation techniques.' *Med. Electron. biol. Engng.* **4,** 1

Pallett, J. E. and Scopes, J. W. (1965). 'Recording respirations in newborn babies by measuring impedance of the chest.' *Med. Electron. biol. Engng.* **3,** 161

Valentinuzzi, M. E., Geddes, L. A. and Baker, L. E. (1971). 'The law of impedance pneumography.' *Med. biol. Engng.*, **9,** 157

Spirometry

Caceres, C. A. (1965). 'Computation for research: a by-product of clinical applications.' *Ann. N.Y. Acad. Sci.* **126,** 926

Gaensler, E. A. (1951). 'An instrument for dynamic vital capacity measurements.' *Science* **114,** 444

Gillet, A. and Lemarchands, H. (1967). 'Use and calibration of the broad-amplitude recorder.' *J. Physiol. Paris,* **59,** 149

Lota, M. J. (1967). 'Portable radio-spirometer for telemetric studies of pulmonary ventilation.' *Archs phys. Med.* **48,** 311

McDermott, M., McDermott, T. J. and Collins, M. M. (1968). 'A portable bellows spirometer and timing unit for the measurement of respiratory function.' *Med. Electron. biol. Engng.* **6,** 291

McKerrow, C. B., McDermott, M. and Gilson, J. C. (1960). 'A spirometer for measuring the forced expiratory volume with a simple calibrating device.' *Lancet* **1,** 149

Nunn, J. F. (1956). 'A new method of spirometry applicable to routine anaesthesia.' *Br. J. Anaesth.* **28,** 440

— and Ezi-Ashi T. I. (1962). 'The accuracy of the respirometer and ventigrator.' *Br. J. Anaesth.* **34,** 422

— and Pouliot, J. C. (1962). 'The measurement of gaseous exchange during nitrous oxide anaesthesia.' *Br. J. Anaesth.* **34,** 752

Rosner, S. W. and Caceres, C. A. (1967). 'The computer analysis of pulmonary function tests.' In *Engineering in the Practice of Medicine,* p. 171, Ed. by B. L. Segal and D. G. Kilpatrick, Baltimore; Williams and Wilkins

Stead, W. W., Wells, H. S., Gault, N. L. and Ognanovitch, J. (1959). 'Inaccuracy of the conventional water-filled spirometer for recording rapid breathing.' *J. appl. Physiol.* **14,** 448

Wilkes, F. C. D., Owen-Thomas, J. B., Swyer, P. R. and Conn, A. W. (1968). 'Evaluation of a respirometer for neonates.' *Br. J. Anaesth.* **40,** 61

Wright, B. M. (1955). 'A respiratory anemometer.' *J. Physiol. Lond.* **127,** 25P

4 – The Measurement of Blood Flow

ELECTROMAGNETIC BLOOD FLOWMETERS

Basically, electromagnetic blood flowmeters operate upon Faraday's well known principle of electromagnetic induction, the blood stream concerned behaving as an electrical conductor. When a conductor is moved in a direction perpendicular to the lines of force of a magnetic field, an e.m.f. is induced in the conductor. If the magnetic field is assumed to be uniform, then the e.m.f. arising from the motion of the conductor is proportional to the product (velocity × field strength).

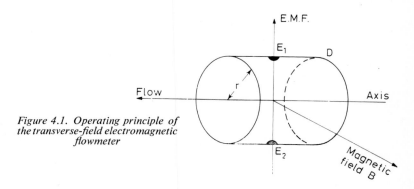

Figure 4.1. Operating principle of the transverse-field electromagnetic flowmeter

The simplest type of electromagnetic flowmeter head is illustrated diagrammatically in *Figure 4.1*, where the cylindrical insulated tube D is fitted with a pair of electrodes E_1 and E_2 at opposite ends of a diameter. A uniform electromagnetic field from an electromagnet is applied in a direction which is mutually perpendicular to both the longitudinal axis of the tube and the electrode diameter. The potential developed at the electrodes is then proportional to the flow velocity. This is the type of arrangement used in a cannulated flow meter head, *Figure 4.2*, the electromagnet polepieces being mounted at right

134

angle ...... tery at either
end. ...... ead is much
short ...... intact blood
vessel ...... to have the
cable ...... bes in order
to pre ...... ns. Cannu-

flow-

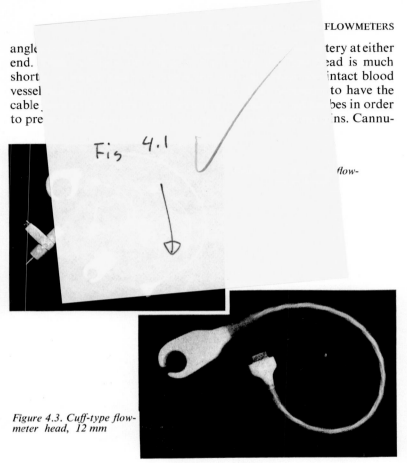

Figure 4.3. Cuff-type flowmeter head, 12 mm

Reproduced by courtesy of Nycotron

lated heads are often used mounted away from an experimental
animal or to measure the flows in a cardiac by-pass and this problem
does not usually arise. Wyatt (1968a, b) in a good review of electromagnetic blood flowmeters makes the point that blood vessels in man
and laboratory animals range in size from a few micrometres up to
50 mm in diameter, with wall thicknesses between 5 and 15 per cent
of the vessel diameter, the flows ranging from a fraction of 1 ml
per minute up to many litres per minute. The smallest reported
vessel whose flow had been measured by this technique had an
external diameter of 1 mm.

In the previous discussion it was assumed that the flow was

135

uniform across the vessel diameter, but in general the flow will be greater along the centre of the vessel and less towards the boundary. This will result in the production of circulating currents in planes normal to the tube axis, *Figure 4.4*, arising from the higher central e.m.f. The output voltage developed across the electrodes is now not the sum of the induced e.m.fs along the diameter alone, but this minus a voltage due to the circulating currents and the resistance of the fluid. In the simple situation with a uniform velocity profile the induced e.m.f. is uniform and there will be no circulating currents. Whereas the flow profile is parabolic for laminar flow, it is almost straight for fully turbulent flow, so that with full turbulence there will be no circulating currents. Thus $E=2a.B.v$. The polarity of the signal depends upon the direction of flow of the blood, so that the system can follow phasic blood flows. It is linear and largely free from errors due to viscosity, density, temperature, conductivity, pressure loss and flow profile (with some restrictions).

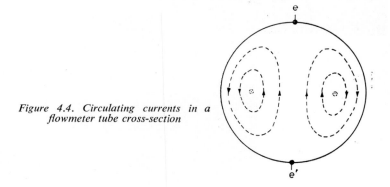

Figure 4.4. Circulating currents in a flowmeter tube cross-section

The equation for the simple, perfect, flowmeter also applies when the fluid velocity is non-uniform provided only that the flow profile possesses rotational symmetry about the tube axis (Shercliff, 1962). This follows because the voltage drop due to the circulating currents is exactly offset by higher induced e.m.fs elsewhere in the cross-section of the tube. It applies for both laminar and turbulent conditions and all others having rotational symmetry. The volume flow is proportional to the velocity for a constant tube cross-section, the relationship to the output voltage being $E=BQ/25\pi d$ micro-volts where B is the flux density in gauss, Q is the volume flow in ml per second, and d is the tube diameter in cm. When the flow profile does not possess a rotational symmetry, a concentration of flow near to the electrodes will produce a large increase in sensitivity while a flow concentration near the side walls will result in a decrease in sensitivity (Goldman, Marple and Scolnik 1963). This situation is illustrated in *Figure 4.5* (Shercliff 1962). With an intact blood vessel there is no need for the pick-up electrodes to penetrate the vessel since the walls will be sufficiently conductive to put the electrodes in contact with the induced e.m.f. The presence of a uniform blood vessel within which there is a rotationally symmetric flow will not affect the condition of rotational symmetry within the tube.

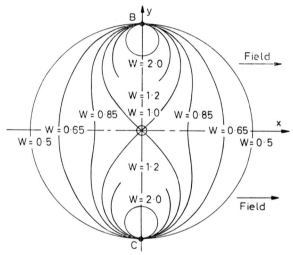

Figure 4.5. The quantity W indicates the ability of flow at various parts of the cross-section to contribute to the output signal (after Shercliff, 1962)

In practical flow heads, the magnetic field is limited in the axial direction by the size of the polepieces or of the coils in the case of coreless heads. The induced e.m.f. steadily falls to zero with distance measured axially from the electrodes, so that circulating currents flow in planes which are parallel to the tube axis and to the electrode diameter, *Figure 4.6*. When these currents flow in the conducting medium between the electrodes they produce in the potential existing between the electrodes a drop which is largely independent of the flow profile and of the conductivity of the blood vessel. However, a variation in sensitivity can arise when different conductivities are present at the boundaries of the flow head, as when the head is immersed in blood and tissue. Ferguson and Landahl (1966) report that with the magnet poles 2·8 tube diameters apart and 3·6 tube diameters wide, the axial insulation bounding the blood vessel must extend for 1·5 diameters on each side of the electrodes in order to reduce sensitivity variations to less than 1 per cent when the head is immersed in 0·9 per cent sodium chloride solution. If the magnetic field is non-uniform over the tube cross-section then a variation of sensitivity can occur with different flow profiles even when the latter possess rotational symmetry (Shercliff, unpublished). This fact is of importance when the need for a miniature head imposes limits upon the field uniformity.

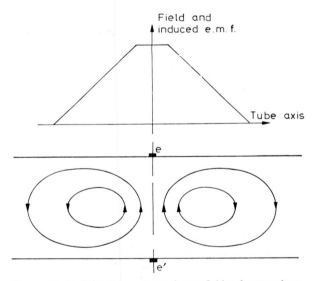

Figure 4.6. End-shorting currents due to field reduction along the axis (after Wyatt, 1968b)

The d.c. field flowmeter

The principle of the d.c. electromagnetic flowmeter for blood flow was employed by Kolin (1936) and Wetterer (1937). Kolin used a field of 1,000 gauss, the voltage produced by the flow being taken from non-polarizable electrodes to a d'Arsonval moving-coil galvanometer. Pulsatile blood flow was later recorded by Kolin and by Wetterer (1937) using a fast-response string galvanometer.

Edgerton (1968) discusses the effect of arterial wall thickness and conductivity upon electromagnetic flowmeter readings. He shows that where the ratio of the inside to outside artery diameter changes during a flowmeter measurement, the sensitivity of the flowmeter changes. The effect can be important where vasodilation or vaso-constriction occurs.

In practice, a number of problems arise with the simple d.c. system. The induced voltage is of the order of microvolts so that a good d.c. amplifier is required, and unwanted electrical noise signals are likely to be troublesome. In addition, large-area non-polarizable pick-up electrodes are needed. A change in the state of polarization of the electrode surfaces can produce a change in the potential difference existing between them which can be interpreted as a change of flow. The problems of d.c. flowmeters are discussed by Feder and Bay (1959), Feder (1959) and Wyatt (1961). The relation-ship between blood velocity and flow-probe output voltage is complicated by the fact that (1) some of the signal is shunted through the conducting wall of the blood vessel, (2) the impedances of the electrodes and the input impedance of the flowmeter affect the signal as does the variable impedance from the blood stream to earth.

A.C. field flowmeters

It is possible to use an electromagnet fed with an alternating or pulsed current instead of a permanent magnet in the flowmeter head. As a result, an alternating signal is developed at the pick-up electrodes. This can now be amplified by an a.c. amplifier followed by synchronous rectification, thus the signal-to-noise ratio should be superior to that of the simple d.c. system. In addition, the repeated reversals of the current at the electrodes do not allow sufficient time for the development of polarization effects. Unfortunately, the a.c. system is not as simple in practice as might appear. The alternating electromagnetic field produced by the energizing magnet coil of the flowmeter head couples with the pick-up electrode circuit, so that a substantial artefact signal is induced in the output circuit of the head, along with the wanted, small, flow signal. The artefact signal, known as the 'transformer effect signal' is 90 degrees out of phase with the flow signal. In a number of electromagnetic flowmeters, the energizing current fed to the electromagnet coils has a sine wave-form. In all electromagnetic flowmeters it is possible to extract the wanted flow signal by using suitable electronic techniques. Details of the arrangements used are given by Cooper and Richardson,

(1959), Richardson (1959), Kolin, Herrold and Assali (1958), Kolin (1959) Kolin *et al* (1964), Thornton and Bejack (1959), Goldman, Marple and Scolnik (1963), O'Rourke (1965), Hoffman *et al* (1960), Ferguson and Wells (1959), Gessner and Bergel (1964), Richardson, Cooper and Ciszczon (1961), Westersten *et al* (1959), Olmsted and Aldrich (1961), Olmsted (1962), Mills (1963), Abel (1959), Elliott, Hoffman and Guz (1963).

With the sinewave flowmeter, the transformer signal is of the same form as the flow signal. However, if a square-wave current is used to energize the electromagnet coils, then the 'transformer effect' signal now consists of two sharp spikes of opposite polarity respectively coincident with the leading and trailing edges of the square wave. During the flat, intervening, portion of the square wave the signal at the pick-up electrodes will be proportional to the blood velocity. After amplification, by suitably gating the circuitry, only the flow signal will be passed, the spikes being ignored. A square wave at 400 Hz is typically used. The use of a square-wave magnet current was reported by Denison, Spencer and Green (1955). Other references to the technique are: Spencer and Denison (1959), (1960) and Scher, Zepeda and Brown (1963).

It is not easy to generate a good square wave of current in the inductive coil circuit. As an alternative the use of a trapezoidal current waveform is described by Yanof (1961) and Yanof, Rosen and Shoemaker (1963). As the repetition frequency of the square wave or trapezoidal wave is increased so the effective frequency response of the flowmeter is extended until a limiting value is reached when the duration of the flow signal is now so short that it is no longer possible to separate the flow signal from the artefact spikes. Brecher (1967) mentions that with a 240-Hz square wave the effective frequency response was from 0–50 Hz for blood flow frequency components. Hirschberg (1967) discusses the design of low-noise input amplifiers for square wave electromagnetic blood flowmeters. Since the input signal at the flow-probe electrodes is only a few microvolts in amplitude, with the usual square wave carrier frequencies in the range 150–200 Hz, the main limitation of the signal-to-noise ratio occurs with the $1/f$ noise generated in the input stage of the amplifier. As an input transformer cannot be used for square wave instruments the input impedance of the amplifier is usually low (1–20 kΩ) Hirschberg found that low-noise bipolar transistors could be used as a satisfactory substitute for valves in the input stages with the probe impedance being less than 20 kΩs. A detailed account of the design of a square-wave electromagnetic flowmeter is that of Hognestad (1966). The waveforms of his instrument are shown in *Figure 4.7*.

A detailed account of the factors affecting the performance of sinewave, square wave and trapezoidal electromagnetic blood flowmeters is the chapter by Wyatt (1971).

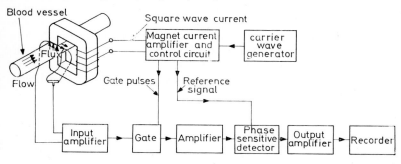

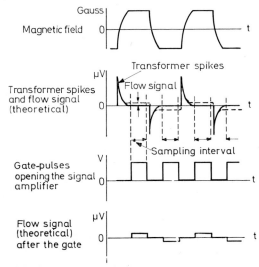

Figure 4.7. Waveforms in a square-wave flowmeter (after Hognestad, 1966)

Zero flow adjustment

When using an electromagnetic blood flowmeter it is necessary to be able to determine accurately the signal corresponding to zero flow.

Unfortunately the signal produced with the magnet turned off is not necessarily the same as that when the flow is zero owing to a number of effects at the electrode-vessel interface (Wyatt, 1961). Occlusion of the vessel concerned distal to the flow probe should stop the flow with a minimal disturbance of the spatial relationship existing between the vessel and transducer. Lightweight plastic snares have been used for this purpose (Beck, Morris and Assali 1965). The problem is more difficult in the case of chronically implanted flow probes. Jacobson and Swan (1966) describe a hydraulic occluder for this purpose. Injection of water into the exteriorized end of the inelastic polyvinyl tube, *Figure 4.8*, expands the silastic tube forcing

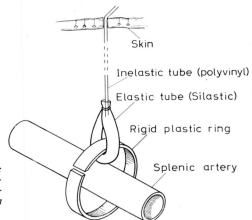

Figure 4.8. A hydraulic occluder for use with electro-magnetic blood flowmeter probes (after Jacobson and Swan, 1966)

the blood vessel against the rigid plastic ring. The occluder has been incorporated into a flow probe head. A balloon occluder is described by Nelson (1967). Jacobson and Swan show that the action of the occluder is identical with that of an arterial clamp. With a gated type of sinewave flowmeter it is possible to adjust the system so that the electrical output corresponds to zero signal input, that is, zero flow. This is accomplished by stopping the magnet drive current. When the flow probe is initially placed around the artery agreement may be obtained between the electrical and mechanical zero flow conditions. However, Jacobson and Swan (1966) report that this correspondence depends markedly upon the spatial relationship between the vessel and probe. This may alter in a conscious animal due to bodily movements, peristalsis or respiration. Arising from

142

this change it is possible to record artefacts in the form of reverse flows. The advantages of cellulose vessels during calibration are stressed by Case, Roselle and Nassar (1966).

The size of the flow head

With electromagnetic flowmeters the output signal is proportional to the velocity of the blood flow and thus to the volume flow if the diameter of the vessel is constant at the site of measurement. It is important that the action of fitting the flow probe around the artery should not significantly occlude the vessel but the probe should be a snug fit in order to reduce movement between probe and vessel to a minimum. In practice, this relative movement can be a source of calibration changes which prove to be troublesome. The larger the number of turns on the probe's electromagnet coils, the larger will be the magnetic field and the flow signal. However, a limit is set by the heat to be dissipated in the coils and the physical size and weight of the probe. Both these factors are obviously important in the case of chronically implanted probes, but the size and weight of the probe are also important in the case of probes used with surgically exposed vessels. An excessive weight of probe and cable will tend to exert traction on to the vessel and may cause the probe to tend to slip off the vessel. In order to cope with a reasonable range of vessel diameters, at least four different flow probes will be needed. The problem is that each head costs of the order of £100.

Calibration of electromagnetic blood flowmeters

For a given vessel diameter under the flow head, the output from the flowmeter is proportional to the volume flow in millilitres per minute. The output signal can be fed into an integrating meter to give the blood volume passing in a given time. With this arrangement it is possible to calibrate the flowmeter by occluding the vessel proximal to the flow head and cannulating the vessel distal to the head. Using a syringe and needle a known volume of blood (20 ml) is injected into the vessel so that it flows under the head. From a knowledge of the integrator reading, a calibration factor can be determined. When this is set up on the calibration control of the flowmeter the flow calibration will be correct (Cappelen and Hall, 1964). Otherwise flow meters can be calibrated by passing steady flows of blood from an elevated reservoir through the vessel and flow head. The volume is determined by measuring the volume collected in a measuring cylinder in a given time.

One method of calibrating a flow probe *in situ* is to arrange a simultaneous measurement of the flow by some other method. Bergel (1968) reports that probes used on the ascending aorta or the pulmonary artery can be calibrated against an indicator dilution method. For smaller vessels Bergel perfuses the entire aorto-iliac system of a dead animal with blood, flow probes being placed around the vessels at suitable points. Once the calibration factor has been established for a particular probe an electrical calibration signal can be injected into the flowmeter. Mills (1968) states that the calibration of his miniature electromagnetic flow probe as determined from *in vitro* studies could be transferred to *in vivo* measurements. This probe was passed into the pulmonary artery of a dog which had an implanted electromagnetic probe around the outside of the artery. With one probe located directly beneath the other, the mean flows agreed within 2 per cent after each system had been independently calibrated and corrections made for the individual frequency responses.

IETIC BLOOD

made in blood flow
w probes. In *Figure*
hown at (a) splenic

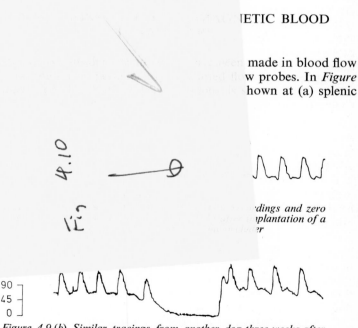

dings and zero
plantation of a
r

Figure 4.9.(b) Similar tracings from another dog three weeks after implanting a combined flow probe and hydraulic occluder

arterial phasic blood flow recordings and the zero flow reading from a conscious dog 2 weeks after implantation of a separate flow probe and hydraulic occluder; at (b), similar tracings from another dog 3 weeks after implanting a combined flow probe and hydraulic occluder. In each case the mean flow signal is shown at the start of the recording. The mean flow is obtained by electronically smoothing the phasic flow signal. The use of miniature electromagnetic flow probes to study coronary flows is described by Khouri and Gregg (1963), Khouri, Gregg and Rayford (1965), and Hepps, Roe and Rutkin (1963). Other applications of electromagnetic flowmeters are those of Elliott, Hoffman and Guz (1963), McDonald *et al* (1965), Meyer *et al* (1963), Mimms and Johnson (1963), Odeblad (1955), Price *et al* (1965), and Weber *et al* (1965).

CATHETER TIP VELOMETER

An important requirement for blood flowmeters arises for a device which is small enough to be incorporated in the tip of a catheter. Mills (1968) describes a miniature electromagnetic flow probe which is mounted inside a Nylon catheter having an outside diameter of 3 mm. When this is inserted into large vessels such as the pulmonary artery or the vena cavae, the blood stream flows around the outside of the catheter. The construction of the device is shown in *Figure 4.10*. Compared with a conventional electromagnetic flow probe, the miniature probe is of an 'inside-out' construction. The electromagnet is formed by the axially wound coil. The voltage induced by

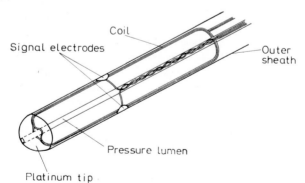

Figure 4.10. Miniature electromagnetic flow probe suitable for insertion into a large blood vessel (after Mills, 1968)

145

the flowing blood cutting the magnetic field is detected between the two electrodes mounted at the sides of the coil. The earthed platinum tip provides entry to a Nylon tube for sensing pressure. Only the electrodes and platinum tip are exposed to blood. The probe is said to respond to velocity in both forward and backward directions with a linear response. The sensitivity remains the same for normal saline and blood so that an *in vitro* calibration can be used *in vivo*. The frequency response is flat to within 5 per cent out to 30 Hz, with a linear phase shift of $1 \cdot 4$ deg/cycle/s^{-1}.

Measurement of urine velocity

It is also possible to use a conventional electromagnetic blood flow-meter to measure urine flow rates during voiding (Cardus, Quesada and Scott, 1963).

THERMAL-TYPE BLOOD FLOWMETERS

The thermal dilution blood flowmeter

The electromagnetic flowmeter is capable of a good frequency response, but requires surgical exposure of the blood vessel of interest in order for the flow probe to be fitted around the vessel. When a frequency response of the order of 4 Hz is sufficient, as for example in recording venous flows, the method of thermal dilution has an application. The measuring head can be placed at the tip of a suitable catheter and passed into the vessel where flow is to be measured. A detailed account of a thermal dilution flowmeter is that of Clark (1968). The instrument was employed to measure blood flow in the veins of the human lower limb. The principle of local thermal dilution is described by Froenk and Ganz (1960) and Dowsett and Lowe (1964). The thermal indicator substance used is normal saline at room temperature. The saline solution is injected via the catheter into the blood stream at a high velocity by means of a power-driven syringe. This results in the production of a local region of thermal mixing. Provided that complete mixing occurs across the blood vessel cross-section, the rate of heat exchange between the saline and blood depends upon the mass flow rate of the blood. The volume flow rate can be determined from a knowledge of the temperature of the indicator and the temperature of the mixed indicator plus blood. The temperatures are measured by means of a pair of calibrated thermistors. The diameter of the flowmeter shown in *Figure 4.11* is 1·4 mm maximum. It is suitable for percutaneous introduction in conscious subjects or for direct insertion into blood vessels exposed during surgery. The flowmeter consists of a long flexible Nylon catheter with a metal probe fixed to one end. An outer catheter with expanding supports is passed over the metal probe, holding the probe in an axial position in the blood vessel. The saline is injected through the inner catheter and emerges through four small orifices in the probe as high velocity jets inclined against

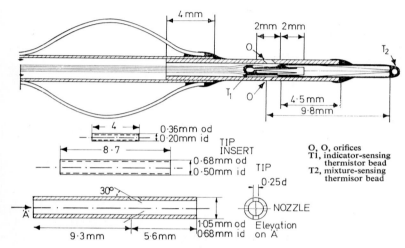

Figure 4.11. Construction of a thermal dilution blood flow probe (after Clark, 1968)

the direction of the blood flow. The temperature of the saline is measured with a thermistor bead mounted within the probe and that of the blood-saline mixture by means of a second thermistor mounted at the tip of the probe. The output from each thermistor bridge circuit is amplified by a chopper-type d.c. amplifier and displayed on a separate channel of a pen recorder system.

The flow pattern in the veins of the lower limb is laminar in both resting and exercising subjects; Clark (1968) quotes a Reynold's number of only 555 for a blood flow of 800 ml/min in a 12-mm diameter vessel. This flow pattern would not give rise to an adequate mixing of the indicator and blood, so that it is arranged to squirt the saline through four small (0·25 mm diameter) orifices at a total volume flow of 1·85 ml/sec, for each jet. Clark quotes a maximum jet velocity of 920 cm/sec with a Reynold's number (based upon the orifice diameter) of 2320. The orifices are inclined in an upstream direction at 30 degrees to the longitudinal axis of the probe.

Consider a quantity of saline at temperature T_s injected into a blood vessel having a steady mass flow rate of $\dot{M}_b$ at a blood temperature of T_b before it mixes with the saline. The mass flow rate of the saline is $\dot{M}_s$, measured, like $\dot{M}_b$, in g/sec. Let $\dot{Q}_s$ and $\dot{Q}_m$ be respectively the rates of heat energy transfer in cal/sec of the saline and mixture of blood and saline. The transfer of mass and heat energy during the mixing process is shown in *Figure 4.12*. When the saline is injected, a transient mixing condition occurs until the temperature of the mixture attains a steady value T_m.

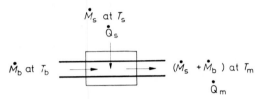

Figure 4.12. The transfer of mass and heat energy during the mixing of the thermal indicator and the blood stream

Subject to the following assumptions, it is possible to derive a simple expression for the volume flow of blood in the vessel:

(1) Steady state conditions have been reached when the temperature T_m is recorded.

(2) A complete mixing of the indicator and blood has occurred across the vessel cross-section.

(3) All the heat transferred from the blood to the saline indicator has taken place within the mixing region.

(4) The injection of the indicator does not alter the inflow of blood upstream of the injection point.

(5) There is no transfer of heat across the wall of the blood vessel into the mixing region.

The quantity of heat contained in a liquid is given by (mass $\times$ specific heat of the liquid $\times$ temperature of the liquid). Thus $\dot{Q}_s = \dot{M}_s . \dot{S}_s . (T_s - T_b)$, where $\dot{Q}_s$ is the rate of heat energy transfer into the system and $\dot{S}_s$ the specific heat of the saline. The rate of excess heat energy transfer past the plane of the mixture temperature thermistor is given by $\dot{Q}_m = (\dot{M}_b + \dot{M}_s).S_m.(T_m - T_b)$, where S_m is the specific heat of the mixture of blood and saline.

For the case of $\dot{M}_s$ having a similar magnitude to $\dot{M}_b$, the specific heat of the mixture is $S_m = (\dot{M}_s.S_s + \dot{M}_b.S_b)/(\dot{M}_s + \dot{M}_b)$.

There is assumed to be no net loss or gain of heat energy, so that $\dot{Q}_m = \dot{Q}_s$.

Hence $\dot{M}_s.S_s.(T_s - T_b) = (\dot{M}_s.S_s + \dot{M}_b.S_b)(T_m - T_b)$

giving $\dot{M}_b = \dfrac{\dot{M}_s.S_s}{S_b} \cdot \dfrac{(T_m - T_s)}{T_b - T_m}$

The volume flow rate of blood is $\dfrac{\dot{M}_b}{P_b} = \dfrac{\dot{M}_s.S_s}{P_b.S_b} \cdot \dfrac{(T_m - T_s)}{(T_b - T_m)}$

where P_b is the density of blood in g/ml.

$(T_m - T_s)$ can be rewritten as $(T_b - T_s) - (T_b - T_m)$ so that the blood volume flow rate can be calculated from a knowledge of the temperatures of the saline indicator, the blood before injection and the mixture of blood plus saline and the mass flow of saline. Clark (1968) took the specific heat of blood as 0·87 cal/g/°C and the blood density as 1·06 g/ml at a haematocrit of 45 per cent, after the results of Mendlowitz (1948). Clark reports that his thermal dilution flowmeter had a frequency response of at least 4 Hz.

Thermal conductivity blood flowmeters

The idea of measuring blood flow based upon the principle that the faster the blood flows the less heat from an external source will be transferred to the blood has been adapted to a wide range of thermal flowmeters since Rein (1929) developed his 'thermostromuhr'. Other references to thermal flowmeters are those of Aschoff and Wever (1956), Felix and Groll (1953), Brill, Hanafee and Norman (1964) and Lawn, Spires and Whitworth (1964). Thermal methods find application to the measurement of local blood flow in the brain. Levy, Stolwijk and Graichen (1967) report the use of a thermal conductivity system for this purpose. The method is based upon the continuous recording of the electrical power required to maintain a given temperature difference between a heated needle probe and an unheated reference probe. The greater the flow of blood, the greater will be the power required to hold the temperature difference constant.

Grahn, Wessel and Paul (1967) describe a linear catheter-tip thermistor flowmeter having a frequency response greater than 100 Hz, and used to record flow patterns in the descending aorta of dogs, obtaining comparable signals to those obtained from a simultaneously recording electromagnetic flowmeter. The flow probe carries three rapid-response micro-thermistors; the velocity sensor RTH1, the temperature sensor RTH2, and the direction sensor RTH3. The thermistors are incorporated into a dual Wheatstone bridge circuit which operates RTH1 at some 5degC above the blood temperature. The bridge acts to maintain the temperature difference constant between RTH1 and RTH2, and senses the direction of blood flow with RTH3. The thermistor dissipation factor d is given by $d = P/t$ where P is the heating power supplied to RTH1 and t is the temperature difference between RTH1 and RTH2. If V is the blood velocity, it is found that $d = A + B.\log V$. Analogue computer circuitry is provided with the flowmeter to solve this equation continuously and provide an output in terms of V. The direction-sensing thermistor produces a reversal of the signal polarity for backward flow.

ULTRASONIC BLOOD FLOWMETERS

Conventional ultrasonic bloodflow meters work upon the principle that there will be a difference in the transit time of ultrasonic radiation propagated through blood when the radiation is travelling upstream or downstream through the blood flow. Piezo-electric crystals are used both to transmit and receive the ultrasonic beam, (*Figure 4.13*). The ultrasonic transmitter and the receiver amplifier are connected alternately to each crystal X_1 and X_2, the changeover occurring 800 times per second. When the transmitter is connected to a crystal, bursts of 3 MHz ultrasound are emitted with a repetition frequency of 12 kHz. Meanwhile the receiver is connected to the other crystal. During the transit of the bursts between the two crystals a ramp voltage generator is started. It is arranged that the height of the ramp is proportional to the transit time of the bursts in the downstream direction. The transmitter and receiver are then interchanged and a second ramp generator used to determine the transit time in the upstream direction. A voltage comparator compares the magnitudes of the two peak ramp voltages and produces a 400 Hz square wave with an amplitude proportional to the blood velocity. The square wave is fed into a synchronous detector circuit to produce a d.c. output voltage which indicates both the magnitude and the direction of flow. The distance between the two crystals is kept constant by the flow-probe mounting. With the blood flow velocities encountered in mammalian vessels the difference in transit times is in the range 2×10^{-10} to 2×10^{-8} seconds. Thus the requirements for sensitivity and stability in the electronic circuits are severe. The pulsed ultrasonic flow meter of Franklin *et al* (1959, 1962) has proved to be more satisfactory than earlier phase-shift systems. Its use to measure the balance between the right and left ventricular output has been described by Franklin, Van Citters and Rushmer (1962).

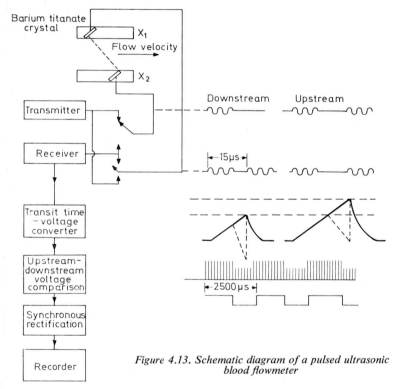

Figure 4.13. Schematic diagram of a pulsed ultrasonic blood flowmeter

The Doppler shift ultrasonic blood flowmeter

A Doppler frequency shift occurs when a source of sound is moving relative to an observer. There is an apparent shift to a higher frequency as the source of sound approaches the observer, and an apparent shift to a lower frequency as the source moves away from the observer. The Doppler-shift blood flowmeter operates by directing a beam of 5 MHz ultrasound on to a moving object such

151

as a blood stream or a foetal heart and monitoring the frequency changes produced in the back-scattered ultrasonic beam. The transmitted and received beams are mixed to produce an output beat frequency signal. With a 5 MHz frequency the ultrasonic wavelength in tissue is about 0·3 mm so that motion at the rate of 3 to 4 cm per second produces a beat frequency of about 300 to 400 Hz. The system can be made compact enough to be implanted for the monitoring of relative blood flow changes in free-ranging animals, the output signal from the flowmeter modulating a radio telemetry transmitter strapped to the animal's back, (Franklin, Watson and Van Citters 1964; Van Citters *et al*, 1965). A description of a Doppler shift flowmeter is that of Franklin, Schlegel and Watson (1963). The Doppler system offers the advantage that it can monitor relative blood flow changes occurring in relatively large blood vessels close to the body surface, for example in the placenta, from outside the body without having to expose the vessel (Plaas 1964).

In the field of obstetrics, the Doppler shift meter has proved to be particularly useful in picking up the foetal heartbeat as early as 10 weeks. The ultrasonic transmitter crystal is coupled to the maternal abdomen with water, or water with a wetting agent. The receiving crystal is mounted coaxially in the probe. The probe is moved around over the abdomen until the monitor loud speaker emits rhythmic pulsations typical of the foetal vascular system.

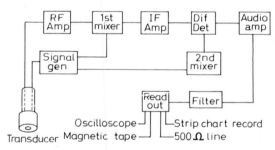

*Figure 4.14. Block diagram of a Doppler-shift ultrasonic
blood flowmeter*

The beat frequencies produced lie mainly in the range 300–400 Hz with a peak at 500 Hz and little above 1 kHz (Callagan, 1967). A block diagram of a Doppler shift meter is shown in *Figure 4.14* and *Figure 4.15* illustrates the formation of the beat frequency from the difference in the transmitted and received frequencies. The sequence

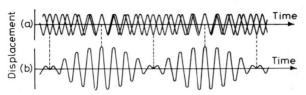

Figure 4.15. The formation of a beat frequency from the difference in the transmitted and received frequencies (after Callagan, 1967)

of events in a foetal cardiac cycle is shown in *Figure 4.16*, taken from Callagan (1967). The signal-to-noise ratio of the ultrasonic trace is normally high, typically in the range 20–40 to 1. In the adult heart, components of the Doppler shift signal can be identified which correspond with the atrial contraction, ventricular contraction and relaxation, as well as to the opening and closing of the atrio-ventricular valves. A comparison of the intracardiac phonocardiograph and Doppler shift tracing is given by Yamakawa and Kitamura (1963). The use of the Doppler method for observation of the foetal

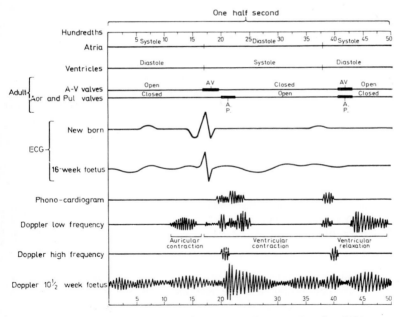

Figure 4.16. Detection of foetal heart beats by an ultrasonic Doppler-shift system (after Callagan, 1967)

153

heart is described by Callagan, Rowland and Goldman (1964), Johnson *et al* (1965), Brown (1971) and Kuah and Embrey (1968). Brown (1967) describes the use of ultrasonics for the localization of the placenta and discusses the application (1968) of ultrasound in relation to the detection of intra-uterine death. Its use as an adjunct to femoral arteriography is discussed by Staple and Brinker (1968) whilst the technique of suprasternal ultrasonography for the measurement of the diameters of the aortic arch, right pulmonary artery and left atrium is dealt with by Goldberg (1971).

OTHER APPLICATIONS OF ULTRASONIC TECHNIQUES TO SURGERY

Pulse-echo systems of ultrasonics used to investigate internal structures of the body are normally based upon either the A-scope or B-scope techniques. In the A-scope technique the transducer generating the ultrasound is placed in the required position on the body surface, for example, the side of the head. The generator is pulsed at regular intervals and sends a pulse of ultrasound into the skull. Some of the ultrasound is reflected back from tissue interfaces and is converted by the transducer into electrical signals which are amplified and fed to the Y-plates of a cathode-ray tube display. The pulsing of the transducer also starts a calibrated timebase so that the time of arrival of the echoes can be calculated. The echoes are delayed by about 13·3 µs for each centimetre of go-and-return path length in soft tissue. Thus it is possible to estimate a displacement of the mid-line structures of the brain, or the growth of a foetal skull. The range of timebase scan times would range from 25 µs for use with the eye to 500 µs for use with a large abdomen. The A-scope gives a one-dimensional display.

In a B-scope, the transducer is moved continuously around the surface of the patient, for example around the abdomen, in an oscillating motion. The cathode-ray tube display now uses a radial timebase, the position of the timebase corresponding to the direction of the ultrasonic beam. Each echo is registered as a bright spot at the appropriate point on the timebase. By continuously photographing the picture as the probe moves, a cross-section of the patient is built up. The probe and the relevant portion of the patient are often placed in a water-bath in order to achieve a good coupling.

Ultrasound is commonly used to localize the mid-line structures of the brain (Ambrose, 1964). The brain mid-line may be displaced from the central position by an asymmetrical space-occupying abnormality such as a haematoma or a tumour. Oksala (1966) has also used the reflection of ultrasound to diagnose abnormalities of the eye, Feigenbaum, Zaky and Waldhausen (1967) to diagnose pericardial effusion, and Schentke and Renger (1966) to diagnose liver disease. In obstetrics, ultrasound is used to estimate foetal head diameters and to visualize the placenta and foetus (Donald and Abdulla, 1967; Sunden, 1964; Wilcocks et al., 1967; Wilcocks and Dunsmore, 1971; Campbell and Dewhurst, 1970). The use of ultra-sound in obstetrics is obviously attractive since even with high doses of ultrasonic irradiation the chromosomal effect, if it is present, is much less than would result from an x-ray examination. Safety aspects of ultrasound are discussed by Bernstine (1969), Bobrow et al. (1971), Boyd et al. (1971) and Hellman et al. (1970). A focused beam of ultrasound has been used to destroy the vestibular end organ in the treatment of Ménières disease, James et al. (1963). It is also possible using ultrasonics to obtain time-motion studies of the heart valves. This has proved of value in the diagnosis of mitral valve disease (Edler, 1966). Ultrasound has been used to investigate space occupying lesions in the urinary tract (Barnett and Morley, 1971) and to detect tumours of the bladder (Kyle et al., 1971).

VENOUS OCCLUSION PLETHYSMOGRAPHY

As a method for the measurement of peripheral blood flow the technique of venous occlusion plethysmography is well established. The principle involved is to arrest completely, for a few seconds, the venous return from the region of interest without directly interfering with the arterial inflow (Greenfield, Whitney and Mowbray, 1963). The venous return is stopped by abruptly inflating a pneumatic cuff to a suitable pressure below the subject's diastolic pressure. The pressure is chosen so that it will occlude all accessible veins, the apparent rate of arterial flow into the limb being unaltered over a fairly wide range of cuff pressures. While the venous return is arrested, a continuous measurement is made of the increase in volume occurring either of the whole limb distal to the point of venous occlusion, or of a segment of limb situated between the point of venous occlusion and a distal cuff inflated so as to cut off the circulation in all vessels. If these arrangements are not used, artefacts may arise due to blood accumulating in the veins of a part of the limb and remaining there. For example, if venous occlusion is accomplished in a forearm by means of a cuff placed above the elbow some of the arterial blood supply to the hand accumulates in the veins of the forearm. Thus in studies on finger blood flow the occlusion must be at the base of the finger and not at the wrist.

The use of a water-filled plethysmograph

The change in volume of the limb is temperature dependent, and for this reason a water-filled plethysmograph is often used, *Figure 4.17* (Greenfield, Whitney and Mowbray, 1963). The subject's forearm is placed inside a thin rubber sleeve contained inside a copper chamber filled with water, which is stirred through holes communicating with a motor-driven paddle in a side chamber. As the limb volume increases so the water level in a vertical tube attached to the chamber rises. This can be measured as an increase in air pressure by means of a sensitive electronic pressure transducer feeding a recorder (Hyman and Winsor, 1966). The whole chamber is surrounded by a circulating water bath whose temperature can be controlled. The plethysmograph is calibrated by adding to or subtracting from the chamber known volumes of water. A typical record is shown in *Figure 4.18*.

The capacitance plethysmograph

A water-filled plethysmograph is bulky and not often convenient to use in cramped conditions, for example, in the operating room. Wood and Hyman (1970) describe a direct reading capacitance plethysmograph for use in venous occlusion plethysmography. In this device, the change in the capacitance between the surface of the limb segment and an encircling flexible screen cuff at a fixed distance from the skin, is related to the fractional change in volume of the part by a simple constant which can be determined from the initial capacitance. Hence, neither a calibration procedure nor the measurement of the segment volume is needed. Wood and Hyman (1970) describe analogue circuits by which the progressive increase in capacitance occurring after venous occlusion is filtered, differentiated and examined for the most consistent part of the curve. The final digital read-out is displayed in units of perfusion, i.e. in ml per 100 ml of tissue per minute. The capacitance measuring cuff which is placed around a forearm or calf consists of a flexible copper wire cloth separated from the limb by a constant thickness layer of polyurethane foam. The active copper screen is separated by another layer of foam from an outer shield electrode which is driven from a unity gain buffer amplifier so that it follows the same potential as the screen.

The mercury-in-rubber strain gauge plethysmograph

It is possible to estimate the change in volume of a limb from a knowledge of the corresponding change in its circumference. This follows since the percentage change in volume of a fixed length cylinder closely approximates to twice the percentage change in its

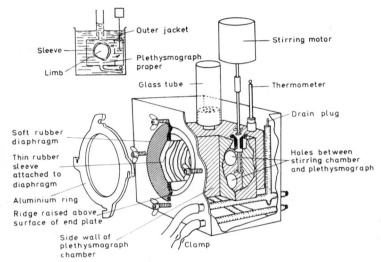

Figure 4.17. Water-filled plethysmograph (after Greenfield, Whitney and Mowbray, 1963)

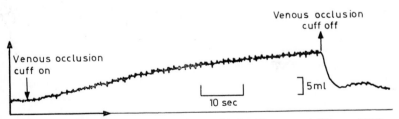

Figure 4.18. Typical plethysmograph record (after Hyman and Winsor, 1966)

circumference if only small changes are considered. This approximation also applies to a limb where the cross-section is not constant provided that the changes are in a uniform proportion along the length. The changes in limb circumference following venous occlusion may be quite small, less than 1 per cent. Whitney (1953) has developed mercury-in-rubber strain gauges which can fit closely the profile of a limb. He calibrates each gauge by approximating the ends of the encircling gauge by a known distance while it is mounted on the limb. A review of the mercury strain gauge technique and its applications is given by Greenfield, Whitney and Mowbray (1963). The use of the gauge offers a number of advantages, including small size, the fact that it can be fitted easily and quickly and is comfortable to wear. Ardill, Fentem and Williams (1968) report on an interesting experiment in which they occluded the circulation to and from the forearm by inflating two cuffs, situated at the wrist and on the upper arm, to 250 mmHg. Two mercury-in-rubber strain gauges were placed on the forearm, the proximal gauge being situated one quarter of the distance from the olecranon to the radial styloid, with the distal gauge 3 to 4 cm distal to it. A volume of 0·9 per cent saline calculated to approximate to the normal resting arterial inflow to the volume of tissue between the cuffs was infused via the brachial artery. In 5 experiments the inflow recorded by the proximal gauge was within 10 per cent of that expected from a knowledge of the rate of infusion and the limb volume between the cuffs. In 2 other experiments it was within 12 per cent. In 5 of the 7 experiments the results obtained from the distal gauge were smaller than those from the proximal gauge.

Brakkee and Vendrik (1966) have pointed out that Whitney's original mechanical method of calibration is rather cumbersome and easily leads to errors. The main reason for this is that the method requires touching of the gauge mounting. This gives rise to almost unavoidable lateral displacements of the rubber tubing. Brakkee and Vendrik found that change in gauge length arising from this manipulation could easily be 20 per cent of the normal calibration displacement. These workers have improved on an electrical calibration technique proposed by Burger et al. (1959). The relative volume change of the limb dV/V is equal to twice the relative change of the limb circumferance dC/C, and this to a first approximation equals the relative change in the gauge length dL/L. Neglecting second order terms, dL/L is one half of the relative electrical resistance change dR/R. Hence, the percentage volume change is equal to the percentage resistance change. Using a Wheatstone bridge circuit, the relationship between the resistance change and the bridge output signal can be calibrated by changing the resistance of one of the other arms by a known percentage. Brakkee and Vendrik show how it is possible to allow in the calibration for the effects of tissue compression. They also provide the circuit for a two channel, mains powered, bridge amplifier for mercury strain gauge plethysmography.

Some other references to the mercury strain gauge technique are those of Celander and Thurnell (1961), Clarke and Hellon (1957), Holling *et al.* (1961), Mason *et al.* (1964) and Strandness and Bell (1965). Sigdell (1969) gives a critical review of the theory of the mercury strain-gauge plethysmograph.

Electrical impedance plethysmography

Since electrical impedance methods have been employed to follow changes in cardiac output, it would seem reasonable to suppose that an impedance method could be used to monitor changes occurring in the volume of a limb following venous occlusion. This has been done by Allwood and Farncombe (1966, 1967), using a tetrapolar system with surface electrodes and transistorized circuitry. Limb volume changes were also simultaneously determined with a water-filled plethysmograph or a mercury-in-rubber strain gauge. Except during intense vasoconstriction or during some intravenous adrenaline infusions which produced a redistribution of blood within the limb segment, there was a good correlation between the methods. As the volume increases, so the measured impedance decreases. Young *et al* (1967) compared an impedance plethysmograph with an electromagnetic flowmeter for recording volume changes in the hind limbs of dogs following venous occlusion. The results justified the use of the impedance method in clinical studies. Young *et al* (1967) find that a tetrapolar arrangement must be used in order to obtain reproducible results.

Kubicek, Patterson and Witsoe (1970) discuss an adaption of the automatically balancing 100 kHz bridge they have used for the measurement of cardiac output by the electrical impedance method for the measurement of leg blood flow. With the subject supine, his ankles are placed on a block of foam rubber approximately 4 inches high. Four disposable aluminized self-adhesive mylar strip electrodes are used. A venous occlusion cuff is placed around the thigh of one leg just above the knee. One strip electrode (No. 1) is wound round the thigh close to the groin side of the cuff. A second electrode (No. 2) is wound round the ankle. These electrodes are connected to the impedance cardiograph described by Kubicek, Patterson and Witsoe (1970) and which supplies these electrodes with a constant current of 100 kHz in frequency. Apart from the ease in making impedance measurements at this frequency, the high frequency removes the risk of producing ventricular defibrillation (Geddes, Baker and Moore, 1969). The two remaining band electrodes (Nos. 2 and 3) are placed approximately 4 inches apart in the central region of the calf. Electrical signals appearing across electrodes 2 and 3 are fed into the voltage input terminals of the impedance cardiograph. The elevation of the limb on the foam rubber ensures a good venous drainage before the occlusion is applied and removes any pressure from electrodes 2 and 3. The radio frequency bridge is then made to balance and the cuff pressure raised to 40 to 50 mm Hg. This occludes the venous outflow from the limb segment and the resultant swelling changes the impedance of the segment and unbalances the bridge causing the impedance output signal dZ to change as shown in *Figure 4.19*. The resultant tracing looks very much like a conventional venous occlusion plethysmogram. The total blood flow per minute into the limb segment has been calculated by Kubicek, Patterson and Witsoe (1970) using the formula $\mathrm{d}V = (pL^2/Z^2_0)\mathrm{d}Z \, 60$,

$$\overline{\mathrm{d}t}$$

where $p = 220$, L is the average distance between electrodes 2 and 3 measured front and back, Z_0 is the initial resting impedance between electrodes 2 and 3, and dZ is the impedance change occurring in the time interval $\mathrm{d}t$ seconds. The volume of the limb segment between electrodes 2 and 3 can be calculated and the blood flow expressed

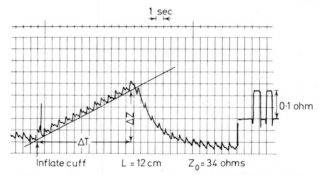

Figure 4.19. Venous occlusion tracing from an electrical impedance plethysmograph with electrodes placed around the calf. The measuring electrodes are separated by 12 cm and the resting impedance of the calf segment is 34 ohms. (Reproduced by courtesy of Instrumentation for Medicine Inc.)

conventionally in terms of ml per minute per 100 ml of tissue. An alternative formula proposed by Kubicek is $\mathrm{d}V = (c^2L/4\pi Z_0)\mathrm{d}Z$ where c is the average circumferance of the limb segment, L is the average distance between electrodes 2 and 3, $\mathrm{d}V$ is the blood flow occurring in a time $\mathrm{d}t$, and Z_0 is the resting impedance between electrodes 2 and 3.

By fitting the impedance cardiograph with two sets of electrode leads, alternate measurements can be made of limb blood flow and cardiac output.

Bashour and Jones (1965) obtained a correlation coefficient of 0·89 for venous occlusion and electrical impedance plethysmographs from opposite normal digits, whilst Mullick, Wheeler and Songster (1970) have found the presence of a baseline impedance change of less than 0·2 per cent on deep inspiration from limb electrodes 2 and 3 to indicate a less than normal venous blood flow change, presumably due to the obstruction of the inferior vena caval pressure. They have used this to detect deep vein thrombosis in post-operative surgical patients.

The use of an air-filled plethysmograph

Mune (1967) has employed an air-filled plethysmograph to record blood flow into the forefoot. A sensitive capacitance manometer was connected to the rubber forefoot bag which was inflated with air to 40 mm water pressure, the outer layer of the bag being relatively firm, the soft inner layer fitting the skin exactly when the bag was inflated. The pressure variations were directly proportional to changes in blood volume.

THIN-FILM RESISTANCE THERMOMETERS

The thin-film thermometer described by Bellhouse et al (1968) has a frequency response extending from zero to about 40 kHz. It is particularly valuable in physiological investigations into the production of turbulent flow patterns in the cardiovascular system. The construction of a needle flow-probe is described in detail by Bellhouse and Bellhouse (1968) and Bellhouse et al (1968) show thin-film probes mounted at the tips of catheters having diameters of 0·025 and 0·090 inch (0·63 mm and 2·25 mm).

Figure 4.20 details the construction of the flow element mounted in the needle probe. The element is formed from a length of hard glass rod which is drawn out in a gas flame; a spherical bead about 0·25 mm in diameter is formed and the rod cut to leave the bead with a stem about 12 mm long. The glass is cleaned with acetone and a narrow strip of platinum paint is painted on to the bead with the strip widening on the back of the sphere where leads will be soldered. Five coats of paint are needed. After each coat, the bead is placed in a furnace at room temperature and raised to 640°C over one hour and held at this temperature for 30 minutes in order to bed the

161

platinum into the glass. The resistance of the finished film is about 15 Ω. Two insulated 39 s.w.g. copper wires are soldered on to the conducting paint with soft solder. The completed element is held in the needle with epoxy resin.

The thickness of the film is about one micrometre. It has a very small thermal capacity, but because of thermal gradients within the substrate, the probe will have a relatively poor frequency response unless the film is operated in a constant temperature mode. By this means thermal waves within the substrate are reduced and a very high frequency response is obtained. Constant temperature operation is achieved by connecting the heated thin-film element in one arm of a Wheatstone bridge circuit whose energizing supply is obtained from the output of a d.c. amplifier, *Figure 4.21*. The temperature of the

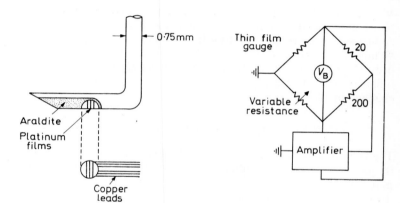

Figure 4.20. Thin-film velocity probe in a hypodermic needle (after Bellhouse and Bellhouse, 1968)

Figure 4.21. Constant temperature feedback bridge (after Bellhouse and Bellhouse, 1968)

element is maintained at a predetermined level, and velocity fluctuations are indicated by fluctuations in the power necessary to balance the bridge. In air, there is a low-frequency effect caused by leakage of heat from the element to the surrounding glass, and this makes a dynamic calibration essential. In fluids such as water and blood which have a higher thermal conductivity the steady state and dynamic calibrations are identical. Bellhouse *et al* (1968) mention the use of a linearizing circuit to straighten the calibration curve, which in any case is not far removed from linearity.

An inherent disadvantage of a single thin-film element is that it is unable to detect a flow reversal. This facility is important in phasic blood-flow studies and can be provided by locating two further elements upstream and downstream of the central element which alone is maintained at a constant resistance. The two outer films are arranged in a bridge circuit and a low current is passed through them. The output from the centre element occurs for flows in both the forward and reverse directions. It corresponds to full-wave rectification of a sinewave flow. However, the frequency response of this probe is good. The output from the bridge circuit containing the outer films is phase sensitive but has an adequate frequency response only up to about 50 Hz. By superimposing the two tracings, the direction of flow for the centre probe can easily be ascertained, *Figure 4.22.*

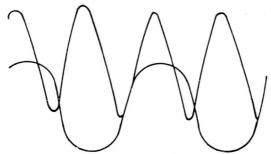

Figure 4.22. Sensing of flow direction. Upper trace, constant temperature probe; lower trace, direction indicator (after Bellhouse and colleagues, 1968)

The heat supplied to a thin-film probe is related to the fluid flow velocity by

$$\frac{i^2 R}{\Delta T} = A\left(\frac{k\sigma^{\frac{1}{3}}}{8}\right)U^{\frac{1}{3}} + B$$

where $i^2 R$ is the heating power supplied to the probe

U is the fluid velocity

ΔT is the difference in temperature of the probe and fluid (typically 5–10°C)

k is the thermal conductivity of the fluid

σ is the Prandtl number of the fluid

8 is the kinematic viscosity of the fluid

B is a constant.

163

REFERENCES

Blood flow meters—electromagnetic

Abel, F. L. (1959). 'Chopper-operated electromagnetic flowmeter.' *I.R.E. Trans. med. Electron.* **6**, 216

Beck, R., Morris, J. A. and Assali, N.S. (1965). 'Calibration characteristics of the pulsed-field electromagnetic flowmeter.' *Am. J. med. Electron.* **4**, 87

Bergel, D. H. (1968). 'The electromagnetic flowmeter.' In *Blood flow Through Tissues and Organs.* Ed. by W. H. Bain and A. Murray Harper. Edinburgh; Livingstone

Brecher, G. A. (1967). 'Types of flowmeters, merits and demerits.' In *Engineering in the Practice of Medicine.* Ed. by B. L. Segal and D. G. Kilpatrick, p. 339. Baltimore; Williams and Wilkins

Cappelen, C. and Hall, K. V. (1964). 'The great saphenous vein used *in situ* as an arterial shunt after vein valve extirpation.' *Acta chir. scand.* **128**, 517

Cardus, D., Quesada, E. M. and Scott, F. B. (1963). 'Use of an electromagnetic flowmeter for urine flow measurements.' *J. appl. Physiol.* **18**, 845

Case, R. B., Roselle, H. A. and Nassar, M. E. (1966). 'Simplified method for calibration of electromagnetic flowmeters.' *Med. res. Engng.* **5**, 38

Cooper, T. and Richardson, A. W. (1959). 'Comparative pulsatile blood flow contours demonstrating the importance of RC output circuit design in electromagnetic blood flow meters.' *I.R.E. Trans. med. Electron.* **6(4)** 207

Denison, A. B., Spencer, M. P. and Green, H. O. (1955). 'A square-wave electromagnetic flowmeter for application to intact blood vessels.' *Circulation Res.* **3**, 39

Edgerton, R. H. (1968). 'The effect of arterial wall thickness and conductivity on electromagnetic flowmeter readings.' *Med. Electron biol. Engng.* **6**, 627

Elliott, S. E., Hoffman, J. I. E. and Guz, A. (1963). 'An electromagnetic flowmeter for simultaneous measurements of pulmonary, arterial and aortic blood flows in the conscious animal.' *Med. Electron. biol. Engng.* **1**, 323

Feder, W. (1959). 'Résumé of D.C. electromagnetic flowmeter group discussion.' *I.R.E. Trans. med. Electron.* **6(4)**, 250

— and Bay, E. B. (1959). 'The D.C. electromagnetic flowmeter and its application to blood flow measurement in unopened vessels.' *I.R.E. Trans. med. Electron.* **6(4)**, 240

Ferguson, D. J. and Landahl, H. D. (1966). 'Magnetic meters: effects of electrical resistance in tissues on flow measurements in an improved calibration for square-wave circuits.' *Circulation Res.* **19**, 917

— and Wells, H. S. (1959). 'Frequencies in pulsatile flow and response of magnetic meters.' *Circulation Res.* **7**, 336

Gessner, U. and Bergel, D. H. (1964). 'Frequency response of electromagnetic flowmeters.' *J. appl. Physiol.* **19**, 1209

Goldman, S. C., Marple, N. B. and Scolnik, W. L. (1963). 'Effects of flow profile on electromagnetic flowmeter accuracy.' *J. appl. Physiol.* **20**, 142

Hepps, S. A., Roe, B. B. and Rutkin, B. B. (1963). 'Coronary blood flow in the intact conscious dog: studies with miniature electromagnetic flow transducers.' *J. thorac. cardiovasc. Surg.* **46,** 783

Hirschberg, H. (1967). 'Design and evaluation of low noise input amplifiers for square wave electromagnetic blood flow meters.' *Digest 7th Int. Conf. Med. and Biol. Engng. Stockholm*

Hoffman, J. I. E., Guz, A., Spotts, R. R. and Weirich, W. L. (1960). 'Stroke volume and cardiac output measurement in the intact animal with an electromagnetic flowmeter.' *Circulation* **22,** 763

Hognestad, H. (1966). 'Square wave electromagnetic flow meter with improved baseline stability.' *Med. res. Engng.* **5,** 28

Jacobson, E. D. and Swan, K. G. (1966). 'Hydraulic occluder for chronic electromagnetic blood flow determinations.' *J. appl. Physiol.* **21,** 1400

Khouri, E. M. and Gregg, D. E. (1963). 'Miniature electromagnetic flowmeter applicable to coronary arteries.' *J. appl. Physiol.* **18,** 224

— Rayford, C. R. (1965). 'Effect of exercise on cardiac output, left coronary flow and myocardial metabolism in the unanesthetized dog.' *Circulation Res.* **5,** 427

Kolin, A. (1936). 'Electromagnetic flow meter: principle of method and its application to blood flow measurements.' *Proc. Soc. exp. Biol. Med.* **35,** 53

— (1959). 'Electromagnetic blood flow meter.' *Science, N. Y.* **130,** 1088

— Herrold, G. and Assali, N. (1958). 'Electromagnetic blood flow meter yielding a baseline without interruption of flow.' *Proc. Soc. exp. Biol. Med.* **98,** 550

— Ross, G., Gaal, P. and Austin, S. (1964). 'Simultaneous electromagnetic measurement of blood flow in the major coronary arteries.' *Nature, Lond.* **203,** 148

McDonald, D. A., Sugawara, H., Engelhardt, W. V. and Attinger, E. O. (1965). 'The form of the arterial flow wave.' *Physiologist Wash.* **8,** 230

Meyer, J. S., Ishikawa, S., Lee, T. K. and Thal, A. (1963). 'Quantitative measurement of cerebral blood flow with electromagnetic flowmeter. Recording internal jugular venous flow of monkey and man.' *Trans. Am. neurol. Ass.* **88,** 78

Mills, C. J. (1963). 'An intraluminal electromagnetic flow meter.' *J. Physiol. Lond.,* **167,** 2

— (1968). 'A catheter tip electromagnetic velocity probe for use in man.' In *Blood Flow Through Organs and Tissues,* p. 38. Ed. by W. H. Bain and W. A. Mackey. Edinburgh; Livingstone

Mimms, M. M. and Johnson, S. (1963). 'Evaluation of canine renal arterial occlusion and hypertension with the electromagnetic flowmeter.' *J. Urol.* **89,** 29

Nelson, P. J. (1967). 'Vascular pneumatic constrictor for *in vivo* calibration of electromagnetic flowmeters.' *J. appl. Physiol.* **22,** 818

Odeblad, E. (1955), 'Electromagnetic measurement of the blood streaming velocity in man.' *Acta med. scand.* **151,** 95

Olmsted, F. (1962). 'Phase detection electromagnetic flowmeter—design and use.' *I.R.E. Trans. bio-med. Electron.* **9,** 88

— and Aldrich, F. D. (1961). 'Improved electromagnetic flowmeter; phase detection, a new principle.' *J. appl. Physiol.* **16,** 197

O'Rourke, M. E. (1965). 'Dynamic accuracy of the electromagnetic flowmeter.' *J. appl. Physiol.* **20**, 142

Price, J. B., Britton, R. C., Peterson, L. M., Reilly, J. W. and Voorhees, A. B. (1965). 'The validity of chronic hepatic blood flow measurements obtained by the electromagnetic flow meter.' *J. surg. Res.* **5**, 313

Richardson, A. W. (1959). 'A simplified electromagnetic flowmeter with high fidelity recording.' *J. appl. Physiol.* **14**, 658

— Cooper, T. and Ciszczon, W. J. (1961). 'A transistorised electromagnetic blood flowmeter.' *J. appl. Physiol.* **16**, 940

Scher, A. M., Zepeda, J. and Brown, O. F. (1963). 'Square wave electromagnetic flowmeter employing commercially available recorder.' *J. appl. Physiol.* **18**, 1265

Shercliff, J. A. (1962). *The Theory of Electromagnetic Flow Measurement.* Cambridge; University Press

Spencer, M. P. and Denison, A. B. (1959). 'The square wave electromagnetic flowmeter: The Theory of operation and design of magnetic probes for clinical and experimental applications.' *I.R.E. Trans. med. Electron.* **6**, 220

— — (1960). 'Square wave electromagnetic flowmeter for surgical and experimental application.' *Meth. med. Res.* **8**, 321

Thornton, W. and Bejack, B. (1959). 'Performance and application of a commercial blood flow probe.' *I.R.E. Trans. med. Electron.* **6**, 237

Weber, K. C., Engle, J. C., Lyons, G. W., Masden, A. J. and Fox, I. J. (1965). 'Calibration and zero flow of electromagnetic flowmeter probes on pulmonary artery and aorta.' *Physiologist, Wash.* **8**, 301

Westersten, A., Herrold, G., Abott, E. and Assali, N. S. (1959). 'Gated sine wave electromagnetic flow meter.' *I.R.E. Trans. med. Electron.* **6**, 213

Wetterer, E. (1937). 'Eine neue Method zur Registerierung der Blustromungsgeschwindigkeit am uneroffneten Gefass.' *Z. Biol.* **98**, 26

Wyatt, D. G. (1961) 'Zero error in induction flowmeters employing a permanent magnet.' *Physics Med. Biol.* **5**, 449

— (1968a). 'Dependence of electromagnetic flowmeter sensitivity upon encircled media.' *Physics Med. Biol.* **13**, 529

— (1968b). 'The electromagnetic blood flowmeter.' *J. Scient. Instrum.*, **1**, 1146

— (1971). 'Electromagnetic blood-flow measurement.' In *IEE Medical Electronics Monographs* 1–6, Ed. by B. W. Watson, p. 181. London; Institution of Electrical Engineers.

Yanof, H. M. (1961). 'A trapezoidal-wave electromagnetic blood flowmeter.' *J. appl. Physiol.* **16**, 566

— Rosen, A. L. and Shoemaker, W. C. (1963). 'Design of an implantable flowmeter transducer based on the Helmholtz coil.' *J. appl. Physiol.* **18**, 227

Blood flow meters—thermal-type

Aschoff, J. and Wever, R. (1956). 'Die Funktionswiese der Diathermie-Thermostromuhr.' *Pflügers Arch. ges. Physiol.* **262**, 133

Brill, J. C., Hanafee, W. N. and Norman, A. (1964). 'A flowmeter for use in angiographic studies.' *Radiology*, **82**, 133

Clark, C. (1968). 'A local thermal dilution flowmeter for the measurement of venous flow in man.' *Med. Electron. Biol. Engng.* **6**, 133

Dowsett, D. J. and Lowe, R. D. (1964). 'Measurement of blood flow by local thermal dilution.' *J. Physiol., Lond.* **172,** 13P

Felix, W. and Groll, H. (1953). 'Die Messung des Blutstromes mit Thermistoren.' *Z. Biol.* **106,** 208

Froenk, A. and Ganz, V. (1960). 'Measurement of flow in single blood vessels including cardiac output by local thermodilution.' *Circulation Res.* **8,** 175

Grahn, A. R., Wessel, H. U. and Paul, M. H. (1967). 'Development of a new linear catheter tip thermistor flow meter.' p. 216. In *Proc. 7th Int. Conf. Med. and Biol. Engng. Stockholm*

Lawn, L., Spires, R. A. and Whitworth, T. G. (1964). 'A simplified thermistor flow meter and thermometer.' *Physics Med. Biol.* **9,** 407

Levy, L. L., Stolwijk, J. A. J. and Graichen, H. (1967). 'Evaluation of local brain blood flow by continuous direct measurement of thermal conductivity.' p. 217. In *Proc. 7th Int. Conf. Med. and Biol. Engng. Stockholm.*

Mendlowitz, M. (1948). 'The specific heat of human blood.' *Science, N. Y.* **107,** 97

Rein, H. (1929). 'Die Thermo-stromuhr.' *Z. Biol.* **89,** 195

Blood flow meters, ultrasonic, and ultrasonic techniques

Ambrose, J. (1964). 'Pulsed ultra-sound illustrations of clinical applications.' *Br. J. Radiol.* **37,** 165

Barnett, E., and Morley, P. (1971). 'Ultrasound in the investigation of space occupying lesions of the urinary tract.' *Br. J. Radiol.,* **44,** 733

Bernstine, R. L. (1969). 'Safety studies with ultrasonic Doppler technique.' *Obstet. Gynec. N. Y.* **34,** 707

Bobrow, M., Blackwell, N., Unrav, A. E., and Bleaney, B. (1971) 'Absence of any observed effect of ultrasonic irradiation on human chromosomes.' *J. Obstet. Gynaec. Br. Commonw.,* **78,** 730

Boyd, E., Abdulla, U., Donald, I., Fleming, J. E. E. Hall, A. J., and Ferguson-Smith, M. A. (1971). 'Chromosome breakage and ultrasound.' *Br. med. J.* **2,** 501.

Brown, R. E. (1967). 'Ultrasonic localization of the placenta.' *Radiology,* **89,** 828

— (1968). 'Detection of intra-uterine death.' *Am. J. Obstet. Gynec.,* **102,** 965

— (1971). 'Doppler ultrasound in obstetrics.' *J. Am. med. Ass.,* **218,** 1395

Callagan, D. A. (1967). 'Ultrasonic Doppler inspection of the fetal heart.' In *Engineering in the Practice of Medicine.* p. 363. Ed. by B. L. Segal, and D. G. Kilpatrick. Baltimore; Williams and Wilkins

— Rowland, T. C. and Goldman, D. E. (1964). 'Ultrasonic Doppler observation of the fetal heart.' *Obstet. Gynec. N.Y.* **23,** 637

Campbell, S., and Dewhurst, C. J. (1970). 'Quintuplet pregnancy diagnosed and assessed by ultrasonic compound scanning.' *Lancet* **1,** 101

Donald, I. and Abdulla, U. (1967). 'Ultrasonics in obstetrics and gynaecology.' *Br. J. Radiol.* **40,** 604

Edler, I. (1966). 'Mitral valve function studied by the ultrasound method.' In *Diagnostic Ultrasound.* Ed. by C. C. Crossman *et al.* p. 198. New York; Plenum Press

Feigenbaum, H., Zaky, A. and Waldhausen, J. A. (1967). 'Use of reflected ultrasound in detecting pericardial effusion.' *Am. J. Cardiol.* **19,** 84.

Franklin, D. L., Baker, D. W. and Rushmer, R. F. (1962). 'Pulsed ultrasonic transit time flowmeter.' *I.R.E. Trans. Biomed. Electron.* **9**, 44
— Van Citters, R. L. and Rushmer, R. F. (1962). 'Balance between right and left ventricular output.' *Circulation Res.* **10**, 17
— Schlegel, W. A. and Watson, N. W. (1963). 'Ultrasonic Doppler shift blood flowmeter : circuitry and practical application.' In *Biomedical Sciences Instrumentation*, p. 309. Ed. by F. Alt. New York; Plenum Press
— Watson, N. W., Van Citters, R. L. (1964). 'Blood velocity telemetered from untethered animals.' *Nature, Lond.* **203**, 528
— Baker, D. W., Ellis, R. M. and Rushmer, R. F. (1959). 'A pulsed ultrasonic flowmeter.' *I.R.E. Trans. med. Electron.* **6**, 204.
Goldberg, B. B. (1971). 'Suprasternal ultrasonography.' *J.Am. med. Ass.* 215, 245
Hellman, L. M., Duffus, G. M., Donald, I., and Sunden, B. (1970). 'Safety of diagnostic ultrasound in obstretics.' *Lancet* **1**, 1133
James, J. A., Dalton, G. A., Hadley, K. J., Freundlich, H. F., Bullen, M. A. and Wells, P. N. T. (1963). 'A new 3-megacycle generator for destruction of the vestibular end organ.' *Acta oto-lar.* **56**, 148
Johnson, W. L., Stegal, H. F., Lein, J. N. and Rushmer, R. F. (1965). 'Detection of fetal life in early pregnancy with an ultrasonic Doppler flowmeter.' *Obstet. Gynec. N.Y.* **26**, 305
Kuah, K. B., and Embrey, M. P. (1968). 'Experience with an ultrasonic foetal pulse monitor.' *Br. med. J.*, **1**, 438
Kyle, K. F., Deane, R. F., Morley, P., and Barnett, E. (1971). 'Ultrasonography of the urinary tract.' *Br. J. Urol.*, **43**, 709
Oksala, A. (1966). 'Development and significance of ultrasonic diagnosis in eye disease.' In *Ultrasonics in Ophthalmology*. Ed. by A. Oksala and H. Gernet. Basle; Karger
Plaas, K. G. (1964). 'A new ultrasonic flowmeter for intravascular application.' *I.R.E. trans. biomed. Electron.* **11**, 154
Schentke, K. U. and Renger, F. (1966). 'Uber die diagnostische Verwertberkeit des Ultraschallhepatograms.' *Z. ges. inn. Med.* **21**, 239
Staple, T. W. and Brinker, R. A. (1968). 'The ultrasonic flowmeter as an adjunct to femoral arteriography.' *Radiology* **90**, 341
Sunden, B. (1964). 'On the diagnostic value of ultrasound in obstetrics and gynecology.' *Acta obstet. gynec. scand.* **43**, Suppl. 6
Van Citters, R. L., Watson, N. W., Franklin, D. L. and Elsner, R. W. (1965). 'Telemetry of aortic blood pressure and flow in free ranging animals.' *Fed. Proc.* **24**, 525
Yamakawa, K. and Kitamura, K. (1963). 'The intracardiac phonocardiograph and the ultrasonic Doppler method.' *Jap. Circul. J.* **27**

Venous occlusion plethysmography

Allwood, M. J. and Farncombe, M. (1966). 'Electrical impedance plethysmography.' *J. Physiol. Lond.* **184**, 63 P
— — (1967). 'Forearm impedance during venous occlusion plethysmography'. *J. Physiol., Lond.* **189**, 33 P
Ardill, B. L., Fentem, P. H. and Williams, R. L. (1968). 'Some observations on the accuracy of blood flow measurement by venous occlusion plethysmography using the mercury-in-rubber strain gauge.' In *Blood Flow Through Organs and Tissues*. Ed. by W. H. Bain and A. M. Harper. p. 25. Edinburgh; Livingstone.

Bashour, F. A., and Jones, R. E. (1965). 'Digital blood flow. 1. Correlative study of the electrical impedance and the venous occlusive plethysmograms.' *Dis. Chest.* **47,** 465

Brakkee, A. J. M., and Vendrik, A. J. H. (1966). 'Strain gauge plethysmography; theoretical and practical notes on a new design.' *J. appl. Physiol.* **21,** 701

Burger, H. C., Horeman, H. W., and Brakkee, A. J. M. (1959). 'Comparison of some methods for measuring peripheral blood flow.' *Physics Med. Biol.* **4,** 168

Celander, O., and Thurnell, G. (1961). 'The "mercury-in-rubber" strain gauge for measurements of blood pressure and peripheral circulation in new-born infants.' *Acta paediat.* **50,** 505

Clarke, R. S. J., and Hellon, R. F. (1957). 'Venous collection in forearm and hand measured by the strain-gauge and volume plethysmograph.' *Clin. Sci.* **16,** 103

Geddes, L. A., Baker, L. E., and Moore, A. G. (1969). 'Hazards in the use of low frequencies for the measurement of physiological events by impedance.' *Med. biol. Engng.* **7,** 289

Greenfield, A. D. M., Whitney, R. J. and Mowbray, J. F. (1963). 'Methods for the investigation of peripheral blood flow.' *Br. med. Bull.* **19,** 101

Holling, H. E., Boland, H. C., and Russ, E. (1961). 'Investigation of arterial obstruction using a mercury-in-rubber strain gauge. *Am. Heart J.,* **62,** 194

Hyman, C. and Winsor, T. (1966). 'An electric volume transducer system for plethysmographic recording.' *J. appl. Physiol.* **21,** 1403

Kubicek, W. G., Patterson, R. P., and Witsoe, D. A. (1970). 'Impedance cardiography as a non-invasive method of monitoring cardiac function and other parameters of the cardiovascular system.' *Ann. N.Y. Acad. Sci.* **170,** 724

Mason, D. T., Braunwald, E., Karsh, R. B., and Bullock, E. A. (1964). 'Effects of ouabain on forearm vascular resistance and venous tone in normal subjects and in patients in heart failure.' *J. clin. Invest.* **43,** 532

Mullick, S. C., Wheeler, H. B., and Songster, G. F. (1970). 'Diagnosis of deep venous thrombosis by measurement of electrical impedance.' *Am. J. Surg.,* **119,** 417

Mune, O. (1967). 'Plethysmography of the forefoot.' *Scand. J. clin. Lab. Invest.* **19,** Suppl. 99, 109

Sigdell, Jan-Erik (1969). 'A critical review of the mercury strain-gauge plethysmograph.' *Med. biol. Engng.,* **7,** 365

Strandness, D. E., and Bell, J. W. (1961). 'Peripheral vascular disease: diagnosis and objective evaluation using a mercury strain-gauge. *Ann. Surg. Suppl.* **161,** 1

Young, D. G., Cox, R. H., Stoner, E. K. and Erdman, W. J. (1967). 'Evaluation of quantitative impedance plethysmography for continuous blood flow measurement. 1. Electrode systems.' *Am. J. phys. Med.* **46,** 1261

— — — — (1967). 'Evaluation of quantitative impedance plethysmography for continuous blood flow measurement. III Blood flow determination *in vivo.*' *Am. J. phys. Med.* **46,** 1450

Whitney, R. J. (1953). 'The measurement of volume changes in human limbs.' *J. physiol. Lond.* **121,** 1

Wood, J. R., and Hyman, C. (1970). 'A direct reading capacitance plethysmograph.' *Med. biol. Engng.* **8,** 59

Thin-film resistance thermometers

Bellhouse, B. J., Schultz, D. L., Karatzas, N. B. and Lee, G. de J., (1968). 'A catheter tip method for the measurement of the pulsatile blood flow velocity in arteries'. In *Blood Flow Through Organs and Tissues* Ed. by W. H. Bain and A. M. Harper, Edinburgh; Livingstone
— and Bellhouse, F. H. (1968). 'Thin-film gauges for the measurement of velocity of skin friction in air, water or blood.' *J. scient. Instrum.* **1,** 1211

5-Recording Electrodes

The choice of the electrodes used for the recording of bio-electric signals from the surface of the body or from muscles requires careful consideration. However good may be the subsequent amplification and recording equipment, if the electrodes are uncomfortable for the patient to wear, or if they are responsible for the generation of artefact signals, then it is unlikely that it will prove to be possible to record satisfactory signals over the required period of time. It is worth stressing the time element, because what may be suitable for use with an unconscious patient during relatively short surgical procedures may not be suitable for use when monitoring for several days may be required in a ward.

Desirable characteristics of electrodes

The most commonly encountered electrodes in studies concerned with surgery and anaesthesia are surface electrodes. These are needed for the recording of the ECG, EEG and impedance changes. The surface properties of such electrodes are important in determining the potential difference existing between the electrode and the underlying electrolyte. It is desirable that this potential difference should be as nearly equal for all electrodes used for a particular measurement from a patient. The contact impedances of the electrodes should also be as low, and as nearly equal, as possible. Any marked difference in the contact impedance of a pair of recording electrodes used in bipolar recording will reduce the in-phase signal rejection ratio of the recording channel. The contact impedance is the impedance at the specified frequency measured beneath the metallic electrode applied to the skin at some point on the patient's body and the tissues beneath the skin at that point.

The discrimination ratio between the wanted antiphase bio-electric signal and the unwanted in-phase interference signal is given by $(R_1/2)(R_2-R_1)$ where R_1 is the total input impedance of the recording amplifier, and R_1 and R_2 are the contact impedances of the electrodes. If $R_i = 2\,M\Omega$ and $R_1 = 5\,k\Omega$ while $R_2 = 4\,k\Omega$, then the discrimination (or rejection) ratio is 1,000.

The voltage presented to the recording channel from the electrodes consists of two main components. One is the contact potential of the order of a fraction of a volt which is relatively constant. It is possible, however, for corrosion effects at the electrodes to generate rapid potential changes which appear as artefacts in an a.c. recording (Flasterstein, 1966). The other is the bio-electric signal which could be up to 1,000 times smaller and varies much more rapidly. In the majority of applications the recording amplifier is only required to respond to alternating signals so that the relatively slowly varying contact potential is ignored. This fact considerably simplifies matters. The problem of stable electrodes is acute when low level d.c. recordings have to be made, for example, of the d.c. electro-oculogram (EOG), where the signals produced by eye movements are of the order of 200 μV (Shackel, 1967). Unwanted signals on the electro-oculogram can arise from the skin potential response (SPR) and from noise generated at the electrode-skin interface. The SPR has been shown to be reduced when perspiration is reduced, and also when the outer horny layer of the skin is removed. The noise generated at the electrode-skin interface arises from the fact that at the interface there is a transition from ionic current flow in the body to electronic current flow in the connecting wires. In order to achieve a stable baseline in the recording, the electrode must have a stable and predictable potential with respect to the electrolyte. For the more exacting requirements as typified by the EOG and EEG it is usual to make use of silver-silver chloride electrodes. Shackel (1967) states that it is possible to attain d.c. drifts on average of less than 50 μV per minute with suction cup silver-silver chloride electrodes.

Reversible electrodes

The contact of a metal electrode with an electrolyte forms a half-cell with a d.c. potential dependent upon the nature of the metal and electrolyte. Two electrodes with a common electrolyte form two half-cells connected in series opposition. With identical electrodes, the e.m.f. of the cell should be zero. If the electrodes are made from dissimilar metals an e.m.f. will exist between them since each metal will assume a different potential with respect to the electrolyte. The completion of an external circuit between the electrodes will cause current to flow. The e.m.f. available depends upon the nature of the metal electrodes, the concentration of ions in the electrolyte and the temperature.

A simple electrolytic cell consists of two copper plates immersed in a solution of copper sulphate. When an external battery is used to drive current through the cell the state of equilibrium existing previously at each electrode is disturbed. At the anode, copper atoms give up electrons and pass into the electrolyte as ions, while copper ions arriving at the cathode acquire electrons and form a deposit of copper. Copper ions are doubly charged, so that each pair of electrons flowing in the external circuit results in the formation of one copper ion and the deposition of one copper atom. Copper is transferred from one electrode to the other and the composition of the electrolyte remains constant. Reversing the current flow simply reverses the transfer of copper, the composition of the electrodes remaining constant. This is a reversible cell. When no current flows, a potential difference will not exist between the electrodes since they each acquire the same potential with respect to the electrolyte.

If both of the electrodes were now replaced with iron electrodes, initially since the electrodes were identical no potential difference would exist between them; however with the passage of current, copper will be deposited upon the cathode and a potential difference will build up and alter the current. This effect is known as polarization. The presence of this potential difference will aid current flow in one direction and oppose it in the other. Small applied potentials may be ineffective in causing current to flow. This arrangement is obviously not a reversible cell. The theory of reversible cells is given by Spiegler and Wyllie (1968).

Silver-silver chloride electrodes

If chemically reactive electrodes are used they must be chosen to be reversible. The major proportion of ions in tissue fluids consists of sodium, potassium, chloride, bicarbonate and protein, with chloride being the most widely distributed. Owing to their reactive nature, sodium and potassium are unsuitable as electrode materials, so that an insoluble chloride offers the best possibility for a stable electrode material, and silver chloride has proved to be acceptable. By taking care with the preparation of the electrodes and selecting them, pairs of silver-silver chloride electrodes can be produced which have potential differences between them of only fractions of a millivolt (Feder, 1963). Venables and Sayer (1963) by selecting silver-silver chloride electrode pairs obtained a standing voltage of not more than

173

0·1 mV with a drift over 30 minutes of about 0·05 mV. Silver-silver chloride electrodes are usually prepared by electrolysis. Two silver discs are suspended in a 5 per cent saline solution, and the electrode to be chlorided connected to the positive pole of a 1·5-V dry cell, the negative pole going to the other electrode. To produce an electrode suitable for EEG recording, current is allowed to flow for about 30 seconds forming a layer of silver chloride upon the surface of the anode. Margerison, St. John-Loe and Binnie (1967) re-commend that re-chloriding should be performed when the current which passes between a pair of silver-silver chloride electrodes immersed in saline exceeds one 1 μA. Geddes, Baker and Moore (1969) recommend a minimum chloriding current density of 5 mA/cm^2 of electrode area. A chloride deposit of 100–500 mA. sec/cm^2 of electrode area gave the lowest electrode-electrolyte impedance.

Polarization over-voltage

With a pair of truly reversible electrodes, there will not be an open circuit potential between them, and the existing potential difference will be unaltered due to polarization effects when a current flows between the electrodes. In practical electrodes the design is such as to minimize both the open circuit potential and the polarization over-voltage (the change in open circuit potential due to current flow). The polarization over-voltage consists of three components Nencini and Pasquali (1968)—the ohmic over-voltage (which is linearly related to the current density), the decomposition over-voltage (which predominates at low current densities) and the concentration over-voltage (which appears at high current densities) (Weinman and Mahler, 1964). These over-voltage components take time to build up. The electrode current-voltage relationship can thus be expressed in terms of a variable polarization impedance having resistive and capacitive components (Weinman and Mahler, 1959). If electrodes showing these properties are used to handle pulses of the order of 2 mV in amplitude and 100 ms wide, then considerable distortion can arise (Nencini and Pasquali, 1968).

An example of a highly polarizable type of electrode is a platinum wire in contact with a saline solution. Current flowing through this electrode may alter its potential considerably since the rate of discharge of ions from the solution is slow at the electrode surface and also there is no rapid supply of ions to the solution.

A detailed account of electrodes suitable for extracellular recording and stimulation is that of Delgado (1964).

ECG electrodes

Undoubtedly, the most commonly recorded electrical signal from patients is the electrocardiogram. Conventional electrocardiographs are supplied with a set of metal plate limb electrodes which are normally held in place by elastic straps. The skin beneath the plates is first cleaned with an ether-meth mixture and a conducting electrode paste or jelly applied to the skin where the plate is to be placed, and the plate rubbed over the jelly to make a good contact before being secured in place. With normal size plates, the contact impedance at 20 Hz with this technique is likely to be of the order of 6,500 Ω for a single electrode. A multipoint electrode of similar size pressed well into the skin would have a contact impedance of the order of 9,000 Ω. Multipoint electrodes *Figure 5.1*, are made from

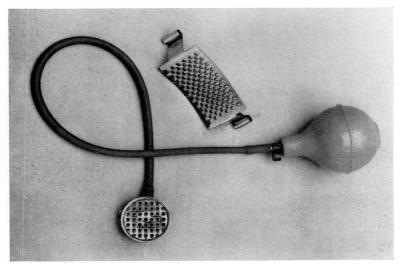

Figure 5.1. Multipoint limb and chest electrodes. (Reproduced by courtesy of Hillier Ltd.)

a stainless steel or rhodium-plated material similar to that used to make a nutmeg grater (Lewes, 1966). In order to obtain the maximum rejection of unwanted in-phase mains frequency signals, it is necessary that not only should the contact impedance of individual electrodes be as low as possible, but they should be as nearly as possible equal. It is also necessary that the input impedance of the recording amplifier should be as high as possible (Geddes and Baker, 1966).

175

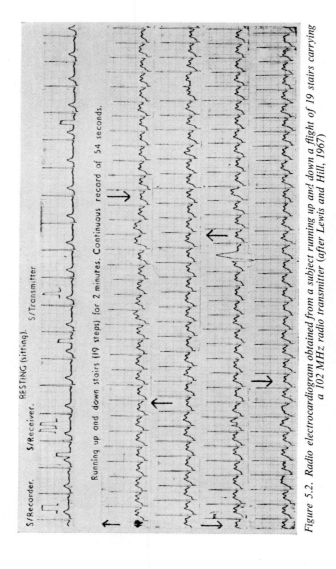

Figure 5.2. Radio electrocardiogram obtained from a subject running up and down a flight of 19 stairs carrying a 102 MHz radio transmitter (after Lewis and Hill, 1967)

176

Suction-cup electrodes are commonly used to record the unipolar chest leads.

Limb electrodes are convenient to use during surgery where the patient's limbs are relatively immobile and the presence of chest electrodes would interfere with the surgery.

With care in applying limb electrodes, there should not be especial difficulty in obtaining contact impedances of the order quoted. If vigilance is relaxed however, a wide spread of values can occur. Schmitt, Okajima and Blaug (1961) measured the contact impedance at 60 Hz of electrodes used in routine electrocardiography. The average value was 2,400 Ω but values up to 40 times this were encountered.

Limb electrodes are not suitable for use when monitoring conscious or semi-conscious patients because of the electromyographic voltages generated by the activity of limb muscles, and there is also the inconvenience to the patient of the trailing leads. In practice, the first factor is not much improved by moving the site of the electrodes to the upper portion of each limb. The great advantage of limb leads lies in the fact that the normal and augmented limb leads are standard and well suited for comparison purposes.

Most patient-monitoring systems employ two or three chest electrodes which are normally stuck on to the skin, a typical siting for three electrodes being over the manubrium, xiphisternum and apex of the heart. This gives a lead which is not dissimilar in appearance from the conventional lead 2. Muscle activity artefact voltages are minimized by placing the electrodes over bony structures. Using a pair of multipoint electrodes stuck to the skin over the manubrium and xiphisternum, Lewes and Hill (1967) were able with this arrangement to obtain a clean ECG by radio telemetry from a subject running up and down a flight of 19 steps (*Figure 5.2*). Of course, the M-X lead is non-standard. Burns and Gollnick (1966) use a floating-mesh ECG electrode during exercise studies.

Since limb electrodes give rise to motion artefacts, Mason and Likar (1966) found electrode sites on the thorax which produced recordings similar to the conventional leads, 1, 2 and 3. They located two of the electrodes on the right and left chest below the clavicles with the third on the anterior axillary line halfway between the costal margin and the crest of the ileum.

The location of the electrodes which gives minimum motion artefacts is not always the best from the diagnostic viewpoint if small changes in the ECG pattern are to be observed.

Gibson *et al* (1962) recommend locating one electrode over the

177

manubrium and a second over the left fifth or sixth interspace at the anterior axillary line when it is required to look for possible alterations in the S-T segment and T wave.

If the subject is not exercising vigorously, a useful form of chest electrode consists of a stainless steel gauze about 1 cm square placed at the centre of a 4 × 4 cm piece of self-adhesive plaster. The skin site is first cleaned with an ether-meth mixture and vigorously rubbed. A little electrode cream is placed on the gauze and the electrode pressed firmly down on the skin (*Figure 5.3*).

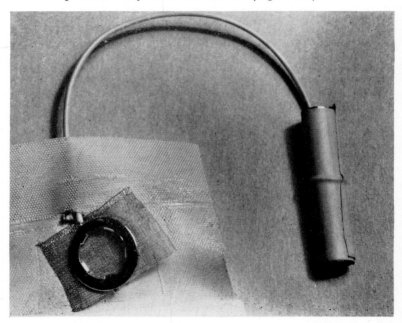

Figure 5.3. Self-adhesive plaster metal gauze ECG electrode. (Reproduced by courtesy of Drachard Ltd.)

Electrode jellies and creams

In the days of low-impedance string-galvanometer ECG recorders, electrode contact impedances of only a few thousand ohms were essential, and abrasive saline electrode creams and jellies were required. Some versions of these will raise a blister on the skin after only 4 hours, while on drying they can leave a deposit which spoils the patient's clothing and perishes rubber straps. Modern electrode creams possess a good conductivity, and will not irritate the skin, even when worn all day. They are colourless and odourless. The jelly must wet the surface of the body and should not contain soap. The preservative used must be chosen to be non-irritant. An average value for the specific resistance of electrode creams is 1,000 Ω cm. This value was obtained by measuring several commercially available creams contained in turn in a measuring cell connected to a 10 Hz Schering bridge, individual results are shown in the Table 5.1.

TABLE 5.1

MEASURED CONDUCTIVITY OF VARIOUS ELECTRODE JELLIES AND CREAMS

Brand	Measured conductivity $(\Omega cm)^{-1}$
Electrode cream, National Aeronautics and Space Administration	12.2×10^{-3}
Cardiopan, Leichti, Berne	8.3×10^{-3}
Redux, Hewlett Packard, Sanburn Division, Walham, Mass.	7.7×10^{-3}
EKG Sol, Burton, Parsons & Co., Washington, D.C.	5.5×10^{-3}
K-Y Lubricating Jelly, Johnson & Johnson Ltd., Slough	3.1×10^{-3}
Electrode Jelly, Data Display Ltd., Liverpool	5.1×10^{-3}
Cambridge Electrode Jelly, Cambridge Instrument Co. Ltd.	10.8×10^{-3}
Cardette Electrode Jelly, Newmark Instrument Co. Ltd., Croydon	3.2×10^{-3}
Electrode Jelly, Smith & Nephew Research Ltd., Harlow	8.5×10^{-3}
Cardioluxe Electrode Jelly, Philips Electrical Ltd.	11.9×10^{-3}

As has been previously mentioned, when using modern ECG recorders which have input impedances in excess of 2 MΩ on either side of earth it is possible to have satisfactory recordings with electrode contact impedances in the range 10 to 20 kΩ. Contact impedances of 3 kΩ or less can be obtained by the use of abrasive creams. Bell, Knox and Small (1939) found that the addition of crushed quartz to green soap reduces the contact impedance measured with soap beneath the electrode by a factor of three after rubbing. Other descriptions of electrode creams are those of Asa *et al* (1964) and Fascenelli *et al* (1966). Montes, Day and Kennedy (1967) discussed the response of human skin to long-term space flight electrodes. They mention that proliferation of bacteria and fungi may occur under the housing of EEG electrodes.

Types of adhesive chest electrodes for monitoring

It has been shown by Kahn (1965) and Boter, Den Hertog and Kuiper (1966) that artefact voltages can be generated as a result of motion at the interface between the metal electrode and the adjacent layer of electrode jelly or paste. In order to stabilize this interface

179

mechanically, both workers recommend the use of a rigid plastic cup containing the electrode and holding the jelly. This is a so-called floating electrode in which the metal electrode does not make contact directly with the skin. Geddes, Baker and Moore (1968) show that for a 10 mm diameter liquid-junction electrode an amplifier input impedance greater than 3 MΩ is required if signal amplitude loss is to be avoided. The cup has a flange to enable it to be fixed to the skin. The cups in both cases are about 1·5 cm in diameter, the side next to the skin in Boter's case being open. Kahn's electrode (produced by Beckman Instruments) has the cup closed on the skin side except for a number of small holes. This cup is filled with jelly using a hypodermic syringe and needle. This particular type of electrode (Beckman) requires a time of the order of half an hour in order to arrive at an acceptably low value of contact impedance. During this period significant amounts of mains hum may be seen on the tracing. In the author's experience this type of electrode should not be employed when it is required to record an ECG in a hurry. Once the contact impedance has stabilized, however, the electrodes work very well and give a stable tracing with the minimum of motion artefacts.

Kahn's electrode is attached to the skin by means of a double-sided adhesive paper ring and can be left in position for several days. Boter's electrode is used in conjunction with a fabric ring and a special non-irritant glue. It has been used to record ECGs from swimmers. However, a skin reaction is likely to occur if the Boter-type electrodes are left in place for more than 24 hours. Rickles and Seal (1968) have evaluated 4 long-term techniques for fixing trans-ducers to the skin. Stomaseal was the best with a mean endurance of 14·7 days on the male sternum.

The Monitron patient-monitoring system, Richardson (1968), uses silver disc electrodes mounted in plastic cups affixed by double-sided sticky rings. Each cup holds a small sponge soaked in agar, the pH being such that skin irritation is not produced. The contact impedance is high, of the order 130 kΩ.

When using cup electrodes, Boter, Den Hertog and Kuiper lay stress on the need to adequately prepare the skin surface by cleaning it with an ether-meth mixture to remove grease, and then abrading the outer horny layer with pumice.

Motion artefacts arising at the electrode-jelly interface can be eliminated by using multipoint electrodes, Lewes (1966), which do not require any electrode jelly or paste. The electrodes are made from a stainless steel multipoint material similar to that used in nutmeg graters. The points painlessly pierce the outer horny layer of the skin. Within a few minutes a layer of perspiration forms beneath the electrode and a contact impedance comparable to that of electrodes using jelly results. It is vital that the electrodes be held firmly pressing on to the skin. Lewes and Hill (1967) in their radio telemetry experiments affixed their multipoint chest electrodes by the fabric ring and glue technique of Boter, Den Hertog and Kuiper. Edwards *et al* (1967) successfully employed silver cup electrodes and double-sided sticky rings to record the ECGs of mountaineers.

An alternative approach is to secure the electrodes by means of a patch of adhesive plaster. The type of plaster must be chosen to minimize skin reaction, and preferably should allow perspiration to pass through it.

Other forms of ECG electrode

For the monitoring of the ECGs of fighter plane pilots, Roman (1966) has developed an extremely light-weight spray-on electrode. The skin is first cleaned with acetone, and a fine wire placed over the site. A conducting paint is then sprayed over the tip of the wire from a spray gun and dried with a jet of warm air. The wires from three chest electrodes are led to a terminal block suspended from the pilot's neck on a light chain. The electrodes are easy and quick to apply and because of their extremely light weight and lack of jelly give rise to minimal motion artefacts. Spray-on electrodes have also been used by Trank, Fetter and Lauer (1968), for recording the ECG of exercising subjects. The impedance of their electrodes fell with time. Another possibility lies in the conducting plastic used by Jenkner (1967) for EEG electrodes. This is Silastic S-2086 by Dow Corning. No paste was required and the contact resistance was the same as with conventional electrodes. The low potential difference generated by sintered silver chloride electrodes also minimizes motion artefact signals.

An interesting development is that of insulated ECG electrodes which rely on capacitive coupling to the subject. They have the advantage of not requiring any conductive paste or jelly and blocking d.c. potentials. When electrodes employing paste are used for extended periods, the paste commences to dry out. This increases the electrode contact impedance and bacterial and fungal growth can occur beneath the electrodes (Montes, Day and Kennedy, 1967). Richardson, Coombes and Adams (1968) used aluminium oxide as the dielectric for insulated electrodes whilst Lagow, Sladek and Richardson (1971) used tantalum oxide. David and Portnoy (1972) used silicon dioxide deposited on a silicon substrate. In order to obtain a sufficiently long time constant for an adequate low frequency response the electrode must be worked into a high input impedance voltage follower circuit. David and Portnoy used a Fairchild μA 740 operational amplifier connected in this configuration mounted in the electrode cup. The input impedance of the circuit is approximately 100 MΩ and the output impedance approximately 5 Ω. The lower cut-off frequency of the electrode system is between 0·01 and 1·0 Hz depending upon the nature of the dielectric and its thickness.

Impedance electrodes

With the two-terminal method for monitoring respiration by impedance changes, it is essential to have a stable contact impedance, otherwise large motion artefacts will result. Baker and Hill (1969) used silver disc electrodes and conductive jelly, the electrodes being held in place with a rubber strap around the thorax. Multipoint electrodes also worked well. Conducting strip electrodes stuck to the skin are useful when impedance changes arising from individual lungs have to be monitored. For experiments designed to follow changes in cardiac output with an impedance technique, Kubicek et al (1966) used flexible metallic band electrodes made by wrapping 4 mm-wide tinned copper braid shielding with a conductive cloth (Velcro Hi-Meg conductive pile V-22-11-WZ) and then sewing the electrodes on to one- or two-inch-wide Velcro backing. The Velcro backing uses Nylon hooks to join its ends. Kuiper and Boter (1968) used a 50 kHz impedance pneumograph to monitor the ventilation by radio telemetry of exercising subjects. They found that silver sheet electrodes (each 60 × 120 × 0·1 mm) gave more reproducible results than did 11-mm diameter disc electrodes. Each type of electrode was glued to the skin. Day and Lippit (1964) describe a long-term electrode system for electrocardiography and impedance pneumography.

EEG electrodes

The amplitude of EEG signals (100 μV or less) calls for low-noise, stable electrodes. A commonly encountered type is the silver stick-on electrode. This consists of a chlorided silver button, slightly domed and about 1 cm in diameter. It has a hole in the centre and a tag at one edge from which runs a flexible connection wire. The electrode is fixed in place on the scalp with collodion, and electrode jelly is forced through the hole from a syringe via a blunt needle. The end of the needle is pressed lightly against the skin and rotated in order to penetrate the outer horny layer. The contact resistance measured with d.c. should not be greater than 5 kΩ for a pair of stick-on electrodes. Clendenning and Auerbach (1964) describe 2 patients suffering from traumatic calcium deposition in skin following prolonged contact with EEG electrode paste.

Electrodes for electromyography

Lippold (1967) describes several types of surface electrodes which are suitable for picking up the electromyographic signals accompanying the activity of specific muscles. These comprise silver disc electrodes which have been chlorided and stuck on to the skin with collodion as in EEG practice, chlorided silver cup electrodes from 3 mm to 20 mm in diameter held in place by suction, or chlorided silver discs 2–10 mm in diameter held in place with sticking plaster. If the electrode is covered with several layers of lint soaked in 10 per cent saline, and waterproof plaster placed on top, then the electrode can remain in place for up to 12 hours without drying producing an appreciable change in the contact impedance.

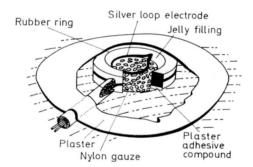

Figure 5.4. Surface-type EMG electrode (after Grieve and Rennie, 1968)

Grieve and Rennie (1968) use the surface electrode of *Figure 5.4* for EMG recordings, the electrodes proving to be viable for at least 26 hours. Each electrode consists of an 8 mm diameter loop of annealed silver wire (0·015 inch diameter) floating in a pool of electrode jelly about 1 mm above the skin. The jelly is contained in a rubber ring through which the ends of the wire pass to run around a groove on the outer surface and away in a silicone rubber sleeve. The ends of the pair of wires are soldered 12 cm away to a screened cable, the joints being protected with rubber sleeves. A disc of Nylon under the rubber ring prevents a metal-to-skin contact forming.

The rubber ring is attached to the skin by a plaster adhesive compound after the site has been rubbed with acetone followed by the removal of surface debris with a razor. A circular plaster is finally used to seal the top of the rubber ring.

When electrodes have to be placed in a specific muscle site, then either monopolar or concentric (coaxial) needle electrodes are used. These commonly have outside diameters of 0·5–0·6 mm and lengths in the range 20–50 mm.

Monopolar EMG electrodes are simply stainless steel electrodes coated with an insulating plastic or varnish except for the tip which is left bare. The EMG signal is taken from between the tip and a reference plate electrode situated on the skin.

Concentric EMG electrodes are made from silver or platinum wire cemented inside a hypodermic needle. The wire tip is bare and made flush with the bevel of the needle. The EMG signal is taken from between the tip of the wire and the shaft of the needle. Basmajian and Stecko (1962) describe a bipolar needle electrode for electromyography.

Scott (1965) has developed an ingenious technique for inserting a fine recording wire into a muscle for EMG recording. The insulated wire is first passed down the lumen and then bent back to pass along the outside of the needle. This is then inserted to the required depth in the muscle. The outer wire is firmly held and the inner wire pulled so that it is cut by the tip of the needle. The needle is now withdrawn leaving the wire in the muscle. The active area is the exposed cross-section at the end of the wire.

Measurement of the contact impedance of recording electrodes

As has been previously mentioned, unless special precautions are taken it is usually desirable to have the contact impedance of surface electrodes with the skin as small as possible. The electrical impedance of the body tissues, as measured beneath the skin, between any pair of electrode sites is quite low of the order of several tens of ohms. However, the impedance of the skin-electrode junction, in comparison with the internal body impedance, is not small. It is the skin-electrode impedance which is known as the contact impedance.

A very crude estimate of the resistance between a pair of electrodes can be made with a conventional d.c. ohmmeter. This method does not measure the individual contact resistances and the d.c. measuring current can give rise to polarization effects at the electrodes which would not be present with a.c. recording. The use of an alternating current avoids polarization, but it must be remembered that at the

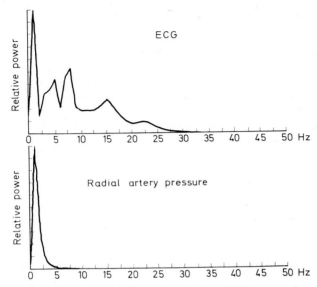

Figure 5.5. Power spectral analysis of a normal ECG averaged over 13 beats, together with the corresponding spectrum for the radial artery pressure

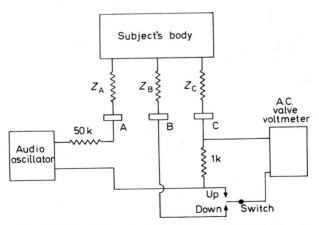

Figure 5.6. Circuit for measuring the contact impedance of a recording electrode

185

higher frequencies the electrode's behaviour is that of a parallel combination of resistors and capacitors and the impedance falls with increasing frequency. A simple a.c. circuit for measuring the contact impedance existing between a pair of recording electrodes is often built into electroencephalographs. When electrodes are to be used for impedance pneumography or plethysmography, the contact impedance measurements should be performed at the frequency with which the electrodes will be used. In the case of the ECG most of the energy is concentrated below 30 Hz, so that 10 Hz is a reasonable frequency at which to measure (Morris, Litman and Groom, 1966). Typical power spectra for a normal human EEG and the corresponding radial artery pressure averaged over 13 beats are shown in *Figure 5.5*.

Referring to *Figure 5.6* A, B, C, are three electrodes placed on the subject's body (often the forearm). The 20 Hz test current enters the subject's body at A and leaves at C returning to the oscillator via the 1 kΩ resistor. With the switch up, the a.c. valve voltmeter reads the r.m.s. voltage developed across the 1 kΩ resistor. The oscillator output is adjusted for a reading on the voltmeter of 100 mV giving a current of 0·1 mA. With the switch down, the voltmeter reading is noted. Assuming that the potential drop across the tissues between A and C is negligible and that the voltmeter draws negligible input current, then since the current is 0·1 mA, each 1 mV read corresponds to 10 Ω of contact impedance at the electrode C. This method offers the advantage that measurements can be performed at specific frequencies. The variation, for typical electrodes, of contact impedance with signal frequency is illustrated in *Figure 5.7(a)*. The variation of the common mode rejection ratio with the degree of electrode contact impedance unbalance is illustrated in *Figure 5.7(b)* (Hill and Khandpur, 1969).

If a knowledge of the frequency is not required, a simpler method is to first note the amplitude of the tracing, say the ECG. A decade resistance box is now connected in parallel with the input to the recording amplifier and the box resistance reduced until the amplitude of the tracing is halved. Then the resistance of the box equals the resistance between the two electrodes. Trouble may be experienced with the pick-up of mains-frequency hum when resistances of several tens of thousands of ohms are used.

Effects of a high electrode contact impedance on the electrocardiogram

The effects produced by a high electrode contact impedance are:

(1) A possible distortion of bipolar leads.

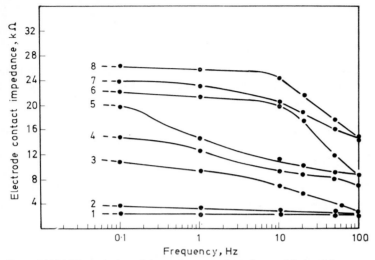

Figure 5.7.(a) The variation of electrode contact impedance with signal frequency;
(1) cup-style self-adhesive electrode of Boter and colleagues (1966); (2) Sanborn
plate electrode with conducting jelly; (3) Newmark plate electrode with
conducting plastic; (4) dry multi-point limb electrode by Hillier Ltd.; (5) dry
multi-point suction chest electrode by Hillier Ltd.; (6) self-adhesive multi-point
chest electrode by Smith and Nephew Ltd. used with conducting jelly; (7) self-
adhesive gauze chest electrode by Drachard Ltd. used with conducting jelly; (8)
dry self-adhesive multipoint chest electrode by Smith and Nephew Ltd.

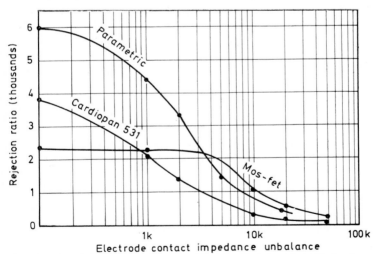

Figure 5.7.(b) The variation of the common mode rejection ratio with the degree
of electrode contact impedance unbalance for three ECG amplifiers

187

(2) A possible distortion of unipolar or augmented unipolar leads.

(3) An increased susceptibility to the pick-up of a.c. mains interference.

The possible distortion effects are most serious in multi-channel ECG recorders, especially when a unipolar lead is being recorded simultaneously with a bipolar lead. In this case contact impedances should not be greater than 5 kΩ and preferably should be around 2·5 kΩ. For single channel ECG recorders, there may not be any significant distortion of the bipolar leads even with contact impedances of many thousands of ohms. The effect of high and unequal contact impedances can be serious in the case of unipolar chest leads or augmented limb leads. The source of the distortion lies in the unbalance of the central terminal caused by the presence of high and unequal contact impedances.

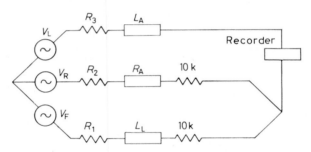

Figure 5.8. Circuit for the measurement of the AVL lead

The circuit arrangement for the measurement of the AVL lead is given in *Figure 5.8*. The voltages V_L V_R, and V_F are the true unipolar voltages existing at the left leg, right arm and left arm respectively. In theory, the recorder should display the voltage difference existing between V_L and the average of V_R and V_F. If the voltages V_R and V_F are connected to a common junction point by equal impedances, then the voltage tapped off at the junction will be the average of V_R and V_F. In this circuit the pair of averaging resistors are shown as each having a value of 10 kΩ, and they are built into the cardiograph. This value is typical of a number of older commercial cardiographs and indeed in some instruments 5 kΩ is used. Suppose that the contact impedances of the right arm and left leg electrodes are denoted by R_2 and R_1. Clearly, if R_1 and R_2 are small in comparison with 10 kΩ then they will have little effect upon the true average of V_F and V_R. When R_1 or R_2 is large and R_1 does not equal R_2 then $(R_1+10,000)$ is quite different from $(R_2+10,000)$ and the voltage at the junction is no longer the true average of V_R and V_F. As R_2 becomes relatively smaller, or R_1 becomes relatively larger, so the potential at the junction approaches that of V_R and the recording takes on the appearance of lead 1 rather than V_L. On the other hand if R_2 becomes relatively large and R_1 becomes relatively small, then the junction approaches the potential of V_F and the recording looks like an inverted lead 3, rather than aV_L. On those aV leads where the pair of electrodes being averaged have nearly the same potential then a poor balance of the averaging circuit will be less significant. For instance, if the bipolar lead 3 record shows only small deflections, then there can be little potential difference between the left arm and left leg. Under these conditions leads 1 and 2 would be similar, with lead aV_R looking like the same thing in reverse and unbalance of the central terminal would have little effect. On the other hand when the signal from lead 2 is large, an unbalance of the central terminal will markedly affect the signal developed in lead aV_L. It would be preferable to use 47 kΩ averaging resistors. The effect of contact impedances in distorting the signals from augmented leads is discussed by King (1964) and Schwarzchild *et al* (1954). The effect of using an electrocardiograph having 4·7k Ω averaging resistors. is illustrated in *Figure 5.9*.

The amount of a.c. mains interference on an ECG tracing depends upon a number of factors. These include the nature of the interference field, the value of the 'common mode rejection ratio' for the cardiograph, the input impedance of the cardiograph, the a.c. potential present on the cardiograph chassis, the leakage resistance to earth and the patient's body capacitance to earth, the magnitude of the impedance between the patient's body and the cardiograph chassis and the imbalance of the impedance between the two active patient electrodes and the input terminals of the cardiograph.

In the conventional limb lead arrangement, one patient electrode, known as the 'indifferent' electrode (usually the right leg) is connected to the chassis of the cardiograph, whilst the other two electrodes (the active electrodes) are connected to the input terminals of the cardiograph. The greater the value of the contact potential present across the contact impedance of the indifferent electrode, the greater is the possible a.c. voltage which can build up between the patient and the cardiograph chassis. This represents the 'common mode' voltage which the cardiograph tries to reject. The rejection produced depends upon the degree of input circuit balance. This is largely determined by the values of the cable capacitance and contact impedance at each input. Inequalities of contact impedance combine with the patient cable capacitance to reduce the common mode rejection to a point where a.c. interference becomes a problem. A measure of susceptibility to a.c. interference is given by multiplying the contact impedance of the indifferent electrode by the difference in the contact impedances of the other two active electrodes. For example if the contact impedance of the indifferent electrode is 5,000 Ω and those of the other electrodes are 5,000 and 4,000 then the a.c. susceptibility factor is $5,000 \times 1,000 = 5$ million. As a practical rule, the factor should be kept to less than 10 million for good results.

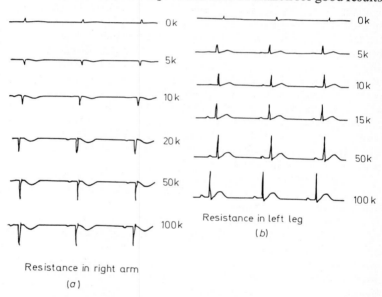

Figure 5.9. The effect of electrode contact impedance unbalance in (a) the right arm lead and (b) the left leg lead, on the AVL recording

Equivalent circuits for the electrode tissue interface

Experiments show that above about 10 Hz the contact impedance of a surface electrode decreases with increasing frequency. The effect can be simulated by the behaviour of a capacitance in parallel with a resistance, this combination being in series with a battery which represents the half-cell potential of the electrode, *Figure 5.10(a)*. An alternative circuit is shown in *Figure 5.10(b)* and some typical values in *Figure 5.10(c)*.

190

Garments for use with electrodes and transducers

In the more comprehensive patient-monitoring systems, it is necessary to affix to the patient a number of electrodes, together with transducers for respiration, temperature and pressure and to run leads back from these to the monitoring console. The secure attachment of the electrodes is a major problem when the monitor operates a heart rate alarm. False triggering is nearly always due to electrode trouble. It is not good practice to have a number of leads trailing from a patient, since tension on these is likely to

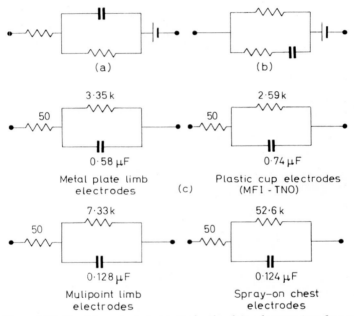

Figure 5.10. Possible equivalent circuits for the electrode-tissue interface as measured with an a.c. bridge

disturb the attached electrodes or transducers. In any case the sight of the leads may be disturbing to visitors. These considerations have led to approaches aimed at utilizing some sort of garment to hold electrodes and transducers and to provide an anchorage for their leads so that only one multicore cable needs be run to the monitor unit.

Richardson (1968) used a modified brassière to hold cup ECG electrodes, and a thermistor temperature probe mounted in the axilla. In practice the garment was not liked by male patients and movement of the patient's torso flexed the garment pulling the electrodes away from the skin and setting off the heart rate alarm. The arrangement is suitable for carefully selected patients who are well nourished—not obese—and have no bony deformities of the chest cage. This requirement precludes the use of a harness in many elderly patients with chest deformities due to infection and malnutrition as a child. The ECG electrodes used with the harness were either of the adhesive ring cup-type or an agar-filled cup-type fixed to the harness by a press-stud. Hill and White (1968) used a disposable

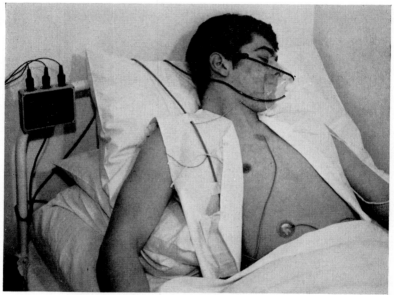

Figure 5.11. Disposable paper waistcoat for connecting to transducers and electrodes (after Hill and White, 1968)

laminated paper jacket which carried a multiway socket, the electrodes together with the temperature and respiration probe being attached independently to the patient. The jacket is loosely fitting and is secured by tapes which can be readily cut. It absorbs perspiration. Perspiration can still be a problem in some patients since it acts to loosen the electrode adhesive. The jacket is fed with a supply voltage of $\pm$ 12 V d.c. It can be put on backwards if the patient is heavy and comatose and cannot be lifted. Such a jacket in use is illustrated in *Figure 5.11.*

The book by Geddes (1972) provides a useful compendium of a wide variety of recording electrodes for the measurement of bio-electric events including surface, subintegumental, intracellular and micropipette electrodes.

REFERENCES

Asa, M. M., Crews, A. H., Rothfield, E. L., Lewis, E. S., Zucker, I. R. and Berstein, A. (1964). 'High fidelity fetal radio electrocardiography.' *Am. J. Cardiol.* **14**, 530

Baker, L. E. and Hill, D. W. (1969). 'The use of electrical impedance techniques for the monitoring of respiratory pattern during anaesthesia.' *Br. J. Anaesth.* **41**, 2

Basmajian, J. V., and Stecko, G. (1962). 'A new bipolar electrode for electromyography.' *J. appl. Physiol.* **17**, 849

Bell, G. H., Knox, J. A. C. and Small, A. J. (1939). 'Electrocardiograph electrolytes.' *Br. Heart J.* **1**, 229

Boter, J., Den Hertog, A. and Kuiper, J. (1966). 'Disturbance-free skin electrodes for persons during exercise.' *Med. Electron. biol. Engng.* **4**, 91

Burns, D. C. and Gollnick, P. D. (1966). 'An inexpensive floating-mesh electrode for EKG recording during exercise.' *J. appl. Physiol.* **21**, 1889

Clendenning, W. E. and Auerbach, R. (1964). 'Traumatic calcium deposition in skin.' *Archs Dermatol.* **89**, 360

David, R. M., and Portnoy, W. M. (1972). 'Insulated electrocardiogram electrodes.' *Med. biol. Engng.*, **10**, 742

Day, J. L. and Lippit, M. W. Jun. (1964). 'A long-term electrode system for electrocardiography and impedance pneumography.' *Psychophysiol.* **1**, 174

Delgado, J. M. R. (1964). 'Electrodes for extracellular recording and stimulation.' In *Physiological Techniques in Biological Research.* p. 89. Ed. by W. L. Nastuk. New York; Academic Press

Edwards, R. H. T., Sluck, D. C., Williams, E. S. and Burgess, P. A. (1967). 'Permanently attached electrodes for high altitude electrocardiograms.' *Bio-med. Engng.* **2**, 544

Fascenelli, F. W., Cordova, C., Simons, D. G., Johnson, J., Pratt, L. and Lamb, L. E. (1966). 'Biochemical monitoring during dynamic stress testing.' *Aerospace Med.* **37**, 911

Feder, W. (1963). 'Silver-silver chloride electrode as a non-polarizable bioelectrode.' *J. appl. Physiol.* **18**, 397

Flasterstein, A. H. (1966). 'Voltage fluctuations of metal-electrolyte interfaces in electrophysiology.' *Med. Electron. biol. Engng.* **4**, 583

Geddes, L. A. and Baker, L. E. (1966). 'The relationship between input impedance and electrode area in recording the ECG.' *Med. Electron. biol. Engng.* **4**, 439

— — (1967). 'Chlorided silver electrodes.' *Med. Res. Engng.* **6**, 33

— — Moore, A. G. (1968). 'The use of liquid-junction electrodes in recording the human electrocardiogram (ECG).' *J. Electrocard..* **1,** 51

— — — (1969). 'Optimum electrolytic chloriding of silver electrodes.' *Med. Electron. Engng.* **7,** 49

Geddes, L. A., (1972). *Electrodes and the Measurement of Bioelectric Events.* New York; John Wiley-Interscience.

Gibson, T. C., Thornton, W. E., Algary, W. P. and Craige, E. (1962). 'Telecardiography and the use of simple computers.' *New Engl. J. Med.* **267,** 1218

Greatbatch, W. (1967). 'Electrochemical polarisation of physiological electrodes.' *Med. Res. Engng.* **6,** 13

Grieve, D. W. and Rennie, R. (1968). 'A method of measuring electromyographic activity for long periods.' *Proc. 2nd European Conf. Med. Electron.* p. 48. London; Hanover Press

Hill, D. W. and Khandpur, R. S. (1968). 'The performance of transistor ECG amplifiers.' *Wld. med. Electron. Instrum. Lond.* **7,** 12

— White, E. (1968). 'The use of a disposable waistcoat to hold electrodes and transducers for patient monitoring.' *Med. Electron. biol. Engng.* **6,** 527

Jenkner, F. L. (1967). 'A new electrode material for multi-purpose biomedical application.' *Electroenceph. clin. Neurophysiol.* **23,** 570

Kahn, A. (1965). 'Motion artefacts and streaming potentials in relation to biochemical electrodes.' *Digest of the 6th Int. Conf. Med. Biol. Engng. Tokyo.* p. 562

King, G. E. (1964). 'Errors in voltage in multi-channel ECG recordings using newer electrode materials.' *Am. Heart J.* **18,** 295

Kubicek, W. G., Karnegis, J. N., Patterson, R. P., Witsoe, D. A. and Mattson, R. H. (1966). 'Development and evaluation of an impedance cardiac output system.' *Aerospace Med.* **37,** 1208

Kuiper, J. and Boter, J. (1968). 'Impedance pneumography of subjects moving freely.' *Progress Report PRI.* p. 45. Utrecht; TNO Medical Physics Institute

Lagow, C. H., Sladek, K. J., and Richardson, P.C. (1971). 'Anodic insulated tantalum oxide electrocardiograph electrodes.' *IEEE Trans. biomed. Engng.*, **BME-18,** 162

Lewes, D. (1966). 'Multipoint electrocardiography without skin preparation.' *Wld. med. Electron. Instrum. Lond.* **4,** 240

— and Hill, D. W. (1967). 'Application of multipoint electrodes to telemetry in patient monitoring and during physical exercise.' *Br. Heart J.* **29,** 689

Lippold, O. C. J. (1967). 'Electromyography.' In *Manual of Psycho-Physiological Methods.* p. 247. Ed. by P. H. Venables and Irene Martin. Amsterdam; North Holland

Mason, R. E. and Likar, I. (1966). 'A new system of multiple lead exercise electrocardiography.' *Am. Heart J.* **71,** 196

Margerison, J. H., St. John-Loe, P. and Binnie, C. D. (1967). 'Electro-encephalography.' In *Manual of Psycho-Physiological Methods.* p. 353. Ed. by P. H. Venables and Irene Martin. Amsterdam; North Holland.

Montes, L. F., Day, J. L. and Kennedy, L. (1967). 'The response of human skin to long-term space flight electrodes.' *J. invest. Dermatol.* **49**, 100

Morris, R. E., Litman, S. and Groom, D. (1966). 'Energy spectrum of the cardiac cycle.' *Proc. 19th ann. Conf. Engng. in Med. and Biol.*

Nencini, R. and Pasquali, E. (1968). 'Manganese dioxide electrodes for stimulation and recording.' *Med. Electron. biol. Engng.* **6**, 193

Richardson, G. A. (1968). 'Experiences with the Monitron system in general medical, intensive care, and surgical wards at University College Hospital.' *Proc. 2nd European Conf. Med. Electron.* p. 10. London; Hanover Press

Richardson, P. C., Coombes, F. K., and Adams, R. M. (1968). 'Some new electrode techniques for long-term physiological monitoring.' *Aerospace. Med.* **39**, 745

Rickles, W. H. and Seal, H. R. (1968). 'Evaluation of four long-term transducer techniques.' *Psychophysiology* **4**, 354

Roman, J. (1966). 'Flight research program—III. High impedance electrode techniques.' *Aerospace Med.* **37**, 790

Russell, B. and Thorne, N. A. (1955). 'Skin reaction beneath adhesive plasters.' *Lancet* **1**, 67

Schmitt, O. H., Okajima, M. and Blaug, M. (1961). 'Skin preparation and electrocardiographic lead impedance.' In *Digest IRE Int. Conf. Med. Electron. New York* Washington D.C.; McGregor and Werner.

Schwartzchild, M. M., Hoffman, I. and Kissin, M. (1954). 'Errors in unipolar limb leads caused by unbalanced skin resistances and a device for their elimination.' *Am. Heart J.* **48**, 235

Scott, R. N. (1965). 'A method of inserting wire electrodes for electro-myography.' *I.E.E.E. Trans. Bio-med. Engng*, 46

Shackel, B. (1967). 'Electro-oculography.' In *Manual of Psycho-Physio-logical Methods.* p. 301. Ed. by P. H. Venables and Irene Martin. Amsterdam; North Holland.

Spiegler, K. S. and Wyllie, M. R. J. (1968). 'Electrical potential differences.' In *Physical Techniques in Biological Research.* p. 227, 2nd ed. Ed. by D. H. Moore, New York; Academic Press

Trank, J., Fetter, R. and Lauer, R. M. (1968). 'A spray-on electrode for recording the electrocardiogram during exercise.' *J. appl. Physiol.* **24**. 267

Venables, P. H. and Sayer, E. (1963). 'On the measurement of the level of the skin potential.' *Br. J. Psychol.* **54**, 251

Weinman, J. and Mahler, Y. (1959). 'The polarisation impedance of stain-less steel recording and stimulating electrodes in saline.' In *Proc. 2nd Int. Conf. Med. Electron. London.* Ed. by C. N. Smythe. London; Iliffe

—— (1964). 'An analysis of electrical properties of metal electrodes.' *Med. Electron. biol. Engng.* **2**, 299

6–Gas and Vapour Analysis

A knowledge of the composition of inspired and expired gas and vapour mixtures is obviously of importance in studies concerned with respiratory physiology, lung function assessment and anaesthesia. Traditional methods of chemical gas analysis have been based on chemical absorption or reaction, but these suffer from the disadvantage of being time consuming and of usually not having provision for an electrical output. Coulometric gas analysers produce an electrical output from a photocell, but the solution through which the gas is bubbled in order to produce a colour change, requires regular renewal. Physical methods of gas analysis are particularly valuable for the analysis of multicomponent gas and vapour streams, and when a continuous analysis is required. Chemical analysers, such as the Lloyd-Haldane (Lloyd, (1958) and Scholander (1947)) are capable of a high accuracy for gases such as carbon dioxide and oxygen and are widely used where a number of discrete samples have to be analysed. The performance of a simple chemical absorption apparatus for carbon dioxide in expired air is evaluated by Nunn (1958). A simplified Haldane chemical gas analyser (Haldane 1920) suitable for routine use with a 're-breathing' method for the estimation of mixed carbon dioxide tension is described by Campbell (1960).

In principle, many different physical properties can be utilized as the basis for a gas analyser, but in practice commercially available analysers concentrate on the measurement of quantities such as thermal conductivity, sonic velocity, paramagnetism, infra-red or ultra-violet absorption or the ratio of charge to mass of ionized molecules. It is proposed to deal first with analysers designed primarily for the analysis of single components of a gas or vapour mixture and then to discuss instruments such as the gas chromatograph and mass spectrometer which can provide a multi-component analysis.

196

PARAMAGNETIC OXYGEN ANALYSERS

The commonly encountered permanent magnets exhibit the property of ferromagnetism. However, other forms of magnetism are known which are not so strong as ferromagnetism. These are paramagnetism and diamagnetism. Oxygen is a paramagnetic substance and it has this property because of the configuration of the orbital electrons in its outer shell. Oxygen is a free radical and has two of its outer shell electrons unpaired. Pauli's exclusion principle requires that paired electrons in the same orbital must possess oppositely directed electron spins and hence their magnetic moments cancel. The two unpaired electrons of oxygen give rise to a magnetic moment and paramagnetism. In the case of both nitric oxide and nitrogen dioxide paramagnetism also arises since these are free radicals. Taking oxygen as 100, the relative susceptibility of nitric oxide is 43.

Pauling, Wood and Sturdevant (1946) describe a simple dumb-bell type of paramagnetic oxygen analyser which has formed the basis of more modern instruments used in medicine. These analysers are used for relatively simple monitoring of atmospheres. For longer term recording in industry a magnetic-wind type of analyser is employed. The analyser of Pauling and colleagues is based upon a cell containing a small glass dumb-bell assembly containing a weakly diamagnetic gas such as nitrogen. The dumb-bell is suspended from a quartz thread between the poles of a powerful permanent magnet. The polepieces are wedge shaped in order to produce a non-linear field. If the gas surrounding the dumb-bell is also nitrogen there will be no force acting on the dumb-bell. If oxygen is added to the gas in the cell the oxygen molecules experience a force which makes them congregate in the region of maximum magnetic field gradient, thus displacing the diamagnetic dumb-bell. The resulting rotation of the suspension turns a small mirror and deflects a beam of light over a scale calibrated in percentages by volume of oxygen or partial pressure of oxygen. The force acting on the oxygen molecules is temperature dependent, and allowance made for this in the calibration or a compensating system used with the magnet (Pauling, Wood and Sturdevant 1946).

A development of the direct reading instrument of Pauling and his colleagues, and Woolmer (1956) is the Servomex analyser type D.C.L. 101 (*Figure 6.1*) which has been evaluated by Nunn (1964). In the D.C.L. 101 analyser the original quartz suspension is replaced with a platinum-iridium suspension which is more robust. A null-balance system is employed, the deflection of the dumb-bell being

197

offset by passing a current through a coil of wire attached to the dumb-bell. The direct current controlled by a helical potentiometer is proportional to the deflecting couple and thus to the oxygen tension of the gas within the cell. The null position is sensed by means of a small mirror attached to the suspension which reflects a beam of

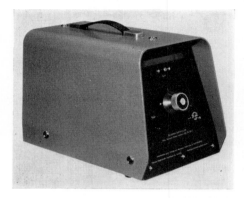

Figure 6.1. Null-balance paramagnetic oxygen analyser. (Reproduced by courtesy of Servomex Controls Ltd.)

Figure 6.2. Direct reading paramagnetic oxygen analyser. (Reproduced by courtesy of Servomex Controls Ltd.)

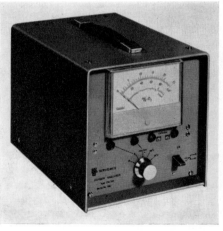

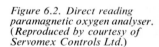

light from a small lamp on to a graduated scale. The analyser requires balancing for each reading, the oxygen tension being read from the 1,000-division dial of the potentiometer, the basic sensitivity being 0·03 per cent oxygen. A stabilized power unit is available to supply the instrument. A temperature-dependent resistor (thermistor) is incorporated to compensate for the effect upon the calibration of changes in the ambient temperature. With the null-balance system the dumb-bell always operates in the same region of magnetic field, so that the effect of changes in the field strength on the linearity of the calibration is eliminated. The analyser's response time is exponential; the 90 per cent response time being less than 8 seconds.

The Servomex type OA150 oxygen analyser (*Figure 6.2*) gives a continuous read-out of 0–25 per cent or 0–100 per cent oxygen, on a meter scale. Displacement of the dumb-bell unbalances the outputs from the pair of photocells, the difference in their output signals being fed to a differential amplifier. This supplies its output current to the dumb-bell coil and thus nulls the deflection, the coil current being shown on the meter. The OA 150 has been evaluated by Ellis and Nunn (1968). They find that it has an adequate sensitivity for clinical purposes (0·25 per cent on the 25 per cent range and 1 per cent on the 100 per cent range) but that an accuracy in excess of that obtainable from a normal Haldane volumetric gas analyser is obtainable by using a digital voltmeter instead of the moving-coil meter.

Paramagnetic analysers are limited in the volume flow rate of gas that can be drawn through the cell, about 150 ml per minute in the case of the OA150 and D.C.L. 101 analysers. The gas stream should also be dried by passage through silica gel or a cold trap. The reading of the analyser depends on the pressure within the cell, and thus on the barometric pressure. Ellis and Nunn (1968) found that for the OA150 the reading was virtually linearly related to the pressure over a range of 0–25 cmH$_2$O.

The motion of paramagnetic molecules into the non-uniform magnetic field gives rise to a phenomenon known as a 'magnetic wind' (Dyer 1947; Linford 1952). The flowing gas can be caused to cool a heated filament and thus to unbalance a Wheatstone bridge circuit. The output voltage from the bridge can be fed to a recorder to give a continuous indication of oxygen concentration changes. A detailed description of a magnetic wind oxygen analyser is given by Medlock (1962).

THERMAL CONDUCTIVITY GAS ANALYSERS

Changes in the composition of a gas stream may give rise to a significant alteration in the thermal conductivity of the stream. As a result, the temperature of a heated filament situated in the stream may rise or fall. In a typical katharometer or thermal conductivity cell, 4 platinum filaments would be employed arranged in a constant current bridge circuit (Jessop, 1966). One of the pairs of filaments (each pair forming 2 opposite arms of the bridge) acts as reference arms for the bridge and serves to compensate for changes occurring in the ambient temperature. The other 2 filaments are situated in the gas stream.

The great drawback to thermal conductivity gas analysis is that it is inherently non-specific, and therefore the simplest analyses occur with binary gas mixtures. More complicated mixtures can be handled by surrounding the reference filaments with the gas stream from which the component to be measured has been removed. When a katharometer is used to measure carbon dioxide in expired air, variations in the proportions of oxygen and nitrogen in the sample stream will have little effect, since they both have almost the same thermal conductivity. Changes in the water vapour content of the stream are eliminated by arranging to saturate the gas fed to both the sample and reference filaments.

A thermal conductivity analyser can be used to follow CO_2 concentration changes in the individual breaths of a patient when there are no gaseous or volatile anaesthetic agents present. A high speed of response is necessary, and this can be obtained by reducing the pressure of the gas surrounding the filaments to a few millimetres of mercury absolute. A good description of the use of thermal conductivity gas analysers in respiratory physiology studies is given by Visser (1957).

INFRA-RED GAS ANALYSERS

The best accuracy with thermal conductivity analysers is achieved with binary or quasi-binary gas mixtures. When it is required to know the composition of a gas stream possessing several components whose proportions can vary widely, then it may be convenient to use infra-red gas analysers in conjunction with an oxygen analyser, nitrogen usually being measured by difference. Infra-red gas analysers depend for their operation upon the fact that many gases and vapours will absorb specific wavelengths of infra-red radiation. As long ago as 1863, infra-red absorption was utilized to measure the carbon dioxide concentration in breath, Tyndall (1863). The main absorption bands for the infra-red radiation arise from vibrational energy changes occurring in the sample molecules. Rotational energy changes must also be taken into account, and in practice it is found that each vibrational energy level has a series of rotational levels associated with it. The vibration-rotation band of

Parallel band of carbon monoxide
at 4·7 μm

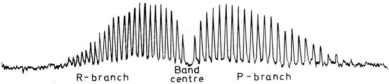

R-branch   Band   P-branch
centre

Figure 6.3. Vibration-rotation infra-red absorption band for carbon monoxide

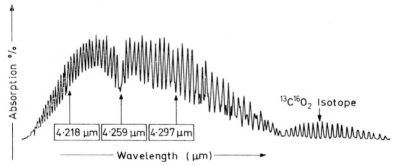

Absorption %

$^{13}C^{16}O_2$ Isotope

4·218 μm 4·259 μm 4·297 μm

Wavelength (μm)

Figure 6.4. Infra-red absorption bands for carbon dioxide

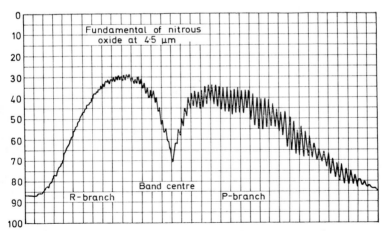

Figure 6.5. Infra-red absorption bands for nitrous oxide

a diatomic molecule should consist of 2 branches, known as the P-branch and the R-branch. *Figure 6.3* illustrates the 2 branches for carbon monoxide showing the fine structure due to rotational energy changes. A similar situation occurs with linear triatomic molecules such as carbon dioxide and nitrous oxide (*Figures 6.4* and *6.5*). It is possible to use a conventional double-beam infra-red spectrometer as a gas analyser by placing a pair of matched gas cells in the beams. One cell is filled with a non-absorbing gas such as nitrogen, and the other with the sample. The difference in optical absorption found between the two cells is a measure of the absorption of the sample at the particular wavelength selected by the dispersive element of the spectrometer.

For medical applications, the most commonly encountered infra-red gas analysers are of the non-dispersive type. Their operating principle is shown in *Figure 6.6*. A double-beam-in-space system uses a pair of hot-wire spirals to form a sample beam and a reference beam of infra-red radiation. A rotating chopping disc, usually driven from a small electric motor, occludes each beam twice per rotation. The resultant chopping frequency lies in the range 2–10 Hz for industrial analysers, and for medical instruments the range would be 20–50 Hz if the analyser had to be fast enough to follow individual breaths. When the opaque portions of the chopper are not in the way, the beams fall one on to each half of a balanced condenser-microphone detector. Basically, this consists of two identical chambers (Luft, 1943), fitted with infra-red transparent windows and separated by means of a thin flexible metal diaphragm. The chambers are each filled to the same absolute or partial pressure of a few centimetres of mercury with the pure gas or vapour to be analysed. Thus the detector of a CO_2 analyser would contain pure CO_2, and that of a halothane analyser would contain pure halothane vapour.

The detector filling can only absorb those infra-red wavelengths which are contained in the absorption bands of the substance to be analysed. Assuming that there is a significant absorption in the sample cell by the component of interest, then the sample beam falling on the detector will be weaker than the reference beam. In the initial setting-up of the analyser the intensities of the sample and reference beams will have been made equal when there is no absorber present in the sample cell. The heating by the detector beams of the detector gas filling will cause the pressure in the reference half of the detector to rise to a higher value than that in the sample half. The diaphragm thus vibrates at the chopping frequency as it is periodically pushed over towards the sample half of the detector. The diaphragm is arranged to form one half of a capacitor. In some instruments, the capacitor is supplied with a constant charge, and the resulting periodic voltage changes at the chopping frequency are amplified by a three-stage tuned amplifier

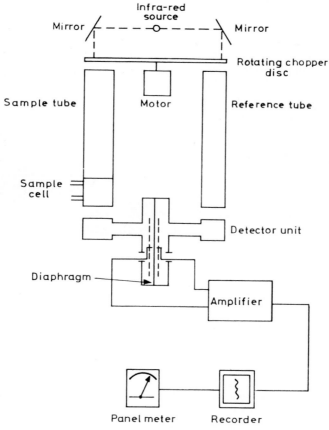

Figure 6.6. Luft-type non-dispersive infra-red gas analyser

having an electrometer input stage. After rectification and smoothing, the output signal is displayed on a meter or recorder calibrated in terms of the concentration of the wanted component. In other instruments, the capacitor forms part of the tuning circuit of a radio frequency oscillator used in an amplitude modulation arrange-

203

ment. This avoids the high values of input resistance required for d.c. electrometer systems and thus helps to minimize noise arising from vibration of input cables and the pick-up of unwanted voltages.

Cross-sensitivity effects arise from the overlapping of absorption bands of the wanted component with those of unwanted components also present in the sample mixture. These effects can be minimized by the use of optical interference filters (Heavens 1955, Francon 1963) to select a band which is clear of overlap, or by placing a gas filter cell in each beam filled with the interfering substance(s). Any wavelengths capable of being absorbed by the interfering substance will be absorbed in the filter cell before it reaches the detector.

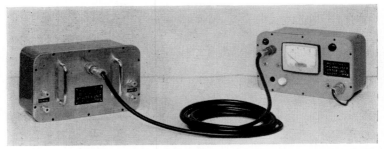

Figure 6.7. Double-beam-in-time infra-red gas analyser using a photoconductive detector. (Reproduced by courtesy of Grubb Parsons Ltd.)

Infra-red gas analysers are of considerable use during anaesthesia and lung function studies. In many cases they can be made fast enough to follow individual breaths. Instruments scaled 0–0·1 per cent CO are widely used for the measurement of lung diffusing capacity. The use of infra-red carbon dioxide analysers is discussed by Collier, Affeldt and Farr (1955), Dubois *et al* (1952) and Hackney, Sears and Collier (1958). Hill (1958) used an infra-red gas analyser to determine the performance of the Fluotec anaesthetic vaporizer. A versatile double-beam-in-time CO_2 infra-red gas analyser using an indium antimonide photoconductive cell in conjunction with all solid-state electronics is described by Hill and Stone (1964a), and a commercial version is shown in *Figure 6.7*. A sparkless pump for use with this instrument in the operating room is described by Hill and Stone (1964b). The analyser is a single-path dual-wavelength instrument. The chopping disc carries two optical interference filters, one set to pass the wavelength at which the component of interest in the sample absorbs, the other set to pass a reference wavelength at which the sample does not absorb. The two wave-lengths pass alternately through the sample cell and common optical path from a single hot-spiral source. Since both beams will be affected, the deposition of pus or dirt on the cell windows will have little effect on the zero setting of the analyser. The design of the instrument is such that the optical portion can be sealed against the ingress of explosive gas mixtures and it can be operated at a distance from the control box. The power supply for the analyser can be either the a.c. mains or a 12 V accumulator. By virtue of its solid-state electronics and detector, the analyser is minimally subject to microphony.

Many organic vapours, such as ethyl alcohol, will absorb strongly at 3·39 μm. This is a wavelength emitted by a helium-neon gas laser. The intense narrow beam generated by the laser can be directed down a long, small diameter, sample cell, so that the sample volume need only be a few millilitres for a cell length of 30 cm. A germanium beam-splitter is placed in the laser beam before the entrance window of the sample cell. By this means a reference beam is produced. A chopping disc is located close to the exit windows of the sample and reference cells. Its segments are arranged so that as one beam is occluded the other is allowed to pass. The beams thus fall alternately upon the detector which is a lead selenide photoconductive cell. The chopping frequency is about 600 Hz. By placing a comb in the reference beam, the relative intensities of the two beams can be made equal in the absence of absorption in the sample cell. When a sample is present, the beams become unbalanced and a signal at the modulation frequency is obtained from the lead selenide detector and fed into a low-noise amplifier and phase-sensitive detector. The reference signal for the phase-sensitive detector is obtained from a lamp and phototransistor, the light shining through the segments of the chopping disc and on to the phototransistor. It is better to work with the ratio of the two beams rather than their difference, in order to cancel out variations in the intensity of the light emitted by the laser.

In order to be able to measure 200 parts per million by volume of alcohol vapour in air, the sample cell length might be 30 cm, whereas in order to measure 10 per cent v/v CO_2 full scale, the cell length would be about 1 mm and the cell volume about 0·25 ml. The cross-section of these small cells is usually oval so that the sample stream quickly flushes out the whole volume and does not leave any stagnant areas. In a good design it is possible to achieve 90 per cent of the full scale deflection in 100 ms with a sample flow of 100 ml per

205

minute. It is possible to record end-expiratory CO_2 concentrations at respiratory rates up to 35 and 40 breaths per minute. A low sampling flow rate is obviously essential when dealing with small children or small animals.

Cormack and Powell (1972) give a detailed account of the techniques they adopted to increase the accuracy of their Luft-type infra-red gas analyser from 0·1 to 0·01 per cent CO_2. The main source of drift was found to be room temperature changes.

THE ULTRA-VIOLET HALOTHANE METER

Halothane vapour exhibits a strong absorption for ultra-violet light around 200 nanometres This fact forms the basis of the simple ultra-violet halothane meter (Robinson, Denson and Summers, 1962). The light source is a 6-watt low-pressure mercury discharge lamp which radiates at 200 nm. This light is passed through a stainless steel sample cell about one inch long and fitted with quartz windows. The emergent light falls on to one of a pair of ultra-violet photocells. The second cell has a V-shaped shutter placed in front of it and monitors the strength of the lamp directly. It is nearer to the lamp than the first photocell, so that the shutter is used to equalize the light intensity falling on each cell. The photocell current of each cell passes through a 10-$M\Omega$ resistor, and the potential differences appearing across each resistor are applied one to each input of a double-triode valve cathode follower. A meter connected between the valve's two cathodes is calibrated 0–5 per cent v/v halothane. Absorption of the ultra-violet light in the sample cell by halothane vapour unbalances the double-triode and deflects the meter. A small sucker pump draws the vapour stream to be sampled through the cell. The halothane meter is particularly useful for monitoring concentrations in circle anaesthetic systems. The effluent should not be returned to the circle since ultra-violet light can decompose halothane vapour, forming irritant products. The meter is virtually unaffected by water vapour (if it is not allowed to condense) and anaesthetic agents other than halothane. Some versions of this instrument suffer from the drawback of possessing a marked drift of the zero.

GAS ANALYSIS BY THE MEASUREMENT OF REFRACTIVE INDEX

Makers of calibrated anaesthetic vaporizers invariably use air as the diluent gas when calibrating their products. They have a need for a

highly stable system for the measurement of single vapour concentrations. Similar considerations apply to the routine measurement
of nitrous oxide–oxygen mixtures delivered by dental and analgesic
gas machines. The method of choice is based upon the measurement
of the refractive index of the mixture (Edmondson, 1957; Hill, 1958).
The refractometer can be calibrated from a knowledge of the refractive index of the gas or vapour concerned, and will hold this
calibration for years. The system is only suitable for binary or quasi-
binary mixtures. Portable refractometers are available which are
very convenient for making spot checks on vaporizers. Hulands and
Nunn (1970) give a good account of possible applications in anaesthesia for portable refractometers.

THE GAS-DISCHARGE NITROGEN METER

The emission of a characteristic purple colour arising from the
presence of nitrogen in a low-pressure gas discharge forms the basis
of the 'nitrogen meter' (Lundin and Akesson, 1954). A rotary oil
vacuum pump draws a sample of the subject's expired air into the
discharge tube which is maintained at an absolute pressure of a few
torr. A d.c. voltage of about 1,500 V applied across electrodes in the
tube excites a purple-coloured discharge if nitrogen is present. The
light output is interrupted by means of a rotating slotted disc and
then passed through optical filters to select the waveband corresponding to the purple colour. The intensity of the light in this
waveband is then measured with a photocell and an amplifier tuned
to the chopping frequency. The light intensity is proportional to the
nitrogen concentration. The nitrogen meter is widely used for the
study of nitrogen wash-out curves in lung function studies, since it is
fast enough to follow the breath-by-breath variations of nitrogen
concentration. Two ranges are normally provided, 0–100 and
0–10 per cent v/v.

MASS SPECTROMETERS

Although comparatively expensive, mass spectrometers offer the
advantage of being able to give a rapid, simultaneous, analysis of
several components in a gas mixture. For example, an analysis
can be given of oxygen, nitrogen, carbon dioxide, and a tracer gas
such as argon, in individual breaths (Fowler and Hugh-Jones,
1957). In a mass spectrometer, a vacuum pump draws a small sample

of the mixture to be analysed into a chamber where the atoms and molecules are ionized by means of an electric discharge, that is to say, they are made to lose one or more of their orbital electrons and become positive ions. The ions are then accelerated by means of an electric field and pass through a powerful magnetic field, the lines of magnetic force lying in a plane perpendicular to their travel. As a result of the interaction of the electric and magnetic fields, the various species of ions follow different curved paths; the radius of a particular path is determined by the ratio of the electrical charge to the mass of the ion concerned. Mass spectrometers measure only mass-to-charge ratios, m/ne, where m is the mass of the ion (atomic, molecular or fragment) and n is the number of electric charges lost or gained during ionization. The majority of ions in a mass spectrometer are singly charged, but some molecules may lose more than one electron without disintigrating. A doubly charged ion with a ratio of $m/2e$ will exhibit an apparent mass one half of the corresponding singly charged ion with a ratio of m/e. The masses of nuclides are conveniently expressed in terms of atomic mass units (a.m.u.). One atomic mass unit is defined as equal to $1/12$ of the mass of the most abundant isotope of carbon. A ^{12}C atom thus has a mass of 12,000 a.m.u. A respiratory mass spectrometer will cover the mass range 2–100 a.m.u.

The individual ionic species fall onto an electrode system which is electrically scanned at regular intervals so that a recorder traces out a series of peaks, each peak being proportional to the number of the ions of that type present in the sample. As a result of the ionization process, the more complicated molecules are broken down to form molecular components each of which produces its own peak on the recorder chart. For gases, the interpretation of the resulting pattern of peaks is usually not difficult, but it can be troublesome in the case of organic molecules, even ethyl alcohol yielding a complicated trace. *Figure 6.8* shows a typical compact mass spectrometer. It can produce a complete gas analysis from a 1-cm³ gas sample at a pressure of 10^{-6} Torr with a sensitivity of 1 part per million. The mass spectrometer is almost the only analyser fast enough to follow oxygen concentration changes occurring in a single breath. Current practice is to use a pair of compact mass spectrometers, one set to analyse for CO_2 and the other for O_2. A portable mass spectrometer designed for respiratory studies in a manned spacecraft is described by Brigden and Roman (1966). Blood gas tensions can be measured *in vivo* by connecting an arterial catheter fitted with a silicone rubber membrane at its tip to a mass spectrometer (Wald *et al.*, 1970). In addition to monitoring O_2, N_2 and CO_2, Wald *et al.* were able to monitor N_2O in blood by monitoring the fragment ion peak (NO) at mass 30 where no other compound normally found in the body produced a response. It is necessary to use the peak at mass 30 because the usual peaks for CO_2 and N_2O coincide at a mass to charge ratio of 44 which is the peak normally used for either CO_2 or N_2O. A membrane-covered catheter is inserted into a blood

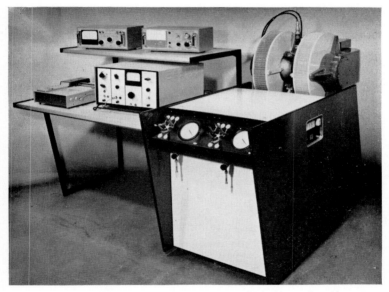

Figure 6.8. Compact mass spectrometer for gas analysis. (Reproduced by courtesy of AEI Ltd.)

vessel and the gas tensions in equilibrium across the membrane measured. A detailed account of the technique is given by Wald *et al.* The mass spectrometer was connected to a nylon arterial catheter terminating in a 0·007 in (0·18 mm) thick silicone rubber membrane. A continuous monitoring of blood O_2, N_2, CO_2 and N_2O tensions was possible. Both N_2O and CO_2 exhibit main peaks at a mass to charge ratio of 44, so that N_2O is monitored by working with the fragmentation peak arising at a mass to charge ratio of 30 corresponding to NO.

209

Quadrupole mass spectrometers

Conventional mass spectrometers suffer from the disadvantage of requiring a bulky electromagnet. The quadrupole mass spectrometer can be much lighter in weight and smaller because it uses only electric fields to achieve mass separation. A practical quadrupole mass spectrometer head consists of four parallel cylindrical rods mounted accurately at the corners of a square (*Figure 6.9*) with opposite rods electrically connected. A radio frequency voltage, together with a d.c. voltage, is placed on the rods. The potentials applied to the two pairs of metal rods are equal in magnitude, but

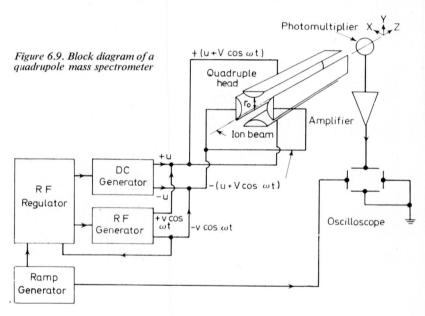

Figure 6.9. Block diagram of a quadrupole mass spectrometer

the d.c. potentials are opposite in sign and the a.c. potentials are arranged to be 180° out of phase. Each pair of rods is separated by a distance $2r_0$. The source of ions is located at one end of the quadrupole array on the z axis. By means of an accelerating voltage, an ion beam is injected through a hole in a diaphragm along the axis of the field and the ratio of the d.c. voltage to the peak a.c. voltage on the rods set equal to 0·17. There then exists only one frequency at which ions of a specific mass-to-charge ratio can travel along the z-axis to be collected at the other end of the head. For singly charged ions the relationship between their mass and the radio frequency is $M = 0\cdot136\ V/r_0{}^2 f^2$, where M is in atomic mass units, r_0 is in cm, and f is in MHz. Ions of other masses undergo increasing oscillations and eventually lose their charges on hitting the rods. Scanning of the mass spectrum can be accomplished by varying the r.f. or d.c. voltage keeping their ratio and f constant. In order for mass separation to occur the ions must spend a sufficient length of time within the quadrupole field to bring about the removal of the unwanted species.

Roboz (1968) gives a good description of the quadrupole mass spectrometer. He describes a typical head as having a rod diameter of 8 mm, a field diameter of 7 mm and a rod length of 200 mm. The r.f. amplitude is 0–800 V, d.c. voltage 0–140 V, r.f. frequency 3–4 MHz, maximum r.f. power 30 W. A stabilization of 1 part in 10^5 for the amplitude and 1 part in 5×10^3 for frequency are minimum requirements. Detection of the selected ions is by means of a low-noise photo-multiplier in order to provide a high sensitivity (down to a few parts per million) and a fast scanning time (100 ms).

Figure 6.10 gives the block diagram of a respiratory quadrupole gas analyser. The quadrupole head is operated under high vacuum conditions with a working pressure of 10^{-6} torr. This is achieved within 30 minutes of start-up by means of an oil diffusion pump backed by a rotary oil vacuum pump. Respiratory gases are sampled through a flexible stainless steel capillary tube which is heated by passing an electric current through it. A separate vacuum pump is employed to pull gas through the capillary at a volume flow of the order of 25 ml per minute. The heated capillary allows a fast response for vapours. Gas from the capillary diffuses through a molecular leak into the ion source of the head. With this type of construction a response time of less than 100 ms is possible for a square wave input of dry air. The flexible capillary is 1 metre long. A typical mass range would be 2–100 a.m.u. The masses of the respiratory gases are nitrogen (28), hydrogen (2), oxygen (32) and carbon dioxide (44). Tracer gases are helium (4), argon (40), and neon (20). The spectrum up to mass 100 can be scanned in 100 ms. The vacuum system is constructed from stainless steel and is fitted with electrical heaters for baking-out absorbed gases. Channels are provided to monitor the amplitudes of 4 or 8 individual mass peaks and to provide electrical outputs so that the individual peaks can be observed on a fast response multi-channel recorder or the spectrum of peaks displayed on an oscilloscope.

A quadrupole mass spectrometer can be set-up to monitor

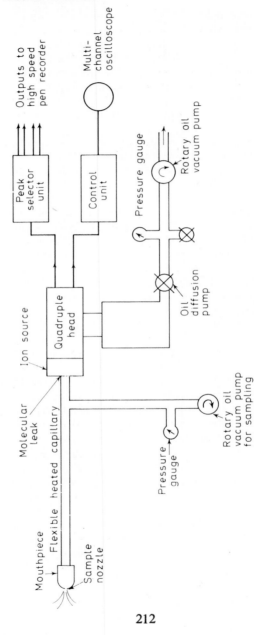

Figure 6.10. Schematic diagram of a quadrupole mass spectrometer designed for respiratory gas analysis

212

simultaneous changes in the concentration of oxygen, nitrogen, carbon dioxide and water vapour in the breath. If the partial pressure of water vapour is known, the fractional concentrations of the gases can be directly determined. Scheid *et al.* (1971) describe an automatic control system for use with a mass spectrometer which corrects for the partial pressure of water vapour in the sample by stabilizing the sum of the mass spectrometer signals for all component gases other than water vapour. It also corrects for pressure changes.

Houseman and Hafner (1971) describe a computer controlled operating and data handling system for a quadrupole mass spectrometer, and Smith and Cromey (1968) describe an inexpensive, bakable, quadrupole mass spectrometer. Bickel *et al.* (1970) have used an analogue computer program for the determination of cardiac output in humans using mass spectrometer analysis of expired air. Adamczyk *et al.* (1966) used a mass spectrometer for the continuous analysis of gaseous compounds excreted by human skin.

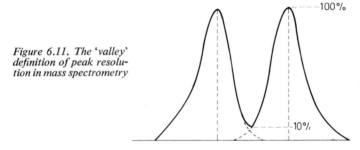

Figure 6.11. The 'valley' definition of peak resolution in mass spectrometry

The resolution of mass spectrometers is usually expressed in terms of the 'valley' definition. Thus, resolution is defined in terms of the highest mass at which two peaks in the spectrum of equal height and differing in mass by one unit exhibit a valley between the peaks not greater than a certain percentage, usually 10 per cent. Referring to *Figure 6.11*, each peak contributes 5 per cent to the valley. A typical quadrupole mass spectrometer would have Unit Resolution (10 per cent valley) up to 100 a.m.u. using its 2–100 a.m.u. range.

GAS CHROMATOGRAPHY

The technique of gas chromatography is proving of great value in the analysis of anaesthetic and respiratory gas mixtures, and for the determination of the contents of gases in blood samples as small as

100 μl. A gas chromatograph is not a continuous analyser and needs to be fed with a series of discrete samples. It is not sufficiently fast to be able to follow individual breath concentrations. However, this is more than compensated by its high sensitivity and versatility.

The heart of a gas chromatograph is the chromatographic column (or columns). This is usually a glass or metal tube, typically six feet long by $\frac{1}{4}$ or $\frac{1}{8}$ inch internal diameter. For the analysis of organic vapours, the column would be uniformly packed with an inert supporting phase such as crushed, sieved firebrick or Celite (a diatomaceous earth) having a typical mesh range of 80–100. This supporting material is coated before packing with 10–30 per cent by weight of a suitable stationary phase. When working with anaesthetic vapours this might be dinonyl phthalate or a silicone fluid. In this case the column is mounted inside a hot-air oven thermostatically controlled at a temperature in the range 70–100°C. The column is perfused with a steady flow of a carrier gas such as helium, hydrogen, argon or nitrogen at a flow rate of the order of 20–60 ml per minute. By means of a rotating plate type of gas sampling valve (Hill and Hook, 1960; Cundall, Hay and Lemunier, 1966) a sample, typically 1 ml or 10 ml, of the gas mixture is injected into the carrier gas stream as it enters the column. The function of the column is to split up the components of the sample in the order of their affinities for the stationary phase. In many cases this is in order of the boiling points of the components. Assuming that the column has the required resolution, it is then necessary to detect the components as they emerge from it.

The flame ionization detector

When trace amounts of organic vapours have to be analysed, it is usual to employ a flame ionization detector (McWilliam and Dewar, 1958). By means of an auxiliary supply of air and hydrogen, a small flame is produced, and the carrier gas emerging from the column is fed into the flame. The presence in the effluent from the column of an organic component causes an increase in the electrical conductivity of the flame. The needle-jet from which the flame burns, together with an outer concentric cylindrical electrode form an ionization chamber. This is polarized with a voltage of the order of 120 V d.c. The resulting ionization current is measured with a vibrating reed or other type of electrometer amplifier and the output displayed on a potentiometric recorder. A suitable hybrid (valve and transistor) amplifier is described by Gabriel and Morriss (1966). Each time the column elutes a separate organic substance the

214

ionization current increases to a maximum value and returns to the small standing current arising from impurities in the carrier gas and a carry-over of stationary phase from the column. Accordingly, for each separate organic substance eluted, the recorder pen traces out a peak on the chart. The area under each peak is proportional to the quantity of that particular substance present in the sample. Measurement of the area beneath the curve can conveniently be accomplished by the use of a digital integrator. In this the voltage feeding the potentiometric recorder of the chromatograph is amplified and fed into a voltage-to-frequency converter. The number of cycles generated by the converter during the passage of the peak is shown on a printing-type counter. With this flame ionization system, sensitivities better than a few parts per million by volume can be attained. For a constant carrier gas flow rate and column temperature, the time elapsing between the injection of the sample and the emergence of a particular peak is characteristic of the sample component concerned. Thus the retention times are used to identify the individual components.

For the analysis of halothane in blood, the halothane is extracted into n-heptane (Butler and Hill, 1961; Wortley et al 1968) or trichloroethylene, and 1µl of the extraction agent containing halothane loaded on to the column which is kept at a temperature of about 80°C. When loading the sample, the needle of the micro-syringe is passed through a rubber septum situated at the column inlet. A suitable column packing is silicone fluid on Celite, the column being about 24 inches long.

Jones et al. (1972) describe a convenient method of gas chromatography for the measurement of methoxyflurane in blood. The methoxyflurane is extracted with silicone fluid. When the extractant is loaded on to the chromatograph, the methoxyflurane peak appears after one minute. The low volatility of the silicone fluid ensures that it is not accompanied by a solvent peak. The response was linear over the range 1–20 mg/100 ml and the coefficient of variation was $\pm 1\cdot 8$ per cent at the 10 mg/100 ml level. Using this technique, specimens can be stored for several days prior to chromatography.

Lowe (1964) describes the use of a flame ionization detector system for the estimation of halothane in blood with the direct injection of 1 µl blood samples. The injection port is run at 50°C. The column is 18 inches long by $\frac{1}{8}$ inch o.d. and operated at 130°C. It is filled with plain 60-85 mesh crushed firebrick saturated with water. The nitrogen carrier gas is also saturated with wet Chromosorb. The halothane peak emerges after only 30 seconds. Calibration is effected using halothane standards prepared in distilled water. The direct injection technique can also be used with biopsy samples.

Jones *et al.* (1972) describe a neat method for the analysis of methoxyflurane (Penthrane) in blood by gas chromatography. The methoxyflurane is extracted from the blood by equilibration with silicone fluid. Because of its non-volatility, injection of the silicone extractant into the gas chromatograph results in a methoxyflurane peak after one minute and this is not accompanied by a solvent peak. The absence of the usual large solvent peak prevents swamping of the methoxyflurane peak and allows a greater throughput of samples. The method also permits the storage of blood samples for several days prior to chromatography. A linear calibration was found over the range 1–20 mg/100 ml and the coefficient of variation in blood at the 10 mg/100 ml level was $\pm 1 \cdot 8$ per cent.

The electron capture detector

The flame ionization detector is sensitive to most organic substances. This makes it attractive for general work, but it has disadvantages, as for example when using heptane as the extraction agent to measure halothane in blood. The heptane is eluted first and gives a very large, broad, peak with the flame detector. The heptane peak thus tends to mask the smaller halothane peak, and also spoils the appearance of the chart record. For halogenated agents such as chloroform, halothane, methoxyflurane and trichloroethylene an exceptionally high sensitivity can be realized by the use of an electron capture detector (Lovelock, 1963). This detector does not give a significant response for heptane. It is not possible to use whole blood injected directly on to the column inlet simply because of the fact that the blood tends to solidify in the fine needle of the micro-syringe when the needle is inside the heated injection port (180°C) of the chromatograph. eBcause of the high sensitivity of the electron capture detector it is possible to dilute the blood 1,000 times with heptane and then inject 1 μl of the heptane containing halothane.

The electron capture detector simply consists of a small-volume coaxial cylinder ionization chamber having a cathode formed from zirconium foil impregnated with tritium (20 mC). Tritium (H_3) is a radioactive isotope of hydrogen and emits weak beta particles. A collecting voltage of about 9 V d.c. is applied across the chamber and the ionization current measured with an electrometer amplifier and recorder. When a halogenated substance enters the chamber it captures some of the free electrons migrating across to the positive central rod anode and diminishes the ionization current, thus giving rise to a negative peak on the recorder chart. For tritium sources of this size in a d.c. mode electron capture detector the calibration curve of halogen concentration against peak height is not linear, but tends to be sigmoid in shape so that a calibration curve has to be used. In spite of this, the electron capture detector offers some important advantages. For the estimation of halothane in blood it can be used with a silicone fluid on Celite column with nitrogen as a non-explosive carrier gas. No additional supplies of hydrogen and oxygen are required as with the flame detector. A detector voltage of only 9 V is required which can be supplied from a dry battery so that the chromatograph can be mounted on one compact trolley for use in the operating room. The response for halothane is about 20 times greater than that for trichloroethylene and about 10 times greater than that for chloroform.

The thermal conductivity detector or katharometer

When it is desired to analyse for inorganic gases such as oxygen, nitrogen, carbon dioxide and nitrous oxide, it is necessary to detect their emergence from the chromatographic column by means of a thermal conductivity cell (katharometer). These gases will not be quantitatively detected by flame or electron capture detectors. Thermistors have been used as the elements of the katharometer, but current (1973) practice favours miniature wire elements. The Wheatstone bridge network of the detector is fed with a constant current, typically 200 mA d.c.

Solid column-filling materials are widely used for gas analysis applications. A column filled with molecular sieve (artificial zeolite) and about six feet long will separate oxygen and nitrogen at 40°C. A suitable sieve is the Type 5A or 13X molecular sieve by the Linde Company. A six feet column of cross-linked polymer beads (Porapak) will separate carbon dioxide and nitrous oxide from (oxygen plus nitrogen). The size of the beads would be typically 80–100 mesh, and the column would be run at about 40°C for this application.

With the polymer bead column run in parallel with an 18-inch column filled with dinonyl phthalate on crushed firebrick it is possible to resolve a mixture of ether, halothane, cyclopropane, oxygen, nitrogen, carbon dioxide and nitrous oxide. An earlier account of this method using activated charcoal instead of the polymer bead column is that of Hill (1960). The combination of a polymer-bead or charcoal column in parallel with a molecular sieve column can be extended to analyse for gases in blood. A known

217

volume of whole blood (100 µl) is added to 0·4 ml of a degassed Van Slyke gas-releasing solution (lactic acid + saponin + ferricyanide + anti-foam). The solution is contained in a sealed reaction vessel which has previously been purged with the chromatograph carrier gas (hydrogen or helium). A magnetic stirrer is used to mix the solution and the blood. During this procedure the carrier gas by-passes the vessel. When all the gases have been liberated, the carrier gas is routed through the vessel to sweep the blood-gases on to the columns. The length of each column and its gas flow is adjusted in order to obtain an optimum resolution of the peaks on the chart. At any instant only one column of the pair is eluting a peak, the other eluting carrier gas to act as a reference for the katharometer. Hydrogen or helium have to be used as the carrier gas as their thermal conductivities are well removed from those of the blood-gases.

Davies (1970) describes a reaction chamber for the analysis of blood gases by means of a katharometer detector gas chromatograph. Eighty micro-litres of blood are required for each analysis, duplicate analyses requiring eight minutes. Calibration for carbon dioxide is carried out using potassium carbonate solutions, for oxygen using room air, and for nitrous oxide by using cylinder nitrous oxide. The reproducibility of the method was found by analysing one blood sample 10 times. The coefficients of variation for oxygen, carbon dioxide and nitrous oxide were in each case approximately 0·5 per cent. Davies compared the oxygen and carbon dioxide contents of whole blood measured by gas chromatography and the manometric Van Slyke method. The correlation coefficient for oxygen was 0·999 and for carbon dioxide it was 0·995.

The preparation of standard gas and vapour mixtures

Most physical methods of gas analysis require calibration by means of standard gas mixtures. For gas mixtures containing only oxygen, nitrogen and carbon dioxide, it is convenient to purchase standard commercial mixtures and to check their accuracy by using a chemical gas analyser such as the Lloyd–Haldane or Scholander. Mixtures of these three gases can also be conveniently made in the laboratory by means of a pair of gas mixing pumps. Each pump consists of a pair of separate phosphor bronze pistons and cylinders running in an oil bath. The relative stroke rate of each piston can be adjusted by means of a set of interchangeable gear wheels, the cylinder outlets feeding a common output manifold. The first pump might be fed with pure oxygen to one cylinder and pure nitrogen to the other. The choice of gear wheels gives a mixture containing from 10 to 90 per cent oxygen in 10 per cent steps. The output from this first pump is supplied to one cylinder of the second pump, the second

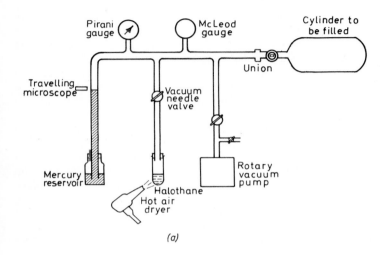

(a)

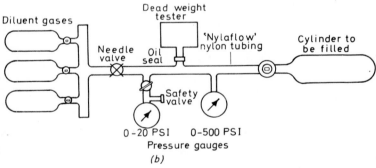

(b)

Figure 6.12. Manifold for filling cylinders with a known pressure of a gas or vapour

cylinder being fed with pure carbon dioxide. The second pump can add from 1 to 10 per cent by volume of carbon dioxide in steps of 1 per cent. A volume flow of about one litre per minute is normally available at pressures near atmospheric. This arrangement is particularly useful for the calibration of blood-gas electrode systems.

For the calibration of infra-red gas analysers or the ultra-violet halothane analyser, sufficiently accurate mixtures of chloroform ether and halothane can be obtained from the appropriate model of an accurate range of vaporizers—such as the 'Vapor' range by Dräger. Alternatively, mixtures in the anaesthetic concentration range can be made up in stainless steel or alloy cylinders under pressure. The cylinder is first evacuated and the required pressure of the vapour placed in it by evaporation from a glass bottle of the liquid connected to the cylinder on a low-pressure manifold (*Figure 6.12*). Once the vapour is in, the required diluent gas can be added by decanting from a full cylinder of gas, or by the use of a compressor. Where possible it is best to use nitrogen as the diluent in order to avoid potentially inflammable or explosive mixtures. An accurate pressure gauge must be used. A description of the method is given by Hill (1961). For lower concentration mixtures, for example of a few hundred parts per million, the cylinders will need to be filled to 2,000 lbf/in² and a compressor will be required. These high-pressure mixtures can take more than 14 days to mix if stored in the vertical position. After filling they should be rolled and stored horizontally. Once mixed they will maintain their composition indefinitely. The pressure of vapour placed in the cylinder should be less than the saturation vapour pressure corresponding to the lowest temperature at which the cylinder is likely to be used, in order to prevent any condensation of the vapour into liquid.

In order to produce low vapour concentrations (down to 0·25 parts per million by volume) for the calibration of gas chromatography detectors, Hill and Newell (1965) found it convenient to make use of a dilution system based upon a continuous slow injector, that is, a power-driven syringe feeding a dilution stage. A full description of possible calibration methods is given by Hill and Powell (1968).

McLaren and Williams (1968) describe an automatic roller gas mixing device for mixing dense gas or vapour mixtures at near atmospheric pressure.

Nunn *et al.* (1970) describe a simple apparatus for the production of known vapour concentrations of volatile anaesthetic agents. A saturating chamber is held at a known temperature in a water bath and the resulting saturated vapour diluted by means of known gas streams. With carrier gas volume flow rates of between 100 and 700 ml per minute, dew point determinations confirmed a saturation of better than 99·5 per cent at the water bath temperature.

REFERENCES

Adamczyk, B., Boerboom, A. J. H., and Kistemaker, J. (1966). 'A mass spectrometer for continuous analysis of gaseous compounds excreted by human skin.' *J. appl. Physiol.*, **21**, 1903

Bickel, R. G., Diner, C. F., and Brammell, H. L. (1970). 'An analog computer program for cardiac output in humans using mass spectrometer analysis of expired air.' *Aerospace Med.* **41**, 203

Brigden, W. E. and Roman, J. (1966). 'Flight research program IV. A small gas analyser for aerospace.' *Aerospace Med.* **37**, 1037

Butler, R. A. and Hill, D. W. (1961). 'Estimation of volatile anaesthetics in tissues by gas chromatography.' *Nature, Lond.* **189**, 488

Campbell, E. J. M. (1960). 'Simplification of Haldane's apparatus for measuring CO_2 concentration in respired gases in clinical practice.' *Br. med. J.* **1**, 457

Collier, C. R., Affeldt, J. E. and Farr, A. F. (1955). 'Continuous rapid infra-red carbon dioxide analysis—fractional sampling and accuracy in determining alveolar CO_2.' *J. Lab. clin. Med.* **45**, 526

Cormack, R. S., and Powell, J. N. (1972). 'Improving the performance of the infra-red carbon dioxide meter.' *Br. J. Anaesth.* **44**, 131

Cundall, R. B., Hay, K. and Lemeunier, P. W. (1966). 'A gas sampling valve for use in vapour phase chromatography.' *J. Scient. Instrum.* **43**, 652

Davies, D. D. (1970). 'A method of gas chromatography for quantitative analysis of blood-gases.' *Br. J. Anaesth.*, **42**, 19

Dubois, A. B., Fowler, R. C., Soffer, A. and Fenn, W. O. (1952). 'Alveolar CO_2 measured by expiration into the rapid infra-red gas analyser.' *J. appl. Physiol.* **4**, 526

Dyer, C. A. (1947). 'A paramagnetic oxygen analyser,' *Rev. Scient. Instrum.* **18**, 696

Edmondson, W. (1957). 'Gas analysis by refractive index measurement.' *Br. J. Anaesth.* **29**, 570

Ellis, F. R. and Nunn, J. F. (1968). 'The measurement of gaseous oxygen tension utilizing paramagnetism: an evaluation of the 'Servomex' OA/150 analyser.' *Br. J. Anaesth.* **40**, 569

Fowler, K. T. and Hugh-Jones, P. (1957). 'Mass spectrometry applied to clinical practice and research.' *Br. med. J.* **1**, 1205

Francon, M. (1963). *Modern applications of Physical Optics.* New York; Interscience

Gabriel, W. P. and Morriss, R. A. (1966). 'A flame ionization meter for gas chromatography.' *J. Scient. Instrum.* **43**, 104

Hackney, J. D., Sears, C. C. and Collier, C. R. (1958). 'Estimation of arterial CO_2 tension by re-breathing technique.' *J. appl. Physiol.* **12**, 3

Haldane, J. S. (1920). *Methods of Air Analysis*, 3rd ed. London; Griffin

Heavens, O. S. (1955). *'Optical Properties of Thin Solid Films.'* London; Butterworths

Hill, D. W. (1958). 'Halothane concentrations obtained with a Fluotec vaporizer.' *Br. J. Anaesth.* **30**, 563

— (1960). In *Gas Chromatography*. Ed. by R. P. W. Scott, London; Butterworths

— (1961). 'The production of accurate gas and vapour mixtures.' *Br. J. appl. Phys.* **12**, 410

— Hook, J. R. (1960). 'Automatic gas-sampling device for gas chromatography.' *J. Scient. Instrum.* **37**, 253

— Newell, H. A. (1965). 'The use of a continuous slow injector for the production of calibration vapour mixtures in the parts per million by volume range.' *J. Scient. Instrum.* **42**, 783

— Powell, T. (1968). *Non-dispersive Infra-red Gas Analysis in Science, Medicine and Industry.* London; Hillger and Watts.

— Stone, R. N. (1964a). 'A versatile infra-red gas analyser using transistors.' *J. Scient. Instrum.* **41**, 732

— — (1964b). 'A transistor-driven gas sampling pump.' *J. Scient. Instrum.* **40**, 421

Houseman, J., and Hafner, F. W. (1971). 'Computer controlled operating and data handling system for a quadrupole mass spectrometer.' *J. Phys. E.* **1**, 46

Hulands, G. H., and Nunn, J. F. (1970). 'Portable interference refractometers in anaesthesia.' *Br. J. Anaesth.* **42**, 1051

Jessop, G. (1966). 'Katharometers.' *J. Scient. Instrum.* **11**, 777

Jones, P. L., Moloy, M. J., and Rosen, M. (1972). 'A technique for the analysis of methoxyflurane in blood by gas chromatography.' *Br. J. Anaesth.* **44**, 124

Linford, A. (1952). 'Measurement of oxygen concentration in gases.' *Coke Gas* **14**, 195

Lloyd, B. B. (1958). 'A development of Haldane's gas analysis apparatus.' *J. Physiol. Lond.* **143**, 5 P

Lovelock, J. E. (1963). 'Electron absorption detectors and technique for use in quantitative and qualitative analysis by gas chromatography.' *Analyt. Chem.* **35**, 474

Lowe, H. J. (1964). 'Flame ionization detection of volatile organic anaesthetics in blood, gases and tissues.' *Anesthesiology* **25**, 808

Luft, K. F. (1943). 'Über eine neue Methode der Registrienden Gasanalyse mit Hilfe der Absorption Ultraroter Strahlen ohne Spektrale Zerlung.' *Z. tech. Phys.* **24**, 97

Lundin, G. and Akesson, L. (1954). 'A new nitrogen meter model.' *Scand. J. clin. lab. Invest.* **6**, 250

McLaren, K. G. and Williams, W. T. (1968). 'Simple automatic magnetic roller gas mixing device.' *J. Scient. Instrum.* **1**, 561

McWilliam, I. C. and Dewar, R. A. (1958). 'Flame ionization detector for gas chromatography.' In *Gas Chromatography.* Ed. by D. H. Desty. p. 142. London; Butterworths

Medlock, R. S. (1962). 'Oxygen analysis.' *Publication TP* 5002, George Kent Ltd., Luton

Munday, C. W. (1958). 'A precision oxygen analyser for chemical plants.' In *Automatic Measurement of Quality in Process Plants.* p. 105. London; Butterworths

Nunn, J. F. (1958). 'The Dräger carbon dioxide analyser.' *Br. J. Anaesth.* **30**, 264

— (1964). 'Evaluation of the Servomex paramagnetic analyser.' *Br. J. Anaesth.* **36**, 366

— Gill, D., and Hulands, G. H. (1970). 'Apparatus for preparing saturated vapour concentrations of liquid anaesthetic agents.' *J. Phys. E.* **3**, 331

Pauling, L., Wood, R. and Sturdevant, C. O. (1946). 'An instrument for determining the partial pressure of oxygen in a gas.' *Science, N. Y.* **103,** 338

Robinson, A., Denson, J. S. and Summers, F. W. (1962). 'Halothane analyser.' *Anesthesiology*, **23,** 391

Roboz, J. (1968). *Introduction to Mass Spectrometry Instrumentation and Techniques*, p. 105. New York; Interscience.

Scheid, P., Slama, H., and Piper, J. (1971). 'Electronic compensation of the effects of water vapour in respiratory mass spectrometry.' *J. appl. Physiol.* **30,** 258

Smith, D., and Cromey, P. R. (1968). 'An inexpensive, bakeable quadrupole mass spectrometer.' *J. Sci. Instrum.*, 1 Ser, **2,** 523

Scholander, P. F. (1947). 'Analyser for accurate estimation of respiratory gases in one-half cubic centimetre samples.' *J. biol. Chem.* **167,** 235

Tyndall, J. (1863). *'On Radiation.'* Rede Lecture, Cambridge

Visser, B. F. (1957). *Clinical Gas Analysis Based on Thermal Conductivity.* Utrecht; Kemink

Wald, A., Hass, W. K., Siew, F. P., and Wood, D. H. (1970). 'Continuous measurement of blood gases *in vivo* by mass spectrography.' *Med. biol. Engng.*, **8,** 111

Woolmer, R. F. (1956). 'The Pauling analyser as an aid to the anaesthetist.' *Br. J. Anaesth.* **28,** 118

Wortley, D. J., Herbert, P., Thornton, J. A. and Whelpton, D. (1968). 'The use of gas chromotography in the measurement of anaesthetic agents in gas and blood: description of apparatus and method.' *Br. J. Anaesth.* **40,** 624

7 –Electrode Systems for Measuring the pH and Oxygen and Carbon Dioxide Tensions of Blood

A knowledge of the acid-base balance condition and of the oxygen and carbon dioxide tensions in the arterial blood is important in the management of many patients. The development of suitable electrode systems, which can be used in clinical situations, yet require only small sample volumes of blood, has made these measurements possible on a routine basis in many centres. However, care is still required in handling the blood samples and in calibrating the apparatus. The most reproducible results are generally obtained if the apparatus is left in the care of a small number of operators who are trained to detect any deviation from normal in its functioning.

Currently, the trend is for the electrode systems for pH, Po_2, and Pco_2 measurements to be mounted on a trolley together with their associated amplifiers and cylinders of calibration gases. The outer jackets of the electrodes are perfused with a stream of water at body temperature from a circulating water-bath. Provision is made for placing blood samples and calibration buffer solutions in the water-bath, and for bubbling calibration gas mixtures through heat-exchanger coils placed in the bath. A small-volume tonometer is usually available in order that blood samples can be readily calibrated with known gas mixtures. With some systems an additional attachment may also be provided to give a read-out directly in terms of oxygen saturation. In effect, the trolley becomes a mobile blood-gas laboratory that can be located close to the operating room, or taken to the bedside in an intensive care ward.

A comparison of four commercial blood-gas analysis systems under working conditions is discussed by Miller and Tutt (1967).

The electrode potential

The idea of an electrode potential leads to an understanding of the mode of action of electrode methods for the measurement of ions in solution. An electrode potential arises at the interface between two material phases. The most usual interface occurs between a metal and a solution. The electrode potential then arises from the passage of ions from the metal into the solution and the combination of metallic ions in the solution with electrons in the metal to form atoms of the metal. When equilibrium is reached between the processes a charged layer exists close to the electrode. The charge facing the electrode is of one sign, whilst that facing the solution is of the opposite sign. Hence the distributed charge is known as an electrical double layer. The double layer acts as a capacitance and contributes to the reduction in the contact impedance of recording electrodes at the higher frequencies.

In order to compare the electrode potentials developed by various combinations of substances it is necessary to have a reference value against which comparisons can be made. Nernst (1912) proposed that the potential of a reversible hydrogen electrode with gas at one atmosphere pressure in equilibrium with a solution of hydrogen ions at unit activity (for example, a 1·184M. solution of HCl at 25°C) shall be taken as zero. Referred to this at 25°C a silver/silver chloride (0·1M KCl) electrode would have an e.m.f. of $+ 0·288V$, while that of a mercury-calomel electrode (0·1M KCl) would be $+ 0·333V$, the hydrogen electrode e.m.f. being taken as zero.

The hydrogen electrode is inconvenient to use in portable instruments and for this reason both mercury-calomel and silver/silver chloride electrodes are widely used as reference electrodes having stable potentials.

MEMBRANE POTENTIAL

An electrode potential also appears when an interface is formed by placing a semipermeable membrane between two liquid phases, the membrane only allowing a reversible transfer of a particular ion. When equilibrium is reached, the potential is proportional to the logarithm of the ratio of the concentrations of the ion to which the membrane is selectively permeable.

The Nernst equation

For a membrane which is perfectly selective for a given ion the potential generated is given by Nernst's equation:

$$E = \frac{-RT}{nF} \log_e \frac{C_1}{C_2}$$

where n is the valence of the ion

R is the gas constant (8.315×10^7 erg per degree per mole)

T is the absolute temperature

F is the Faraday (96,500 coulombs required to convert one equivalent of an element to an equivalent of ions)

C_1 and C_2 are the concentrations of the given ion on either side of the membrane.

This form of the equation is only true for very dilute solutions. For stronger solutions the Nernst equation is expressed in terms of the ionic activity:

$$a = C \times V$$

where a = the activity of the given ion

C = the concentration of that ion

V = the activity coefficient.

$$\text{Thus } E = \frac{-RT}{nF} \log_e \frac{a_1}{a_2}$$

The availability of selectively permeable membranes gives rise to a potential which is proportional to the effective concentration of the ion concerned. It is now possible to consider the use of a glass membrane in a pH electrode in order to obtain an e.m.f. proportional to hydrogen ion concentration.

ELECTRODE SYSTEMS FOR MEASURING pH OF BODY FLUIDS

The basic components of a pH meter are shown in *Figure 7.1*. The sample solution S whose pH is to be measured is placed in a beaker or cuvette, and a pair of electrodes, IE and RE, placed in the solution. The electrodes and the solution can be considered as forming a battery whose e.m.f. is pH sensitive. The battery has a high value of internal resistance in many cases, so that its e.m.f. is measured by means of an electrometer E, the output meter of the electrometer being calibrated in terms of pH units. The indicator electrode IE is made to be responsive to the H^+ ion concentration of the sample, that is, to the pH. The reference electrode RE provides a constant reference potential against which changes in the potential developed by the indicator electrode can be recorded.

226

The pH-sensitive glass electrode

Laboratory pH meters almost invariably use a glass electrode as the indicator electrode (Eisenman *et al* 1966). The glass electrode may be regarded as a membrane electrode in which current transfer between the solutions separated by the membrane is dominated by the

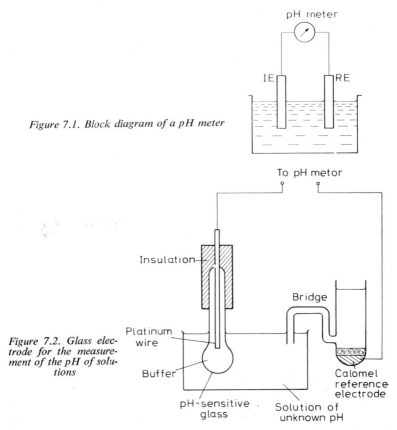

Figure 7.1. Block diagram of a pH meter

Figure 7.2. Glass electrode for the measurement of the pH of solutions

hydrogen ion, the membrane acting as though it was only permeable to hydrogen ions. Referring to *Figure 7.2*, at one end of the tubular electrode is blown a thin-walled bulb. The bulb contains a buffer solution, usually of pH 1, that is a solution having a known, stable, pH value. A platinum wire dips in the buffer and is connected by means of a highly insulated, low leakage, screened cable to the input terminal of the pH meter. The upper end of the glass electrode is sealed to prevent leakage of the buffer. When the glass electrode is placed in the sample solution, a d.c. potential arises between the inside and the outside surfaces of the glass bulb. The magnitude of the potential is proportional to the difference in pH existing between the buffer solution B inside the bulb and the sample solution S. It is assumed that this potential arises from an ion exchange occurring at the surfaces of the glass bulb, the exchange being controlled by the concentration of H^+ ions present in each solution. The wall of the

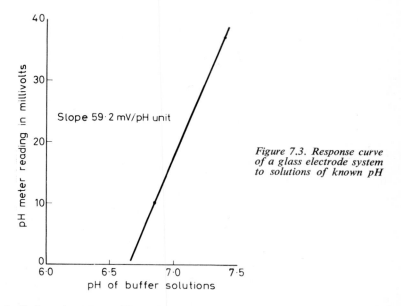

Figure 7.3. Response curve of a glass electrode system to solutions of known pH

bulb functions as a pH-sensitive glass membrane. The membrane need not necessarily be shaped in the form of a bulb, it can be flat or a tubular capillary as required. The response obtained from a glass electrode system for various values of sample pH is given in *Figure 7.3*. The graph is a straight line having a slope of 59·2 mV per pH unit. The slope is dependent upon the absolute temperature of the sample, and increases by 0·34 per cent/degC. In practice, the sensitivity of a pH electrode should be checked at regular intervals by means of buffer solutions of known pH. If the sensitivity has become noticeably diminished, the electrode should be etched or changed.

The membrane of a glass electrode is slightly sensitive to ions other than H^+, especially to Na^+ ions. This is known as the salt error, and reduces the response from the electrode when it is placed in samples having high values of pH and high Na^+ concentrations. Modern types of pH-sensitive glasses are very much less sensitive to other ions than were the older types. On the other hand, glasses have been developed which have a deliberately enhanced sensitivity to ions such as sodium and potassium. Electrode systems are available for the measurement of these ions. Khuri, Agulian and Harik (1968) describe glass ultra-micro electrodes for the measurement of pH, sodium and potassium, in fluid samples as small as 0·01 ml. They can be used both *in vivo* and *in vitro*.

It is often found that when a glass electrode has been in use for two months or more, then its sensitivity and speed of response may diminish. This situation arises from the fact that the surface of the glass membrane has become inactive due to a depletion of metal ions. It then forms a screen which partly covers an active layer of the glass. The effect is more noticeable when the electrode is used with solutions which contain protein. The manufacturer of the electrode provides instructions on how to etch the electrode surface clean in order to restore the sensitivity. This can be done a number of times. The electrode must be carefully rinsed between use with different samples in order to avoid contaminating one sample or buffer with another.

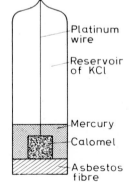

Figure 7.4. Calomel reference electrode

Platinum wire

Reservoir of KCl

Mercury

Calomel

Asbestos fibre

The calomel reference electrode

A calomel reference electrode is nearly always used in conjunction with a glass electrode. Referring to *Figure 7.4*, the lower end of the calomel electrode is formed by an asbestos fibre or ceramic plug.

229

This serves as a liquid junction between the saturated KCl solution within the electrode and the sample solution. The tubular body of the electrode holds a reservoir of saturated KCl solution, and into this is immersed a cylinder of calomel (HgCl). A blob of mercury and a platinum wire serve to make contact with the calomel. The wire connects to a lead going to the reference electrode terminal of the pH meter. The pores of the ceramic plug or fibre must not be allowed to become blocked, and the calomel electrode should be held at a constant temperature in order to maintain a constant potential.

In some forms of glass electrode, the reference electrode is contained in the interior of the glass electrode. This may consist of a simple silver–silver chloride electrode immersed in an inner solution which has a controlled concentration of Cl^- ions.

The carbon dioxide electrode described by Severinghaus (1962) also uses a calomel reference electrode. For this reference electrode 0·1 molar KCl solution was used rather than a saturated KCl solution. Severinghaus states that such an electrode should read $+91$ mV when compared with a standard saturated calomel electrode.

pH meters

The output voltage from a glass electrode is normally zero when the solution in which it is immersed is nearly neutral, that is, having a pH in the region of 7. For acid solutions a positive output is obtained, and this becomes negative (*Figure 7.3*) for alkaline solutions. The output voltage changes by about 60 mV for each pH unit change. The pH electrode has an internal resistance of the order of 100 to 1,000 MΩ. For this reason the millivoltmeter used with the electrode must have a high input resistance, typically 10^5 MΩ in order to prevent loading the electrode by more than 1 per cent. A d.c. precision potentiometer (Hill, 1965) is well suited to the accurate measurement of millivoltages. However, it has an input resistance of only a few ohms. A simple 'impedance converter' is then needed to couple the output from the pH electrode system into the potentiometer. This can consist of a battery-powered electrometer valve. It is connected as one arm of a bridge, a sensitive galvanometer being connected between its anode load and the slider of a potentiometer forming part of a voltage-divider resistor chain connected between the H.T. lines. The galvanometer is provided with a shunt resistor which can be switched in to give a reduced sensitivity for use during the initial balancing procedure. A two-position, high-insulation switch enables the grid of the valve to be either earthed or connected to the lead from the glass electrode. The reference electrode is connected via the output terminals of the precision d.c. potentiometer to earth. The polarity of the voltages produced by the electrodes and the potentiometer is arranged to be opposite. With the grid earthed, the potentiometer connected to one side of the galvanometer is adjusted to make the galvanometer read zero. The grid is then connected to the glass electrode and the resulting deflection of the galvanometer nulled by adjusting the output controls of the d.c. precision potentiometer. When this happens, the magnitude of the e.m.f. produced by the electrodes is equal to that read off from the calibrated dials of the potentiometer. A calibration curve is constructed of mV against pH by the use of buffer solutions of known pH. The author used such an arrangement to measure blood pH values for a number of years.

Commercial pH meters are usually calibrated in terms of pH units, but also often have a mV scale. Meters used to measure the pH of urine samples may be portable, and use an electrometer valve system on the lines of that just described, with a multi-turn helical potentiometer in place of the d.c. precision potentiometer. The pH meters for use with blood work operate over a limited range of pH and one well-known model by Electronic Instruments Ltd. uses a vibrating reed electrometer arrangement (Hill, 1965). The output from the electrodes is applied across the plates of a capacitor having a high insulation resistance. One plate is kept vibrating by an electrical drive at a few hundred hertz. The varying plate separation produces across the capacitor an a.c. voltage which is passed though a low-leakage capacitor and amplified by an a.c. amplifier whose output is then rectified and displayed on a meter calibrated in terms of pH units. The input resistance of this system is high since it depends on the quality of the insulation of the capacitors, and zero drift is small since an a.c. rather than a d.c. amplifier is employed. A variable zero control and a sensitivity control are provided so that the pH meter can be set up on buffer solutions of known pH. Automatic temperature compensation can be provided by means of a resistance thermometer element which is inserted in the sample solution. As the temperature of the solution increases, so the resistance of the thermometer element also increases. It is arranged that this increase in resistance reduces the gain of the amplifier to hold the sensitivity of the pH electrode system sensibly constant over a stated temperature range. A pH meter for use with blood should be able to detect changes of 60 μV (0·001 pH units).

Bates and Covington (1968) state that over the past decade considerable efforts have been devoted to three areas of biological pH studies. These are (1) improvements in the accuracy of measurement of blood pH; (2) the development of techniques for *in vivo* acid-base studies and (3) the development of micro-pH electrodes suitable for intracellular measurements. Bates and Covington summarize the main published work in this field since 1964.

BUFFER SOLUTIONS FOR USE IN BLOOD pH MEASUREMENTS

Convenient buffer solutions for use with blood samples are the two phosphate buffers—0·025 molar potassium dihydrogen phosphate: 0·025 molar disodium hydrogen phosphate (Bates and Acree, 1945) and 0·01 molar potassium dihydrogen phosphate: 0·04 molar disodium hydrogen phosphate (Semple, Mattock and Uncles, 1962). These have pH values at 38°C of 6·840 and 7·416 and at 20°C of 6·881 and 7·429 pH units respectively (Bates 1962, Bates and Guggenheim, 1960).

TEMPERATURE COEFFICIENT OF BLOOD: EFFECT OF THE ACID-BASE STATE

In the absence of cellular metabolism or damage, a change in the temperature of blood *in vitro* will give rise to a reversible change in the acid-base state of the blood. Rosenthal (1948) found a linear relationship existing between changes in blood temperature and pH over the range 18 – 38°C. The blood samples used had a pH at 38°C which lay in the range 7·25 to 7·45. Rosenthal found the temperature coefficient for the pH of blood to be 0·0147 pH units/degC.

Burton (1965) found during his studies on the acid-base balance of patients undergoing cardiac surgery under profound hypothermia that his measured values for the temperature coefficient of blood differed significantly from the mean value quoted by Rosenthal (1948). In order to investigate the effect, Burton took seven samples of human blood and either allowed these to sediment at 4°C or lightly centrifuged them at this temperature at which metabolism was negligible (Gambino, 1961). Small quantities of saline, hydrochloric acid or sodium bicarbonate were then added to the plasma layer so that, following re-suspension of the cells, there was a 1 part in 200 dilution of the blood in all fractions. A range of base excess of

$+ 10$ to $- 14$ milli-equivalents per litre was produced for the samples. Samples of 1 ml were taken from each of the seven fractions and nine different respiratory states were obtained by equilibration at 38°C, 30°C and 20°C with mixtures containing respectively 3·64, 5·18 and 7·62 per cent v/v CO_2 in oxygen. Within these limits of CO_2 tension and base excess, a linear relationship was found between the temperature coefficient of blood pH and the log of P_{CO_2}. The slope and position of pH: P_{CO_2} buffer lines were altered by changes in temperature. Changes in metabolic state produced by the addition of acid or alakli did not significantly alter the relationship.

Burton mentions that when the temperature of the water-bath containing the electrodes was altered, care was taken to ensure that the salt bridge connecting the capillary glass electrode to the calomel reference electrode was fully saturated with potassium chloride at the new temperature of measurement. This minimizes any variation in junction potential arising from changes in the potassium chloride concentration (Semple, 1961).

Adamsons et al (1964) have also shown that the temperature coefficient of blood pH is dependent upon both the pH of blood measured at 38°C and the metabolic state of the blood.

Dawson, Ostrander and Gray (1967) discuss the design of a new electronic circuit giving an improved performance and temperature control with ion-sensitive electrodes. A square-wave pulsed metal oxide silicon field effect transistor replaces the more usual chopped electrometer pre-amplifier. Cowell, Band and Semple (1967) give the design of a rapid-response pH meter which can follow the rapidly fluctuating signals from a fast-response pH electrode. A noise level of 0·001 pH units with a baseline drift of better than 0·001 pH units per hour is achieved with a response time of 2 ms for an input resistance of between 10^{10} and 10^{11} ohms. Band and Semple (1967) have used a glass electrode mounted in a modified intra-arterial needle to monitor arterial blood pH continuously. At flow rates greater than 2 ml/minute through the needle, the time for 90 per cent response was about 40 ms.

THE CARBON DIOXIDE ELECTRODE

The design of a practical electrode for the direct measurement of the partial pressure (tension) of carbon dioxide in blood has been given by Severinghaus and Bradley (1958). It is modified from that of Stow, Baer and Randall (1957). The CO_2 electrode is basically a pH-sensitive glass electrode arranged to measure the pH of a very thin film of an aqueous sodium bicarbonate solution. The solution is separated from the blood (or gas) sample by a polytetra-fluoroethylene (Teflon) membrane. This is permeable to carbon dioxide gas molecules, but not to ions which might affect the pH of the bicarbonate solution.

The mode of action of the CO_2 electrode is illustrated in *Figure 7.5*. The bicarbonate solution is held between the dome-ended glass electrode and the Teflon membrane by a matrix consisting of a thin layer of Cellophane, glass wool, or sheer Nylon stocking. The matrix layer is stretched over the end of the glass electrode and held in place by a rubber band. In one design the Teflon membrane is held in place over the end of a Perspex tube by means of a rubber O-ring.

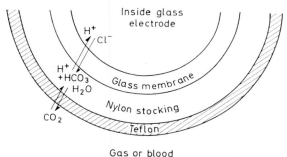

Figure 7.5. The mode of action of the carbon dioxide electrode

The tube is then inverted and a few millilitres of sodium bicarbonate solution added to the rear of the Teflon. The pH glass electrode with its Cellophane covering is then gently inserted into the Perspex tube and brought up to the rear of the Teflon, gentle agitation being employed to remove any remaining air bubbles from around the tip of the electrode. In addition to the pH-sensitive glass electrode, a reference calomel electrode is also required and this is mounted in the electrode housing in contact with electrolyte. Teflon is a good insulating material, so that the inside of the CO_2 electrode is completely insulated from both the cuvette and the water-bath.

When carbon dioxide gas molecules dissolve in the sodium bicarbonate electrolyte layer, the carbon dioxide reacts with the water to form carbonic acid, thus lowering the pH of the solution. The pH falls by almost one pH unit for a tenfold increase in the carbon dioxide tension of the sample. Hence the pH change is a linear function of the logarithm of the CO_2 tension. This relationship holds,

234

if a glass-wool matrix is used, over the range 0·2 to 100 per cent CO_2. However, if Cellophane is used, the relationship becomes non-linear for CO_2 concentrations below about 1.5 per cent. The maximum sensitivity in terms of pH change for a given change in CO_2 tension is obtained by using a bicarbonate concentration of about 0·01 moles/litre. The sensitivity is reduced to about one half when pure distilled water is used as the electrolyte. On the other hand it falls gradually when bicarbonate concentrations greater than 0·1 moles/litre are used since the concentration of carbonate ions now becomes significant. The response time is reduced with more dilute electrolyte, so that if a loss of sensitivity of the order of 5 per cent can be tolerated, there may be advantages in reducing the strength of the electrolyte to 0·001 moles/litre.

The response time of the CO_2 electrode is of the order 0·5 to 3 minutes, depending upon the amount of pH change involved, the thickness of the Teflon membrane, the direction of the pH change, the bicarbonate concentration, and the presence of a catalyst of the hydration reaction of CO_2. The speed of response is greater for an increasing Pco_2 than it is for a decreasing Pco_2. The enzyme carbonic anhydrase (present in red blood cells) can be added to the electrolyte in order to reduce the response time of the electrode. However, it does not remain active for more than a few days at body temperature. Of the other possible membrane materials, polyethylene is reliable but is considerably slower than Teflon. Rubber and Silastic (silicone rubber) membranes tend to become waterlogged and slow, and drifts in the electrode calibration may become troublesome.

The response time of a 1-ml thick Teflon membrane alone is quoted by Severinghaus as being about one minute to reach 95 per cent of the final CO_2 equilibrium value. The Cellophane spacer used beneath the Teflon membrane has been shown to be responsible for slowing the response time of the electrode, particularly at low values of Pco_2, and also to give rise to non-linearity of the calibration curve at the low Pco_2 end. The use of a piece of sheer Nylon stocking reduces the response time and improves the linearity of the electrode. It is also possible to use powdered glass-wool for the spacer layer and this offers the advantage of a rapid response time. The response is considerably faster in an electrode with glass-wool than it is in an electrode with no spacer at all. Thus the glass-wool is catalysing the reaction of CO_2 with water. With a 3/8 mil thick Teflon membrane and glass-wool powder it is possible to achieve a 95 per cent response time of 20 seconds. The response time of the catalytic electrode is now set almost entirely by the response time for the membrane itself, one minute in the case of a 1 mil thick Teflon membrane.

Calibration of a CO_2 electrode

To avoid cooling and drying of the electrode, calibration gas mixtures should not be run through the cuvette of the electrode for long periods. The gas mixtures should also not be run at a slow flow rate through a long piece of plastic or rubber tubing, since under these circumstances they may lose CO_2 before reaching the cuvette. If an extensive calibration is being carried out, then the cuvette should be periodically flushed through with a dilute detergent-anti-foam mixture in order to keep the membrane moist. Normally the output meter used with the CO_2 electrode will be calibrated directly in terms of P_{CO_2} in mmHg, a typical range being 15–150 mmHg. Two calibration gas mixtures are employed. The first is flushed through the cuvette and the instrument set to read this value. The second mixture is next flushed through and the sensitivity control altered to make the reading correct. The first gas mixture is now replaced in the cuvette and the procedure repeated until both mixtures read correctly on the scale.

If a sensitive pH meter is only available for use with the CO_2 electrode, two known gas mixtures should be placed in turn in the cuvette and the pH readings R_1 and R_2 noted. Let the corresponding CO_2 percentages for the mixtures be $\%_1$ and $\%_2$. Then the sensitivity of the electrode system S is given by $S=(R_1-R_2)/(\log\%_1-\log\%_2)$. Suppose that an unknown sample contains $x\%$ CO_2 where $\%_1 > \%x > \%_2$. Then $\log\%x=(R_x-R_2)/S+\log\%_2$ or $\log\%x=\log_1-(R_1-R_x)/S$. The P_{CO_2} of the sample is then found by multiplying $\%x$ by (barometric pressure—water vapour pressure at the temperature of the sample). An approximate calibration may be obtained by plotting on semi-log graph paper. P_{CO_2} or percentage of CO_2 is plotted on the logarithmic scale against instrument readings on the linear scale. There should be no difference in reading between equivalent blood and gas samples.

Handling of blood samples for the CO_2 electrode

The cuvette of the electrode should be filled with a gas mixture containing a P_{CO_2} of about the same value as is to be expected from the blood sample before this is injected. A large difference between the gas and blood P_{CO_2} may require that additional blood is passed through the electrode. If pure CO_2 has been used for checking the sensitivity, the cuvette should be carefully washed out in order to remove any dissolved CO_2 from the cuvette walls and membrane. The blood sample is taken, without air bubbles, into a heparinized syringe and immediately capped, agitated, and stored in a water-bath kept at the electrode temperature. The cuvette volume of the Severinghaus CO_2 electrode is about 0·1 ml and the minimum blood sample volume needed is about 0·3 ml. After filling the cuvette slowly, an interval of 10 seconds is allowed for residual gas to diffuse from the walls and membrane, and then an additional 0·5 ml of blood passed through. The lower stopcock of the cuvette is then closed, but the upper one is left open in order to eliminate pressure changes occurring in the cuvette. One to two minutes is allowed for equilibrium to be complete before the reading is taken.

Freshly drawn blood at body temperature continues to use oxygen and therefore to produce carbon dioxide. Thus its oxygen tension will fall and its carbon dioxide tension rise (Severinghaus, 1959; Nunn, 1962). The process of metabolism can be retarded by storing the blood samples in iced water in a Dewar flask. Lunn and Mapleson (1963) found that this treatment limited changes in the carbon dioxide tension of whole blood to within $2\frac{1}{2}$ per cent of the initial value for periods of at least two hours and possibly up to four hours. After storage, the cells and plasma must be re-mixed by rolling the syringe between the hands, (Severinghaus, 1960; Nunn, 1962).

Effects of temperature changes on the CO_2 electrode

It is necessary that the temperature of the electrode be held constant to within $\pm 0·1$ degC by means of an efficient thermostatically controlled water-bath system. This follows since the combined effects of temperature changes upon the sensitivity of the pH electrode and upon the P_{CO_2} of the blood sample amount to a total variation in sensitivity of 8 per cent per degC.

P_{CO_2} electrode read-out

Essentially, the requirements for the CO_2 electrode amplifier are those of a sensitive pH meter. The entire range of CO_2 concentration from 1 per cent to 100 per cent v/v is covered in a range of less than 2 pH units. The associated pH meter should be such that it can be read to within 0·001 pH unit. In order to avoid loading the glass electrode, the input resistance of the meter should be at least 1,000 MΩ. The latest types of instruments for blood-gas analysis are provided with an in-line digital display of the output from the electrode concerned.

237

Dynamic response of the CO_2 electrode

Lunn and Mapleson (1963) discuss the performance of the CO_2 electrode in detail. It can be assumed that the chemical reaction within the bicarbonate solution and the response time of the pH measurement system are rapid compared with the overall response time of the electrode, also that the bicarbonate solution and the gas in the cuvette are each perfectly mixed. That this is true follows from the size of the cuvette and the diffusion coefficient of carbon dioxide in gas and water. The cabon dioxide tension of the bicarbonate solution will then respond to a small step change in the carbon dioxide tension of the sample in an exponential fashion with a time constant equal to the product of the capacity of the bicarbonate solution for carbon dioxide and the resistance of the Teflon membrane to the diffusion of carbon dioxide. In practice, Lunn and Mapleson (1963) found that for a gas sample the time constant of the CO_2 electrode depended upon the carbon dioxide tension of the bicarbonate solution. Above a bicarbonate CO_2 tension of 50 mmHg. the time constant was constant at 0·2 minutes. However, for lower tensions the time constant increased rapidly, being approximately 5 minutes for a tension in the bicarbonate solution of 1 mmHg. In each a 0·01 molar bicarbonate solution was used without a catalyst. For a small step change in the CO_2 tension of the sample a simple exponential response was observed from the electrode. In the case of liquid samples the response was a two-part exponential. With blood samples having a CO_2 tension up to 120 mmHg in which metabolism prevents any fall in carbon dioxide tension, it was found that an exponential response occurred for the first minute or two, and then the response slowed down giving a second, longer time constant. This effect may be due to the fact that the turbulance produced by the sample injection keeps it well mixed for a minute or two and then diffusion through the liquid becomes a serious limitation to the speed of response.

The use of a CO_2 electrode to estimate the CO_2 content of whole blood

Severinghaus (1962) mentions that by diluting whole blood in the ratio 20 : 1 with 0·01 molar hydrochloric acid, both the bicarbonate and carbamino CO_2 of the blood are converted to free CO_2 in solution. This can then be measured with a CO_2 electrode. The blood can be diluted anaerobically by means of a 20-ml syringe, a 1-ml syringe and a three-way stopcock. The dead-space of the 1-ml syringe and stopcock are first filled with the hydrochloric acid. The remaining stopcock dead-space is then washed out with blood and exactly 1 ml of blood put into the 1-ml syringe. The stopcock is closed and its dead-space washed out with hydrochloric acid from the 20-ml syringe. The volume of HCl in the syringe is set at 19 ml and the stopcock turned to connect together the 1-ml and 20-ml syringes. The contents of the syringes are mixed by pushing the plungers alternately. The P_{CO_2} of the mixture is measured by means of the CO_2 electrode. The system is standardized by means of a solution containing exactly 25 mM/litre of sodium carbonate. The CO_2 content of the sample blood is given by multiplying the observed blood P_{CO_2} : carbonate solution P_{CO_2} ratio by 25. It is important to make the standard solution from sodium carbonate and not from sodium bicarbonate since the latter contains both carbonate and water. Before weighing out the carbonate it should be heated to 150°C for two hours in order to drive off water.

Linden, Ledsom and Norman (1965) use 0·1 molar hydrochloric acid, the 20 ml of acid being added to 1 ml of blood as before. The acid destroys the erythrocytes and releases the carbon dioxide carried in combination in the blood. Let v ml of blood containing A millimoles/litre be mixed with V ml of 0·1 molar hydrochloric acid. Then the CO_2 content of the mixture is $C_{CO_2} = A.v/(V+v)$ millimoles at the particular P_{CO_2} and 38°C. The Bunsen solubility coefficient α expresses the number of millilitres of gas which will dissolve in 1 ml of the liquid concerned at 0°C and a partial pressure of 760 mmHg. Under the conditions of NTP, one millimole of carbon dioxide occupies a volume of 22·6 ml. At 38°C (311°K) this volume becomes $22·6 \cdot \dfrac{311}{273}$. Hence the mixture of blood and hydrochloric acid holding all its carbon dioxide in the dissolved state contains $\dfrac{22·6(A.v)}{(V+v)} \cdot \dfrac{311}{273}$ of gaseous CO_2/litre at a pressure of P_{CO_2}. However, what is required for the solubility coefficient is the volume of gas dissolving in 1 ml of solution under the conditions of 38°C (311°K) and a partial pressure of 760 mmHg. This is $(760/P_{CO_2}) . (311/273)22·6(A.v)/1000(V+v) = V_1$. Now, $\alpha = V_1$ so that $P_{CO_2} = (760 . 311 . 22·6 . A.v)/[1000 . 273 . \alpha(V+v)]$ mmHg. Rearranging, the CO_2 content $A = [P_{CO_2} . 1000 . 273 . \alpha(V+v)]/(760 . 22·6 . v . 311)$ millimoles per litre. Provided that the same syringes and tap are used, v and V are constants for the apparatus working at a constant temperature of 38°C. Hence $A = K.P_{CO_2}$ millimoles per litre. The P_{CO_2} electrode exhibits a logarithmic response between P_{CO_2} and the pH. Thus $A = KP_{CO_2} = k$ antilog pH or $\log A = k_1 pH$. That is to say there is a linear relation-

239

ship between the logarithm of the content of carbon dioxide in the blood and the pH as recorded by the electrode.

The constant k_1 was determined by Linden, Ledsom and Norman using a series of solutions of anhydrous sodium carbonate having concentrations of 25, 20, 15, 10, 8, 7·14, 6 and 5 millimoles per litre. These were made up in water which had been distilled, re-boiled, and stored under soda lime. The graph of log C_{CO_2} against pH showed a linear relationship for CO_2 concentrations in the range 25–8mM/litre and there appeared to be a second line covering the range 8–5. Using dog arterial blood, Linden, Ledsom and Norman (1965) obtained a good agreement between CO_2 contents determined by the traditional technique of Van Slyke and Neill (1924) and the use of the P_{CO_2} electrode. The average content agreed to within ± 0.32 mM. The average difference was 0·081 mM, the P_{CO_2} electrode system giving the higher result.

Kelman (1967) describes a digital computer program to convert the carbon dioxide tension into whole blood CO_2 content at various temperatures and in the presence of metabolic acidosis or alkalosis.

CATION ELECTRODES

The availability of membrane materials which are selectively permeable to a particular ionic species has led to the production of electrodes which are responsive to particular ions such as Na^+ and K^+. Eisenman, Rudin and Casby (1957) devised a glass electrode made from a mixture of sodium, aluminium and potassium oxides at pH 7·6. The electrode was insensitive to calcium, magnesium, ammonia and lithium ions except when these were present in unusual concentrations. Freidman et al (1959) used a flow-through cuvette sodium electrode to continuously record the concentration of sodium in the femoral arteries of dogs. They were able to detect sodium concentration changes of only a few milli-equivalents per litre produced by the action of pressor and depressor agents.

Moreton (1970) mentions that cation electrodes designed for intracellular use present difficulties due to the high specific resistance of the glass, 10^8–10^9 ohms. It is thus difficult to insulate the non-active portion of the electrode. If the cation-sensitive micro-electrodes are stored for several weeks in saline, their resistance falls by several orders of magnitude. The cation response is also improved. Moreton has shown that the same result can be produced in as little as 24 hours by raising the temperature to 90°C. The fall in resistance from about 150 meg-ohms to about 1 meg-ohm is due to the uptake of water by the glass.

POLAROGRAPHIC ELECTRODES FOR THE MEASUREMENT OF THE OXYGEN TENSION OF BLOOD

Basically, the technique of polarography is used in the oxygen electrode to produce an electrical current by means of the electrochemical reduction of oxygen, $O_2 + 4e^- = 2 \times 0^{--}$. For a constant concentration of oxygen in the solution to be measured, the amount

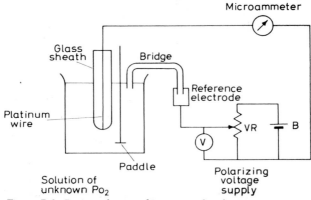

Figure 7.6. Basic polarographic system for the measurement of blood oxygen tension

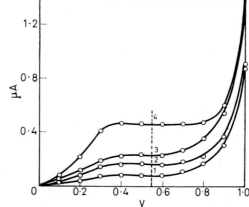

Figure 7.7. Calibration curves for an oxygen electrode placed in solutions of known oxygen tension (after Gleichmann and Lübbers, 1960)

of oxygen reduced and hence the current will depend on the value of the potential applied to the polarizable electrode. *Figure 7.6* shows a simple polarographic system. A potentiometer VR allows a pro-

241

portion of the voltage from a mercury battery B to be applied across the polarographic cell consisting of a platinum cathode and a silver/silver chloride anode immersed in the solution whose oxygen tension is to be measured. The cell current (of the order of 1 μA) is measured by means of the sensitive microammeter. A typical calibration curve is given in *Figure 7.7* (Gleichmann and Lübbers 1960). The curve was obtained from four known gas mixtures, and passes through the origin. CO_2 had no effect on the current obtained for oxygen. Up to some 400 mV, increasing the polarizing voltage applied across the cell will cause a corresponding increase in the cell current. However, from 400 to 800 mV there is a plateau region and the current changes little with increasing voltage. Under these conditions each oxygen molecule reaching the surface of the platinum cathode will be almost instantly reduced, the reduction current then being proportional to the amount of oxygen reaching the electrode per unit time. In general, the current is proportional to the oxygen availability of the electrode while in the sample, and not necessarily to the oxygen tension of the sample. The main condition that must be observed to ensure that the electrode current is proportional to the oxygen tension of the sample is that the oxygen must be transported to the cathode only by diffusion. In a homogeneous sample the amount of oxygen transported to the anode by diffusion will depend upon the difference in oxygen tension of the sample and that existing at the anode surface. Since the oxygen at the anode surface of a correctly working cell is zero, the cell current will be proportional to the oxygen tension of the sample. A constant zone of diffusion is established in front of the anode surface.

The development of a suitable platinum electrode for the measurement of the oxygen tension of blood has taken some 60 years. The main trouble has been in the poisoning action on the electrode of blood cells and proteins. Bartels (1951) measured the oxygen tension of whole blood by means of a dropping mercury electrode in which the cathode surface was constantly renewed. However, each blood sample required a separate calibration curve. The platinum electrode is more convenient to use in principle, but requires frequent cleaning in order to remove protein deposits, Inch (1958). Davies and Brink (1942) showed that bare platinum electrodes could be used for oxygen tension measurements when the platinum surface was protected by an agar or collodion membrane.

The Clark electrode

Although the membrane-covered electrodes were more stable and more accurate than the bare electrodes, they suffered from the disadvantage that the cell current had to traverse both the membrane and the sample before reaching the reference electrode. Clark (1956) placed both the platinum cathode and the reference electrode behind the membrane so that the membrane would completely insulate the electrodes from the sample. The cell was now virtually unaffected by the characteristics of the blood sample other than its oxygen tension. The oxygen consumption of the original Clark-type electrode is by no means negligible. The blood sample used with this electrode must be stirred or agitated, otherwise the reading from the electrode

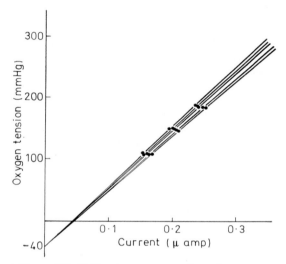

Figure 7.8. Calibration curves used to obtain a calibration constant for an oxygen electrode. Curve taken at 2-hourly intervals (after McConn and Robinson, 1963)

will diminish with time owing to the depletion of oxygen by the action of the electrode in the immediate vicinity. Sproule *et al* (1957) agitated the blood by producing a rhythmical pressure on a rubber tube, and Kreuzer, Watson and Ball (1958) oscillated the electrode system. Severinghaus and Bradley (1958) used a Clark-type electrode together with a rotating magnet in the sample cuvette to produce stirring. A detailed description of the use of a Clark-type oxygen electrode is given by Bishop (1960). McConn and Robinson (1963) found that with a Clark-type electrode, the ratio of the current obtained for water equilibrated with air, to the zero or background current, is a constant. A series of calibration curves for the same electrode, *Figure 7.8*, had a common point of intersection on the oxygen tension axis, that is to say, that zero electrode current was not given by a solution having zero oxygen tension, but occurred at a definite oxygen tension (the intercept) which McConn and Robinson called the 'electrode constant'. From a knowledge of this constant for a particular electrode it is possible to rapidly calibrate the electrode, using water equilibrated with air. A blood oxygen tension can then be determined in eight minutes. The electrode used by these workers was a Model B48A by Electronic Instruments Ltd., the current given for water equilibrated with air being 200 nA and the current from a solution having zero oxygen tension being 40 nA. With this electrode the background current was not a negligible proportion of the normal working current as stated by Severinghaus and Bradley (1958). By using a series of calibration gases, McConn and Robinson showed that when the straight line calibration curves were produced backwards they did not pass through the origin, but intersected the oxygen tension axis at a negative value (*Figure 7.8*.) A true zero current of less than 10 nA could be obtained by deoxygenating the electrolyte of the electrode by bubbling nitrogen through it for 30 minutes and then placing the electrode in water redistilled from alkaline pyragallol.

Mapleson *et al.* (1970) have shown that the response time of Clarke-type electrodes can be variable from day to day, and that, on the average, the response is considerably slower than had hitherto been suspected. With the electrodes and membranes used by them, 100 per cent response occupied more than 10 minutes and the response was different for different blood tensions. Although the system was fundamentally linear, incomplete response leads to a considerable apparent non-linearity and hysteresis. The incompleteness of response can be corrected mathematically.

When an oxygen electrode is used on-line for the continuous recording of blood oxygen tension, the need to heparinize the effluent stream of blood introduces a dilution effect on both the blood pO_2 and pCO_2 tensions. Dell'Osso (1970) provides a method of calculation which allows for this effect.

The requirements for a fast response and a calibration which is independent of the blood flow are mutually contradictory for membrane-covered blood oxygen tension electrodes. A theoretical evaluation is compared with results from practical electrodes by Schuler and Kreuzer (1967).

In respiratory studies when a mass spectrometer is not available there is a need for a fast response oxygen electrode. Friesen and McIlroy (1970) achieved an 80 milli-second response time by using a 3 micro-metre thick polytetrafluoroethylene (Teflon) membrane. By manually stretching the membrane to just below its breaking point a 40 milli-second response time was obtained and this was adequate for alveolar sampling during heavy exercise.

Clark and Becattini (1967) have designed a balanced portable m.o.s. field-effect transistor amplifier for use with a Clark-type oxygen electrode (*Figure 7.9*). Heitmann, Buckles and Laver (1967)

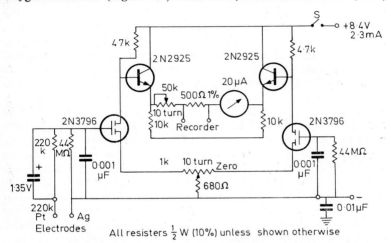

Figure 7.9. Field effect transistor amplifier for use with a Clark-type oxygen electrode (after Clark and Becattini, 1967)

have analysed the performance of commercially available membrane-covered oxygen electrodes in terms of the residual current, sensitivity, response time and linearity. A glycerin-water mixture was used for calibration purposes. It gave an identical reading to blood having a haematocrit of 40. Hahn (1969) describes the use of a field effect transistor operational amplifier having a digital voltmeter output to measure the current from an oxygen micro-cathode. Ganfield and Laughlin (1969) used a pair of low-cost plastic field-effect transistors in front of an operational amplifier in a simple arrangement to measure oxygen electrode currents.

Parker, Key and Davies (1971) describe a useful catheter-tip oxygen transducer using a silver-lead galvanic cell. A diamel-coated wire of 150 μm diameter is positioned and sealed within a lead cylinder with epoxy resin (Araldite resin AY105 with hardner HT972). The silver-lead assembly is sealed into the end of an etched polytetrafluoroethylene tube of 0·8 mm outside diameter. Contact to the lead cylinder is made by cold welding an insulated copper wire to the back of the lead cylinder. Both the silver and the copper wire are connected to a miniature autoclavable plug. The assembly is dipped into a saturated solution of K_2CO_3 and $KHCO_3$ and allowed to dry and then fitted into a cap of polytetrafluoroethylene having a wall thickness of about 25 μm. This is sealed onto the polytetrafluoroethylene catheter containing the wires using silicone rubber adhesive, the contact surfaces having previously been etched. It is also possible to use a polyvinyl chloride membrane which is easier to produce. At this stage the cell is inactive. It is activated when required by holding the tip in steam for two minutes. To sterilize the device it is autoclaved at 134°C for three minutes. This provides both activation and sterilization. After activation the cell consists of a silver cathode and a lead anode in contact with a thin film of saturated K_2CO_3 and $KHCO_3$. Oxygen is reduced at the cathode according to the equation $O_2+2H_2O+4e^-\rightarrow4(OH^-)$. At the anode, lead is converted to lead hydroxide according to the equation $2Pb+4(OH^-)\rightarrow2Pb(OH)_2+4e^-$. The electrons released flow through the external load resistor (2·2 kΩ) of the cell, the current flowing being proportional to the rate of reduction of oxygen at the silver surface. A typical sensitivity would be about 1 nano-ampere per mm Hg Po_2. Parker, Key and Davies (1971) describe a suitable operational amplifier circuit for displaying the cell current on a potentiometric recorder.

The use of an oxygen electrode to measure the oxygen content of whole blood

In a similar fashion to the Pco_2 electrode it is possible to make use of an oxygen tension polarographic electrode to measure the oxygen content of a sample of whole blood. The method is given in detail by Linden, Ledsom and Norman (1965). Half a millilitre of blood is diluted with 20 ml of a solution of saponin and potassium ferricyanide, using the two-syringe technique employed in the measurement of carbon dioxide content with a Pco_2 electrode. The solution consists of 6 g of potassium ferricyanide and 3 g of saponin per litre of distilled water, it is made freshly each day and stored in a 500-ml bottle partially immersed in a water bath at 38°±1degC. Adding the solution to the blood sample produces haemolysis and the release of oxygen from combination with the haemoglobin. The oxygen remains in a physically dissolved state in the solution and its tension is then measured with the polarographic electrode.

Once the oxygen is in physical solution the tension and concentration are linked by the Bunsen solubility coefficient α. This is defined as ml O_2 at NTP/ml solution at a partial pressure of 760 mmHg. If V ml of saponin-ferricyanide solution be used and the oxygen tension of this solution be P_s mmHg then the oxygen content of this volume is $\alpha \cdot V \cdot (P_s/760) \cdot (311/273)$ ml. The oxygen content provided by the v ml of blood is obtained by difference, that is, in v ml of blood there are $\alpha (311/273)(P_m/760)(V+v)(-P_s/760)(v)$. In 100 ml of blood there will be $(100/v) \cdot \alpha \cdot (311/273)(1/760) \cdot [P_m - P_s \cdot V/(V+v)]$ ml/100 ml. Since α, V and v are constants, the oxygen content $Co_2 = K[P_m - P_s \cdot V/(V+v)]$ ml/100 ml, where K is a constant. The factor $v/(V+v)$ represents the dilution of the oxygen dissolved in the saponin-ferricyanide solution occurring as the result of the addition of v ml of blood. Linden found this to have a value of 0·975 by filling the two syringes and three-way tap with water and weighing.

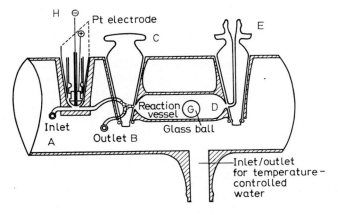

Figure 7.10. Apparatus for the determination of the oxygen content of 25-microlitre blood samples (after Lübbers, 1966)

Linden and his colleagues determined the value of the constant K by analysing nine samples of dog blood of varying oxygen content with the manometric technique of Van Slyke and Neill (1924), and also taking readings on each blood with the oxygen electrode arrangement.

Lübbers (1966) states that the polarographic method for the measurement of the oxygen tension of whole blood was first described by Baumberger (1940) who used a dropping mercury electrode. Lübbers describes a micro-apparatus for the determination of both oxygen tension and content from a 25-microlitre blood sample. This is shown in *Figure 7.10*. The whole apparatus is first filled with a solution of sodium ferricyanide and the oxygen tension of this solution measured with the polarographic electrode H. Then chamber D is closed off by means of stopcocks C and E. After flushing through the capillary tube AB, this is filled with the blood sample and its oxygen tension measured. Stopcocks C and E are then opened and 25 μl of blood pushed into chamber D by means of a micro-syringe, and C and E shut. The blood and ferricyanide solution are mixed together by rolling the glass ball G around the chamber. The oxygen tension of the mixture is measured and the oxygen content calculated.

Solymar, Rucklidge and Prys-Roberts (1971) describe a neat stainless steel cell for the routine determination of blood oxygen content using a polarographic oxygen electrode. Each measurement takes 4 to 5 minutes.

Polarographic electrodes for measurement of tissue oxygen tensions

A need exists for a relatively simple method for the determination of tissue oxygen tensions both in experimental animals and man. This need was particularly apparent to radio-biologists concerned with the effect of oxygen in increasing the sensitivity of tumours to ionizing radiation. By means of a local extracorporeal circulation it is possible to drop the oxygen tension of the surrounding well-perfused tissue while leaving the poorly perfused tumour at a relatively higher oxygen tension. For this type of work, a simple polarographic electrode consisting of a gold or platinum wire 0·004 inch in diameter covered in epoxy resin except for the tip and mounted inside a hypodermic needle may be used (Montgomery and Horwitz, 1950; Montgomery, 1957; Johansen and Krog, 1959). The reference electrode can consist of a chlorided silver plate covered with ECG electrode paste and strapped on to an arm or leg. Each electrode pair is polarized at 600 mV and the polarographic current recorded with a simple battery-powered electrometer on the lines of that described by Cater, Phillips and Silver (1956). These electrodes are calibrated by placing them in a physiological saline solution equilibrated with air at the start and finish of the experiment.

The electrode is used in the tissue without any protective membrane so that poisoning by protein will occur. However, a change in calibration of up to 10 per cent is normally acceptable over a period of an hour or two. Cater, Phillips and Silver describe a bare noble metal electrode, and Cater and Silver (1961) describe an ultra-micro-needle electrode in which the cathode surface area is of the order of 1–5 μm^2. Electrodes of this size retain the rapid response of the larger electrodes, but do not appear to suffer from many of the disadvantages, that is, they can be made insensitive to stirring, they consume extremely small amounts of oxygen, and they cause little mechanical damage to tissues on insertion. They are still affected by the electrophoretic deposition of protein and are easily damaged. Silver (1966) describes a micro-electrode of the Clark type, based upon a 25–50-μm platinum wire electropolished down to a 1 μm tip and fused into a thin glass insulation. The cathode is covered with a thin membrane of the histological mountant DPX and used with a silver reference electrode mounted in the same assembly as the cathode.

Walker *et al* (1968) describe a membrane-covered flush-type oxygen electrode developed for the measurement of the tissue Po_2 of human foetal scalp.

Fuel cells

Weil, Sodal and Speck (1967) report the use of a modified solid oxide fuel cell to analyse the oxygen concentration of gases. The cell is linear from 1·0 to 99·6 per cent v/v oxygen. Continuous or single breath analysis is possible since the cell's time constant is only 0·2 seconds. A comparison between the modified Westinghouse Type 203C cell and a Scholander apparatus gave a mean difference between the two methods of 0·008 per cent v/v with a standard deviation of 0·015 per cent v/v.

Catheter-type oxygen electrodes

A demand exists for an oxygen polarographic electrode whose dimensions are sufficiently small that the electrode can be mounted at the tip of a catheter for *in vivo* work. The use of a Clark-type of electrode is necessary in order to obtain a calibration which is stable over extended periods. Beneken Kolmer and Kreuzer (1968) describe a catheter-tip electrode which has an outer diameter of only 2 mm, *Figure 7.11*. The central platinum cathode 300 μm in diameter is insulated by a plastic (polyvinyl chloride) or glass tube. The outer silver anode supports a Teflon membrane 3 or 6 μm in thickness which is held in place by a silver ring. The electrolyte is a phosphate buffer solution of pH approximately 9. The length of the electrode assembly is 10 mm. The current output of the electrode is about 4 μA for a 300-μm diameter cathode in 100 per cent oxygen at 37°C. The calibration curve is said to be linear up to 100 per cent oxygen with a constant environmental temperature, and it passes through the origin. The calibration varies from electrode to electrode, but for an

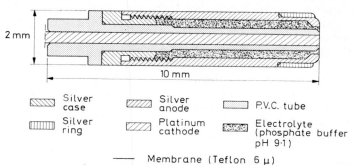

⬚	Silver case	⬚	Silver anode	⬚	P.V.C. tube	
⬚	Silver ring	⬚	Platinum cathode	⬚	Electrolyte (phosphate buffer pH 9·1)	

—— Membrane (Teflon 6 μ)

Figure 7.11. Construction of oxygen catheter electrode (after Beneken Kolmer and Kreuzer, 1968)

individual electrode it remains within 2 per cent over 34 days. When used in the gas phase its reading is not influenced by the presence of CO_2, ether, trichloroethylene, halothane or N_2O. The electrode is polarized with 800 mV.

The particularly interesting property of the electrode, apart from its small size is its fast speed of response, 0·20–0·25 seconds for a 95 per cent deflection with a change in concentration between 0–100

Figure 7.12. Normal respiratory curves for O_2 and CO_2 obtained with an oxygen electrode and infrared gas analyser (after Beneken Kolmer and Kreuzer, 1968)

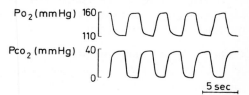

per cent in both directions. This is two to three times longer than that obtained with a mass spectrometer. *Figure 7.12* shows breath-by-breath alveolar oxygen tensions recorded with the electrode and alveolar CO_2 recorded using an infra-red gas analyser. With the electrode it is also possible to detect cardiogenic oscillations present on the alveolar portions of the oxygen tension tracing. It has been ascertained that these oscillations are in fact due to P_{O_2} changes and not due to a mechanical effect of pressure or flow on the electrode.

This electrode arrangement can also be used for the continuous recording *in vivo* of blood oxygen tension (Kreuzer, Harris and Nessler 1960). When used in gas streams, rapid diffusion ensures that there is no flow dependency for linear gas velocities from 0–312 cm per second. However, with liquids the calibration is flow dependent, above flow velocities of 8–10 cm/s the P_{O_2} reading becomes constant. Kreuzer and colleagues report that static pressures in the range 0–120 cm H_2O did not affect the output of the electrode, but that rapid pulsating pressures did.

Computer programs

Cohen (1969) describes a computer program which interprets acid base parameters to within the 95 per cent confidence limits. It defines the primary single or mixed disturbance and estimates the degree of compensation. It can be adapted to existing programs which read the raw data and compute the acid base parameters thus automating both the calculations and the interpretation of the results. Jalowayski *et al.* (1968) have written a computer program to calculate oxygen saturation, oxygen content, base excess, buffer base and standard bicarbonate from P_{O_2}, pH and P_{CO_2} measurements, and have applied it to both adult and foetal bloods. Kelman (1968) describes a computer program for the production of O_2–CO_2 diagrams. The parameters considered are the subject's haemoglobin concentration, body temperature, non-respiratory acid-base state, mixed venous blood composition, the inspired gas concentration and the barometric pressure. Kelman (1967) also provides correction factors to be applied to measured blood-gas tensions and pH. These cover temperature differences between the measuring electrodes and the patient and metabolic changes occurring in the sample during the period between sampling and analysis.

REFERENCES

pH topics

Adamsons, K., Daniel, S. S., Gandy, G. and James, L. S. (1964). 'Influence of temperature on blood pH of the human adult and newborn.' *J. appl. Physiol.* **19**, 897

Astrup, P. and Schroder, S. (1956). 'Apparatus for anaerobic determination of the pH of blood at 38 degrees centigrade.' *Scand. J. clin. lab. Invest.* **8**, 30 B

Band, D. M. and Semple, S. J. G. (1967). 'Continuous measurement of blood pH with an indwelling glass electrode.' *J. appl. Physiol.* **22**, 854

Bates, R. G. (1962). 'Revised standard values for pH measurements from 0° to 95°C.' *J. Res. natn. Bur. Stand.* **664,** 179

— and Acree, S. F. (1945). 'pH of aqueous mixtures of potassium dihydrogen phosphate and disodium hydrogen phosphate at 0°C to 60°C.' *J. Res. natn. Bur. Stand.* **34,** 373

— and Covington, A. K. (1968). 'Behaviour of the glass electrode and other pH responsive electrodes in biological media.' *Ann. N.Y. Acad. Sci.* **148.** 67

Burton, G. W. (1965). 'Effects of the acid-base state upon the temperature coefficient of pH of blood.' *Br. J. Anaesth.* **37,** 89

Collis, J. M. and Neaverson, M. A. (1967). 'Arterialized venous blood: a comparison of pH, P_{CO_2}, P_{O_2} and oxygen saturation with that of arterial blood.' *Br. J. Anaesth.* **39,** 883

Cowell, T. K., Band, D. M. and Semple, S. J. G. (1967). 'A fast-response pH meter.' *J. appl. Physiol.* **22,** 858

Dawson, J. B., Ostrander, G. K. and Gray, T. J. (1967). 'New electronics for glass electrodes.' *Med. Electron. biol. Engng.* **5,** 591

Eisenman, G., Mattock, G., Bates, R. and Friedman, S. M. (1966). *The Glass Electrode.* London; Wiley.

Gambino, S. R. (1961). 'Collection of capillary blood for simultaneous determinations of arterial pH, CO_2 content, P_{CO_2} and oxygen saturation.' *Am. J. clin. Path.* **35,** 175

Hill, D. W. (1965). *Principles of Electronics in Medical Research.* London; Butterworths

Khuri, R. N., Agulian, S. K. and Harik, R. I. (1968). 'Internal capillary glass microelectrodes with a glass seal for pH, sodium and potassium.' *Pflügers Arch. ges Physiol.* **301,** 182 B

Miller, J. N., and Tutt, P. (1967). 'A comparison of four blood gas analysis systems in working conditions.' *Bio-med. Engng.* **2,** 456

Nernst, W. (1921). *Theoretische Chemie.* 8th ed. Stuttgart; Enke

Norman, J., Ledsome, J. R. and Linden, R. J. (1965). 'A system for the measurement of respiratory and acid-base parameters in blood.' *Br. J. Anaesth.* **37,** 466

Nunn, J. F. (1962). 'The undressing of pH.' *Lancet.* **1,** 803

Robinson, J. S. (1962). 'pH and P_{CO_2} measurements in blood.' *Br. J. Anaesth.* **34,** 611

Rosenthal, T. B. (1948). 'The effect of temperature on the pH of blood and plasma *in vitro*.' *J. biol. Chem.* **173,** 25, 116, 117 B

Semple, S. J. G. (1961). 'Observed pH differences of blood and plasma with different bridge solutions.' *J. appl. Physiol.* **16,** 576

— Mattock, G. and Uncles, R. (1962). 'A buffer standard for blood pH measurements.' *J. biol. Chem.* **237,** 963, 116, 117 B

CO_2 electrodes

Bartels, H. and Reinhardt, W. (1960). 'Einfache methode zur Sauerstoffdruckmessung im Blut.' *Pflügers Arch. ges. Physiol.* **271,** 105 B

Fatt, I. (1964). 'Rapid-responding carbon dioxide and oxygen electrodes.' *J. appl. Physiol.* **19,** 550

Gambino, S. R. (1961). 'Collection of capillary blood for simultaneous determinations of arterial pH, CO_2 content, P_{CO_2} and oxygen saturation.' *Am. J. clin. Path.* **35,** 175

Gleichmann, U. (1960). 'Fortlaufende Messung des Kohlensauredruckers im arteriellen Blut.' *Pflügers Arch. ges. Physiol.* **272**, 57B

— Lübbers, D. W. (1960). 'Die Messung des Kohlensauredruckers in Gasen und Flüssigkeiten mit der P_{CO_2} Elektrode uniter besonderer Berucksichtigung der Gleichzeitigen Messung von P_{O_2}, P_{CO_2} und pH im Blut.' *Pflügers, Arch. ges Physiol.* **271**, 456 B

Hertz, C. H. and Siesjo, B. (1959). 'A rapid and sensitive electrode for continuous measurement of P_{CO_2} in liquids and tissue.' *Acta physiol. scand.* **47**, 106, 115

Kelman, G. R. (1967). 'Digital computer procedure for the conversion of P_{CO_2} into blood CO_2 content.' *Resp. Physiol. Neth.* **3**, 111

Lunn, J. N. and Mapleson, W. W. (1963). 'The Severinghaus P_{CO_2} electrode: A theoretical and experimental assessment.' *Br. J. Anaesth.* **35**, 666

Nunn, J. F. (1962). 'Measurement of blood oxygen tension: handling of samples.' *Br. J. Anaesth.* **34**, 621

Robinson, J. S. (1962). 'pH and P_{CO_2} measurements in blood.' *Br. J. Anaesth.* **34**, 611

Severinghaus, J. W. (1959). 'Recent developments in blood O_2 and CO_2 electrodes.' In *pH and Blood Gas Electrodes*. Ed. by R. F. Woolmer. London; Churchill

— (1960). 'Methods of measurement of blood and carbon dioxide during anaesthesia.' *Anesthesiology*, **21**, 717 C

— (1962). 'Electrodes for blood and gas P_{CO_2}, CO_2 and blood pH.' *Acta anaesth. scand.* Suppl. **11**, 207C

— Bradley, A. F. (1958). 'Electrodes for blood P_{O_2} and P_{CO_2} determination: *J. appl. Physiol.* **13**, 515

Snell, F. M. (1960). 'Electrometric measurements of CO_2 and bicarbonate ion.' *J. appl. Physiol.* **15**, 729 B

Stow, R. W., Baer, R. F. and Randall, B. F. (1957). 'Rapid measurement of the tension of carbon dioxide.' *Archs phys. Med. Rehabil.* **38**, 646

Oxygen electrodes

Adams, A. P. and Morgan-Hughes, J. O (1967). 'Determination of the blood-gas factor of the oxygen electrode using a new tonometer.' *Br. J. Anaesth.* **39**, 107 C

Bartels, H. (1951). 'Potentiometrische Bestimmung des Sauerstoffdruckes im Vollblut mit der Quecksilbertropfelektrode.' *Pflügers Arch ges. Physiol*, **254**, 107 B

Baumberger, J. P. (1940). 'The accurate determination of haemoglobin, oxyhaemoglobin, and carbon monoxide haemoglobin (or myohaemoglobin) by means of the dropping mercury electrode.' *Am. J. Physiol.* **129**, 109, 308

Beneken Kolmer, H. H. and Kreuzer, F. (1968). 'Continuous polarographic recording of oxygen pressure in respiratory air.' *Resp. Physiol. Neth.* **4**, 109

Bishop, J. M. (1960). 'Measurement of blood oxygen tension.' *Proc. R. Soc. Med.* **53**, 90, 177

Bradley, A. F., Stupfel, M. and Severinghaus, J. W. (1956). 'Effect of temperature on P_{CO_2} and P_{O_2} of blood *in vitro*.' *J. appl. Physiol.* **9**, 201 B

Cater, D. B., Phillips, A. F. and Silver, I. A. (1956). 'Apparatus and techniques for the measurement of oxidation-reduction potentials, pH and oxygen tension *in vivo*.' *Proc. Ry. Soc., B.* **146**, 90 B 289

Cater, D. B. and Silver, I. A. (1961). 'Electrodes and microelectrodes used in biology.' In *Reference Electrodes*. Ed. by D. J. G. Ives and J. G. Janz. New York; Academic Press

Clark, L. C. (1956). 'Monitor and control of blood and tissue oxygen tensions.' *Trans. Am. Soc. artif. Internal Organs.* **2**, 41, 93

— Becattini, F. (1967). 'An inexpensive portable solid-state amplifier for use with the Clark oxygen electrode.' *Ala. Jnl. med. Scis.* **4**, 337

Davies, P. W. and Brink, F. jun. (1942). 'Micro-electrodes for measuring local oxygen tensions in animal tissues.' *Rev. scient. Instrum.* **13**, 524

Dell'Osso, L. F. (1970). 'An iterative method for calculating the effects on blood P_{O_2} of dilution with heparin saline solutions.' *Med. biol. Engng.* **8**, 595

Fatt, I. (1964). 'Rapid responding carbon dioxide and oxygen electrodes.' *J. appl. Physiol.* **19**, 550

Friesen, W. O., and McIlroy, M. B. (1970). 'Rapidly responding oxygen electrode for respiratory gas sampling.' *J. appl. Physiol.* **29**, 258

Ganfield, R. A. and Laughlin, D. E. (1969). 'Plastic f.e.ts. for physiological measurements.' *J. appl. Physiol.* **27**, 141

Gleichmann, U. and Lübbers, D. W. (1960). 'Die Messung des Sauerstoffdruckers in Gasen und Flüssigkeiten mit der Pt-Elektrode unter besonderer Buruchsichtigung der Messung im Blut.' *Pflügers Arch. ges. Physiol.* **271**, 431 B

Hahn, C. E. W. (1969). 'The measurement of oxygen microcathode currents by means of a field-effect transistor operational amplifier system with digital display.' *J. scient. Instrum.* **2**, 48

Hedley-Whyte, J. and Laver, M. B. (1964). 'O_2. Solubility in blood and temperature correction factors for P_{O_2}.' *J. appl. Physiol.* **19**, 901

— Radford, E. P. and Laver, M. B. (1965). 'Nomogram for temperature correction or electrode calibration during P_{O_2}, measurement.' *J. appl. Physiol.* **20**, 785

Heitmann, H., Buckles, R. G. and Laver, M. B. (1967). 'Blood P_{O_2} measurements: performance of microelectrodes.' *Resp. Physiol. Neth.* **3**, 380

Inch, W. R. (1958). 'Problems associated with the use of the exposed platinum electrode for measuring oxygen tensions *in vivo*.' *Can. J. Biochem. Physiol.* **36**, 1009

Johansen, K. and Krog, J. (1959). 'Polarographic determination of intravascular oxygen tensions *in vivo*.' *Acta physiol. scand.* **46**, 106, 228

Kreuzer, F., Harris, E. D. and Nessler, C. G. (1960). 'A method for continuous recording *in vivo* of blood oxygen tension.' *J. appl. Physiol.* **15**, 77

— Watson, T. R. and Ball, J. M. (1958). 'Comparative measurements with a new procedure for measuring the blood oxygen tension *in vitro*.' *J. appl. Physiol.* **12**, 65 B

Laver, M. B. and Seifen, A. (1965). 'Measurement of blood oxygen tension in anaesthesia.' *Anesthesiology*, **26**, 73 C

Linden, R. J., Ledsome, J. R. and Norman, J. (1965). 'Simple methods for the determination of the concentrations of carbon dioxide and oxygen in blood.' *Br. J. Anaesth.* **37**, 77

Lübbers, D. W. (1966). 'Methods of measuring oxygen tensions of blood and organ surfaces.' In *Oxygen Measurements in Blood and Tissues and their Significance*, p. 103. Ed. by J. P. Payne and D. W. Hill, London; Churchill

McConn, R. and Robinson, J. S. (1963). 'Notes on the oxygen electrode.' *Br. J. Anaesth.* **35,** 679

Mapleson, W. W., Horton, J. N., Ng, W. S., and Imrie, D. D. (1970). 'The response pattern of polarographic oxygen electrodes and its influence on linearity and hysteresis.' *Med. biol. Engng.* **8,** 585

Morgan, F., Kettel, L. J. and Cugell, D. W. (1966). 'Measurement of blood Po_2 with microcathode electrode.' *J. appl. Physiol.* **21,** 725

Montgomery, H. (1957). 'Oxygen tension of peripheral tissue.' *Am. J. Med.* **23,** 697

— and Horwitz, O. (1950). 'Oxygen tension of tissues by the polarographic method.' *J. clin. Invest.* **29,** 120

Nunn, J. F. (1962). 'Measurement of blood oxygen tension: handling of samples.' *Br. J. Anaesth.* **34,** 621

— Bergman, N. A., Bunatyan, A. and Coleman, A. J. (1965). 'Temperature coefficients for Pco_2 and Po_2 of blood *in vitro*.' *J. appl. Physiol.* **20,** 23

Parker, D., Key, A., and Davies, R. (1971). 'A disposable catheter-tip transducer for continuous measurement of blood oxygen tension *in vivo*.' *Bio-med. Engng.*, **6,** 313

Polgar, G. and Forster, R. E. (1960). 'Measurement of oxygen tension in unstirred blood with a platinum electrode.' *J. appl. Physiol.* **15,** 706 B

Rhodes, P. G. and Moser, K. M. (1966). 'Sources of error in oxygen tension measurement.' *J. appl. Physiol.* **21,** 729

Schuler, R. and Kreuzer, F. (1967). 'Rapid polarographic *in vivo* oxygen catheter electrodes.' *Resp. Physiol. Neth.* **3,** 90

Silver, I. A. (1966). 'The measurement of oxygen tension in tissues.' In *Oxygen Measurements in Blood and Tissues and their Significance*, p. 135. Ed. by J. P. Payne and D. W. Hill. London: Churchill

Solymar, M., Rucklidge, M. A., and Prys-Roberts, C. (1971). 'A modified approach to the polarographic measurement of blood O_2 content.' *J. appl. Physiol.* **30,** 272

Sproule, B. J., Miller, W. F., Cushing, I. E. and Chapman, C. B. (1957). 'An improved polarographic method for measuring oxygen tension in whole blood.' *J. appl. Physiol.* **11,** 365

Van Slyke, D. D. and Neill, J. M. (1924). 'The determination of gases in blood and other solutions by vacuum extraction and manometric measurement.' *J. biol. Chem.* **61,** 116 B, 523

Walker, A., Phillips, L., Powe, L. and Wood, C. (1968). 'A new instrument for the measurement of tissue Po_2 of human fetal scalp.' *Am. J. Obstet. Gynec.* **100,** 63 B

Weil, J. V., Sodal, I. E. and Speck, R. P. (1967). 'A modified fuel cell for the analysis of oxygen concentration of gases.' *J. appl. Physiol.* **23,** 419

Cation electrodes

Eisenman, G., Rudin, D. O. and Casby, J. U. (1957). 'Glass electrode for measuring sodium ion.' *Science* **126,** 831

Friedman, S. M., Jamieson, J. D., Hinke, J. A. M., and Friedman, C. L. (1959). 'Drug-induced changes in blood pressure and in blood sodium as measured by a glass electrode.' *Am. J. Physiol.* **196,** 1049

Moreton, R. B. (1970). 'Cation selective microelectrodes for intracellular measurements: Rapid hydration by high temperature storage.' *Med. biol. Engng.* **8,** 89

Tonometers

Adams, A. P. and Morgan-Hughes, J. O. (1967). 'Determination of the blood-gas factor of the oxygen electrode using a new tonometer.' *Br. J. Anaesth.* **39,** 107

Fahri, L. E. (1965). 'Continuous duty tonometer system.' *J. appl. Physiol.* **20,** 1098

Kelman, G. R., Coleman, A. J. and Nunn, J. F. (1966). 'Evaluation of a microtonometer used with a capillary glass pH electrode.' *J. appl. Physiol.* **21,** 1103

Laue, D. (1951). 'Eine neues Tonometer zur raschen Aquilibrierung von Blut mit verschieden Gastrucken.' *Pflügers Arch. ges. Physiol.* **254,** 142

Thornton, J. A. and Nunn, J. F. (1960). 'Accuracy of determination of P_{CO_2} by the indirect method.' *Guy's Hosp. Rep.* **18,** B 45 203

Computer programs

Cohen, M. L. (1969). 'A computer program for the interpretation of blood gas analysis.' *Computers biomed. Res.* **2,** 549

Jalowayski, A., Lauterbach, R., Smith, B. E., and Modell, J. H. (1968). 'A computer method for determination of acid-base and oxygenation variables in adult and infant blood samples.' *J. Lab. clin. Med.* **71,** 328

Kelman, G. R. (1967). 'Correction factors to be applied to measured blood gas tensions and pH.' *Bio-med Engng.* **2,** 362

— (1968). 'Computer program for the production of O_2–CO_2 diagrams.' *Resp. Physiol.,* **4,** 260

8 – The Measurement of Cardiac Output by Indicator Dilution Methods and Impedance Measurements

The cardiac output is defined as the quantity of blood pumped by the left ventricle into the aorta per minute. It can be measured directly by placing an electromagnetic or ultrasonic flow probe on the aorta or pulmonary artery in order to measure the stroke volume, and multiplying this by the heart rate. Since this approach requires surgery, the cardiac output in patients is commonly measured by indirect methods. From the viewpoint of electronic equipment, the indicator dilution methods are of particular interest.

PRINCIPLES OF THE INDICATOR DILUTION METHOD

In this technique, a small amount of an indicator substance such as a dye or a radioisotope is injected into a large vein or preferably into the right side of the heart itself. The indicator is passed rapidly through the right heart, the lungs, the left heart and then into the arterial circulation. The appearance of the bolus of indicator in a peripheral artery is detected by means of a suitable recording system. The output of the detection system is displayed on a chart recorder to give the cardiac output curve shown in *Figure 8.1*. The bolus of indicator is injected at the point shown. After the elapse of the appearance time of several seconds the output of the detector rises to a maximum and then falls off. The appearance time corresponds to that required for the fastest particles of indicator to travel to the detector via the shortest route. Before the detector output has time to return to zero a fraction of the indicator injected will have passed through some of the peripheral vessels and returned a second time through the heart. This results in the curve describing a second or re-circulation peak. In order to calculate the cardiac output, the detector output must be calibrated in terms of indicator concentration and the primary peak extrapolated on to the baseline (*Figure 8.1*).

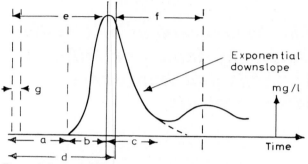

Figure 8.1. Dye dilution curve (a) appearance time; (b) peak concentration time; (c) disappearance time; (d) median circulation time (time to complete one half of the primary curve area); (e) build-up time; (f) recirculation time; (g) duration of injection

Assuming that the primary curve has been continued on to the baseline, the area under the curve is calculated, and the mean concentration of the indicator in the arterial blood determined for the duration of the complete curve. If this is 2·5 mg/l of blood, for example, and the duration of the curve was 10 seconds when 5 mg of indicator had been injected, then the passage of $\dot{Q}.\frac{10}{60}$ litres of blood would be required within 10 seconds to carry the 5 mg of dye, where $\dot{Q}$ is the cardiac output in litres per minute. The cardiac output must then be given by $5 = 2\cdot5 \, . \, \dot{Q}/6$, that is, $\dot{Q} = 12$ litres per minute. It is seen that the cardiac output is given by:

$$\frac{\text{mass of indicator injected (mg)}}{\left(\begin{array}{l}\text{average concentration of indicator in mg} \\ \text{per litre of blood for duration of curve}\end{array}\right) \times \begin{array}{c}\text{curve} \\ \text{duration} \\ \text{in seconds}\end{array}} = \frac{\text{mg}}{\begin{array}{c}\text{area} \\ \text{under} \\ \text{curve}\end{array}}$$

The cardiac output in litres per minute is given by:

$$\frac{\text{mg of dye injected} \times 60}{\text{area under curve in (mg per litre} \times \text{seconds)}}$$

The use of dye dilution methods

A commonly encountered method of estimating cardiac output is based upon the use of a dye as the indicator substance. The dye now usually chosen is indocyanine green (Cardio Green) described by Fox and Wood (1957). This dye has the advantage that it absorbs light in the 800 nm region of the spectrum where both reduced and oxygenated haemoglobin have the same optical absorption. It is thus not necessary to have the patient breathe oxygen while the dye curve is recorded as was necessary with some blue dyes. The dye concentration in blood can thus be measured with the infra-red photocell of a two-wavelength oximeter (Chapter 12), and no compensation is necessary for changes occurring in the haemoglobin opacity. The dye is rapidly cleared from the circulation so that repeated cardiac output determinations are possible, only about 3 per cent remaining in the circulation 20 minutes after injection. It appears to be mainly excreted by the liver in the bile, (Wheeler, Cranston and Miltzer (1958); Cherrick et al (1960). The use of semiconductor photocells has made possible the construction of compact, lightweight dye cuvettes. The cuvette volume can be as small as 0·01 ml. A venous catheter is introduced into the right atrium and a bolus of dye injected from a syringe which may be fitted with electrical contacts in order to produce an injection mark on the chart paper of the dye densitometer. In adults 5 mg of Cardio Green dye per injection is typical in a 1 ml volume. For children the dose is reduced to 2·5 mg. Meanwhile a constant flow rate of blood, typically 0·4 ml/s, from an artery such as the femoral or radial is withdrawn through the cuvette by means of a motor-driven syringe (*Figure 8.2*). The chart recorder attached to the densitometer describes the dye curve, a convenient chart speed being 5 mm

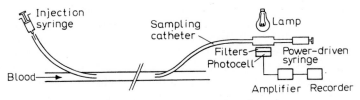

Figure 8.2. Apparatus for recording dye curve

per second. This is the most accurate arrangement, but it is also possible to detect the dye by means of shining a beam of light through the pinna of the ear on to a photocell (Payne, 1960). This method is of use for routine determinations in children. The volume of the bolus of dye is chosen to be smaller than the volume of the oximeter into which it is injected. The bolus is immediately followed with an injection of saline to wash it into the circulation. Some operators do not use a saline flush.

Hamilton (1962) discusses the shape of the dye curve. He prefers to regard the left heart as a simple reservoir and assumes that a volume of blood within it is completely mixed with the dye. During the rising phase of the primary peak of the curve the concentration is built up as more dye enters the heart than leaves, and at the peak, dye is entering and leaving at about the same rate. During the down-slope of the curve very little dye is entering the left heart, and the concentration of dye in the blood leaving the left heart follows a simple exponential form due to the wash-out process. The amount of dye washed out per unit time is thus proportional to the dye concentration present at that time in the left heart reservoir. The prolongation of the exponential curve to cut the time axis will enclose an area describing the time concentration relationships of all the dye on its first passage round the circulation and will not include any of the second circulation. When the dye curve is re-plotted with the dye concentration (Y-axis) on a logarithmic scale and the time (X-axis) on a linear scale the exponential down-slope of the curve becomes a straight line and this is projected downwards to cut the baseline and the area under this curve calculated.

Calculation of the area under the dye curve without recirculation

Once the exponential downslope of the dye curve has been determined using a semi-logarithmic plot and carried on to the baseline the required area under the curve can be measured in arbitrary units by counting squares, or more conveniently by the use of a planimeter. The units required for the area under the curve for use in the cardiac output calculation are mg/litre seconds. Suppose that the recorder connected to the dye densitometer deflects by 50 mm when a cali-bration dye concentration of 6 mg/litre is passed through the cuvette, and that the chart speed is 5 mm per second. If a rectangle of dimensions 50×25 mm is drawn on the chart close to the dye curve, then this area is equivalent to 30 mg/litre seconds. By running the planimeter around this area a calibration factor is found to convert the planimeter reading for the dye curve into mg/litre seconds. When the dye curve area in these units is divided by the time in seconds from the start to the finish of the curve without circulation, the result will be the mean concentration of dye in mg/litre. An approximation, to the area under the curve can be obtained by summing the dye concentrations occurring at one second intervals from the start to the finish of the curve, Payne (1960).

A number of alternative methods can be used, particularly when a digital computer is available. Shubin, Weil and Rockwell (1967) note the times at which the dye curve has fallen to 70 per cent and 40 per cent of the peak concentration. Let these times be T_{70} and T_{40} respectively, while T_0 is the time at which the dye curve starts to rise. The area required under the whole curve is given by

$$\int_{T_0}^{\infty} Cdt = \int_{T_0}^{T_{70}} Cdt + \int_{T_{70}}^{T_{40}} Cdt + \int_{T_{40}}^{\infty} Cdt$$

where C is the dye concentration at time t. Shubin and his colleagues show that

$$\int_{T_{70}}^{\infty} Cdt = 2 \cdot 3 \int_{T_{70}}^{T_{40}} Cdt$$

The areas under the curve from T_0 to T_{70} and from T_{70} to T_{40} are calculated by the computer using the well-known trapezium rule of numerical analysis. That is to say, by dividing the areas up into a large number of rectangular strips and then summing the areas of the strips. The area found from T_{70} to T_{40} is multiplied by $2 \cdot 3$ and added to the area found from T_0 to T_{70} to yield the area under the whole curve.

It can also be shown that the area under the curve from the time T_{peak} at which the peak concentration occurs is given by

$$\int_{T_{\text{peak}}}^{\infty} Cdt = \tau C_{\text{peak}}$$ where C_{peak} is the peak concentration and τ is the time constant of the exponential downslope of the dye curve. The time constant is determined as the time taken for the curve to fall from 90 per cent of the peak value to $33 \cdot 3$ per cent of the peak value. The area $\int_{T_0}^{T_{\text{peak}}} Cdt$ is found as before by summing strip areas and τC_{peak} added to it.

Warner and Wood (1952) approximate the raw dye curve by a triangle the apex of which coincides with the point of the peak dye concentration. The sides of the triangle are respectively a line drawn between the apex and the start of the upslope of the curve, the baseline and a line drawn from the apex closely following the downslope before recirculation and produced to meet the baseline. The area under the dye curve without recirculation is then taken to be equal to $1 \cdot 324$ times the area of the triangle. Kelman (1966) has found that this triangular approximation consistently overestimated the area under the dye curve. Dow (1955) derives the empirical formula $A = PC \cdot PCT/(3 \cdot 0 - 0 \cdot 9PCT/AT)$ where A is the area under the dye curve, PC is the peak concentration, PCT is the time interval from the injection of the dye to the peak concentration, and AT is the time interval from the injection to the start of the rise of the curve. Thorburn (1961) discusses the use of the forward part of the dye curve to derive the area under the whole curve. He obtained a good measure of agreement with Dow's method.

Calibration of the dye densitometer

The concentration axis of the dye curve can be calibrated by making up a series of standard dye concentrations in blood and drawing them through the cuvette. The zero adjustment of the densitometer and recorder is first set using a 10-ml sample of the patient's blood to which has been added 0·4 ml of distilled water. Cardio Green is supplied at a concentration of 5 mg/100 ml. One millilitre of this stock solution is added to 7 ml of distilled water to produce a concentration of 0·625 mg/ml. This is dilution A; 4 ml of A is then diluted with a further 4 ml of water to give dilution B (0·312 mg/ml); 4 ml of B is added to 4 ml of water giving dilution C (0·156 mg/ml). In a similar fashion dilutions D (0·078 mg/ml) and E (0·039 mg/ml) are prepared. Adding 0·2 ml of A to 5 ml of blood gives a calibration concentration of 24·05 mg/litre. Using the other dilutions with 5 ml aliquots of blood gives concentrations of 12·025 mg/l, 6·0125 mg/l, 3·000 mg/l and 1·500 mg/l. A total of 35 ml of blood is used. This method can require more blood than can be spared from an animal. An alternative approach is to use a micro-syringe to inject a known volume of dye solution into a flowing stream of water which is pulled through a U-tube containing glass beads to act as a mixing chamber, the effluent from the chamber being drawn through the cuvette. This dynamic method is described by Emanuel et al (1966). Cardiac output can then be calculated from the formula:

$$\dot{Q}_b = \frac{A_c \times i \times Q_c}{i_c \times A}$$

where $\dot{Q}_b$ is the cardiac output in litres per minute

$\dot{Q}_c$ is the volume flow rate through the densitometer cuvette in litres per minute

A is the area (mg per litre × seconds) contained by the primary dye curve of the patient

i is the volume of dye solution injected into the patient

i_c is the volume of the same dye solution injected into the mixer during the calibration

A_c is the area under the calibration dye curve (mg per litre × seconds)

CARDIAC OUTPUT COMPUTERS

The calculation of the area under the dye curve without re-circulation becomes tedious if there are a number of determinations to be made. For this reason there are now available a number of special-purpose analogue computers designed to give a meter or recorder reading directly in terms of cardiac output, and digital computer programs to calculate cardiac output.

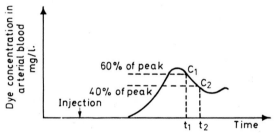

Figure 8.3. Dye curve concentrations used by analogue computer

The theory of the Sanborn Model 130 analogue cardiac output computer (Uhrenholdt, 1967) will be given to indicate an analogue approach. Referring to *Figure 8.3*, let C_1 and C_2 be the dye concentrations at times t_1 and t_2 on the exponential down-slope of the dye curve. The area under the curve from $t=t_1$ to $t=\infty$, is given by:

$$\int_0^\infty C_1\exp(-kt)=\frac{+1}{k}\cdot C_1\exp(-kt_1)=C_1/K=\text{area }(D+E)$$

where k and K are constants

Similarly, the area under the curve from $t=t_2$ to $t=\infty$ is equal to

$$\int_0^\infty C_2\exp(-kt)=\frac{+1}{k}\cdot C_2\exp(-kt_2)=C_2/K=\text{area }E$$

Let the dye concentrations C_1 and C_2 be in the ratio $x : 1$, that is $C_1 = xC_2$ then area $E = C_1 K/x$

$$\text{Area } D = C_1/K - C_1/Kx = C_1 \frac{x-1}{Kx}$$

$$\text{so that area } (D+E) = \frac{(x-1)}{x} \text{ area } D$$

The procedure used by the analogue computer for determining the total area A under the dye curve without re-circulation is as follows. The computer first integrates the dye concentration (proportional to the densitometer output voltage) with respect to time from $t=0$ to $t=t_1$. This gives the area B. The integration sensitivity is then multiplied by a factor $(x-1)/x$ and integration continued at the enhanced rate for the time interval (t_2-t_1). At $t=t_2$, the total output from the integrator is proportional to the wanted area A. In the Sanborn Model 130 cardiac output computer C_1 is taken as 60 per cent of the peak value and C_2 as 40 per cent of the peak. Thus $C_2 = \frac{2}{3}C_1$ giving $(x-1)/x = 3$. Area $A = (B+D+E) = (B+3D)$. The circuitry automatically increases the rate of integration three-fold from $t=t_1$ to $t=t_2$. At $t=t_1$ the computer generates a voltage equal to C_1/x, and compares this continuously with the diminishing voltage proportional to C, at the same time integrating at the faster rate. When the voltage proportional to C becomes equal to the pre-set value of C_1/x integration is stopped. The total output from the integrator is displayed and this must be multiplied by a factor in order to convert it to cardiac output.

ESTIMATION OF BEAT-BY-BEAT CHANGES IN STROKE VOLUME

In clinical practice, when frequent determinations of cardiac output and stroke volume are required, the use of indicator dilution methods becomes time consuming and impractical. Warner *et al* (1953) describe a method based upon the measurement of central aortic pressure. The relationship used is $SV = k \cdot P_{md}(1+S_a/D_a)$ where SV is the stroke volume of the heart, k is a constant, S_a is the systolic pressure area (the mean pressure that acts at the periphery of the arterial bed during systole multiplied by the duration of systole), D_a is the diastolic pressure area (the mean pressure at the periphery during diastole multiplied by the duration of diastole), U is the total volume of blood in all arteries extending from the aortic arch to the arterioles at the end of systole minus the volume of this arterial bed at the end of the previous diastole. Since no blood enters the aorta from the left ventricle during diastole, the diastolic drainage is equal to this increment in the volume of the arterial bed which is present at the end of systole. The corresponding increment in mean pressure between the end of diastole and the end of systole multiplied by a constant of proportionality is equal to the increment in volume. Thus, $P_{md} \times k = U$. In order to estimate P_{md} from the central arterial pulse pressure, the time of transmission of the pulse wave from the aorta to the periphery of the arterial tree must be taken into account. Since it is impossible to measure this time of transmission to each point at the periphery of the arterial bed, it is calculated by multiplying the time of transmission between two recording points such as aorta to femoral artery or brachial to radial arteries by a constant c which is chosen to give a reasonably acceptable resting, supine value for the mean time of transmission (100 to 110 milliseconds). The ratio S_a/D_a and the value for P_{md} can be measured directly from the central pressure pulse. The constant k relating change in pressure to change in volume is found from a measurement of cardiac output with a dye-dilution technique, and U calculated, together with a mean value for k using the mean of the values for P_{md} from the pressure pulses during the dye curve and the value of U. Then stroke volume can be found for any beat using the measured ratio of S_a/D_a for that beat.

The method of Warner *et al* (1953) depends upon a determination of the position of the dichrotic notch and this may be difficult in the case of patients in shock.

Pulse contour methods for following stroke volume changes

In patient monitoring schemes there is a requirement to be able to follow stroke volume changes on a beat-by-beat basis. The electrical impedance technique offers one possibility of doing this and digital computer programs have been written to calculate the stroke volume from the impedance waveform in real time. However, few centres have as yet the necessary equipment. It is much more likely that an arterial pressure recording will be available and many workers have investigated the possibility of obtaining an index of the stroke volume from the pulse contour. The simplest approximation is to correlate the pulse pressure (systolic-diastolic) with the stroke volume. Herd, Leclair and Simon (1966) found that the difference (mean pressure-end diastolic pressure) measured in the ascending aorta of dogs gave a useful index of stroke volume over the range 50–150 per cent of the control cardiac output. A calibration constant is obtained by running a dye curve. The scatter of the data points was about twice as much if the femoral artery (mean-end diastolic) pressure was used. Significantly greater scatter was obtained in the relationship between stroke volume and pulse pressure measured either in the ascending aorta or femoral artery. A more complicated approximation can be obtained from a knowledge of the volume-pressure relationships for the various parts of the aortic system and deriving a cardiac ejection curve which satisfies the contour of the aortic pressure pulse. The stroke volume is given by $SV = U + SD$ where U is the arterial uptake and SD the systolic drainage. The methodology is discussed by Opdyke (1952).

A number of analogue and digital computer systems now exist for detecting arrhythmias in the ECG on the basis of detecting departures from a dominant rhythm, ventricular extrasystoles being distinguished on the basis of a broadened QRS complex (Bushman, 1967; Horth, 1969). Such an arrangement can be run in parallel with the stroke volume monitoring to check on abnormal stroke volumes.

THE USE OF A RADIOACTIVE INDICATOR

Veall and Vetter (1958) describe in detail the use of radio-iodinated human serum albumin (RISA) labelled with iodine-131. The concentration of radio-iodine required is set by the volume injected and the sensitivity of the recording equipment. A concentration of 50 μc per ml is usually adequate. The protein concentration needs to be about 2 per cent v/v in order to avoid errors arising from adsorption on the glassware.

The radioactivity detection system consists of a scintillation counter fitted with a two inch diameter crystal of thallium-activated sodium iodide. Veall and Vetter mention that in order to obtain reasonably accurate values for the cardiac output the counter should be preceded by an efficient collimator. This requires the use of a larger dose of radioactivity and makes the positioning of the counter critical if it is also to be used for the determination of the pulmonary circulation time. For these reasons, Veall and Vetter recommend the use of a collimator having a cylindrical aperture 2·5 cm in diameter by 5 cm deep. The complete counter assembly is mounted in a counterbalanced stand so that it can be conveniently positioned over the heart of a supine patient. The scintillation counter is connected via a low-capacity coaxial cable, which also carries the e.h.t. supply, to a pulse amplifier and discriminator and then to a linear ratemeter. This should have a range covering about 1,000 counts per second, full scale. A time constant of 0·5 second is needed during recording, with provision for increasing this to cover 5 to 20 seconds for use during the calibration procedure. The provision of a 'backing-off' control for the zero setting is required to enable the residual counts from previous injections to be offset during the taking of serial cardiac output measurements. The ratemeter feeds either a potentiometric or moving-coil recorder having a speed of response of at least 0·5 second for full scale deflection with a chart speed of 5 mm per second.

It is first necessary to prepare a standard solution for calibration purposes of 5 ml of an approximately 1 : 1000 or 1 : 1500 dilution of the radioactive protein solution to be injected. The value of the dilution needs to be known accurately and this can be found by injecting a known weight of solution into, say, a one litre volume of water. A 5 ml syringe-full of the dilutant is actively counted by placing it in a jig a suitable distance from the face of the scintillation counter. It is usually possible to adjust the response of the scintillation counter in terms of count rate by altering either the setting of the pulse height analyser or discriminator circuit or the value of the e.h.t. voltage applied to the counter. Before giving the injection, it is first necessary to check that the recorded curve will not exceed the full scale deflection of the recorder. For this purpose, the standard solution is placed in the aperture of the collimator with the counter inverted and the adjustments made to produce about 75 per cent of full scale deflection. In order to be able to extract the maximum amount of information from the dilution curve, it is desirable that it be double peaked (*Figure 8.4*) so that the collimator should be located in the region of the apex and directed to view both halves of the heart. With the ratemeter time constant set at 0·4 seconds, an accurately known volume of the labelled albumin solution–approximately 1 ml (10 micro-curies)—is injected smoothly and as rapidly as possible into an arm vein and a timing mark made on the recorder chart. After allowing 5 to 10 minutes to elapse in order to obtain a uniformly mixed blood level, a record is obtained on the chart of the equilibrium count rate with the ratemeter switched to a longer time constant (10 seconds), and simultaneously with the reading a 5 ml blood sample is obtained. In the case of some cardiac patients, for example, with mitral valve incompetence or a low cardiac output, a greater length of time will have to be allowed for mixing to occur. The activity of the sample is determined by counting it in the jig used for the standard solution. The haemotocrit of the sample

267

is also measured and corrected for trapped plasma as described by Chaplin and Mollinson (1952).

In order to reduce the uptake of the radio-iodine by the thyroid gland, potassium iodide may be administered orally. Uhrenholdt (1968) administered 750 mg of potassium iodide orally before and then four days after the radio-cardiogram, for which the injected dose was 45–55 μCi of ^{131}I RISA.

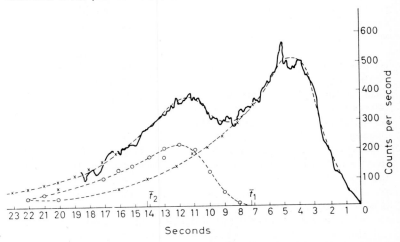

Figure 8.4. Double-peaked cardiac output curve obtained by external scintillation counting of ^{131}I labelled human serum albumin passing through the right and left heart

Let V = volume of RISA injected in ml

D = dilution of the injectate to produce the standard solution

S = activity of standard in counts per minute per 5 ml

Then the counts per minute per ml of ^{131}I injected = $V . D . \dfrac{S.}{5}$

Let E = activity in counts per minute over the heart at the time of drawing the blood sample

B = activity of blood sample in counts per minute per 5 ml.

To calculate the area under the whole dilution curve define a known area bounded by a rectangle with sides of X seconds and Y counts per second over the heart.

This area $A = (X \cdot Y) \times 60 \times 200 \times B/E$. The factor 200 converts from the blood sample volume of 5 ml to litres and the factor 60 converts from seconds to minutes. By planimetry it is determined that the area under the dilution curve$=f\times A$. For a particular patient (*Figure 8.4*) the following values were found: $V=0\cdot582$ ml, $D=873$, $S=14\cdot149$, $E=7646$, $B=1420$, $X=5$ seconds, $Y=400$ counts per second, $f=3\cdot03$.

Cardiac output in litres per minute$=\dfrac{(V\times D\times S/5)\times 60}{f\times X\times Y\times 60\times 200\times B/E}$

The injected dose $(v\times D\times S/5)=0\cdot582\times873\times14149/5=14\cdot3\times10^5$
Area under curve$=3\cdot03\times240\times10^5\times1420/7646=135\times10^5$
Cardiac output$=14\cdot3\times60/135=6\cdot4$ litres per minute.

The analysis of double peaked radiocardiograms

In the calculation of the cardiac output from a radiocardiogram, it is necessary to use the total area under the curve, that is under both peaks if two peaks are present. Depending on the shape and position of the collimator used only a single peak may be found. The boundary of the area is given by the projection of the exponential downslope of the single peak or of the left heart peak if two are present, to cut the baseline at 1 per cent of the initial peak activity. In the case of a double peaked curve, it is necessary to use the total area under the curve, since the height of the final equilibrium plateau is derived from activity emanating from both the right and left halves of the heart (Shipley *et al.*, 1953).

The contribution of the right heart curve to the total area is found by extrapolating the exponential down slope of the right heart curve to cut the time axis at a point corresponding with 1 per cent of the peak concentration (*Figure 8.4*). Subtracting the amplitudes of the right heart curve from that of the total curve yields the separate peak due to the left heart only. For both the right and left heart curves, the mean transit time $\bar{t}$ is calculated from the formula $\bar{t}=\Sigma C_n t_n \mathrm{d}t/\Sigma C_n \mathrm{d}t$ where C_n is the activity in counts per minute per litre of blood at time t_n (Hamilton *et al.*, 1932; Zierler *et al.*, 1962). If $\bar{t}_L$ and $\bar{t}_R$ are the time intervals corresponding with the mean transit times for the right and left heart curves, then $(\bar{t}_L—\bar{t}_R)$ is the central mean transit time or CMTT. The central blood volume (CBV) is given by the product of the cardiac output and the CMTT (Gott *et al.*, 1961; Johnson *et al.*, 1964). When a clear dip occurs between the two peaks of the radiocardiogram, this is likely to coincide with the peak of radioactivity in the lungs. More accurately, a second isotope (^{125}I) can be used in conjunction with a second scintillation counter to obtain a lung activity curve (Johnson *et al.*, 1964). On this basis, the CMTT can now be divided into arterial (right heart peak-to-lung peak) and venous (lung peak-to-left heart peak) portions. In patients with severe heart disease whose radiocardiograms are flattened in appearance, this approach will not be possible unless a separate lung activity curve is available. The ratio A/H (Shipley *et al.*, 1953) should also be calculated. H is the activity expressed in terms of counts per minute per litre of blood corresponding with the equilibrium plateau of the radiocardiogram, and A is the total area under the radiocardiogram in counts per minute per litre of blood × seconds. Both the cardiac output and the central blood volume should also be normalized on the basis of the patient's body surface area. Another useful parameter is the ratio $CMTT/\dot{Q}$. For patients with normal hearts this would be less than unity (Johnson *et al.*, 1964).

For each radiocardiogram, the build-up time (from the start of the rise of the curve to the time of the peak) was noted for the right heart peak. With this information, it is possible to perform a compartmental analysis on the curve (Valentinuzzi *et al.*, 1971, 1972). In this technique, the circulation lying between the sites of injection and detection of the indicator is assumed to consist of N identical compartments connected in series. Each is taken to have the same time constant and to be perfused with the same volume flow. The usual Stewart-Hamilton formula for cardiac output in litres per minute is $\dot{Q} = m \times 60/A$, where m is the activity injected in the case of a radiocardiogram and A is the area under the curve. This can be adapted to read $\dot{Q} = \dfrac{m \times 60 \times \alpha}{C_p \times t_p}$ where C_p is the peak activity and t_p is the build-up time for that peak. The constant α is related to the number of compartments assumed to lie between the sites of injection and detection. *Figure 8.5* shows the relationship between N and α_N. Thus, knowing the cardiac output, it is possible to determine α_N and hence N. It should be mentioned that the value of alpha corresponding with $N=1$ was extrapolated by iteration based upon the use of successive ratios of the values of α_N and also on the assumption that these ratios tend towards a constant value. The expression for calculating α_N is

$$N = \frac{1}{(N-2)!} (N-1)^{(N-1)} \exp[-(N-1)]$$

Since this expression only has meaning for integer values of N, adjacent points were joined by straight lines in order to allow for interpolation. A similar procedure should be adopted for the left heart curve, but now the build-up time for the left heart peak is taken as $(t_{pL}-\text{CMTT})$, the time of occurrence of the left heart peak now being found from the left heart curve and not the total curve.

If a two-channel recorder is available, one channel should be used to display the radiocardiogram, and the other to give an indication of the patient's heart rate as obtained from a photo-electric peripheral

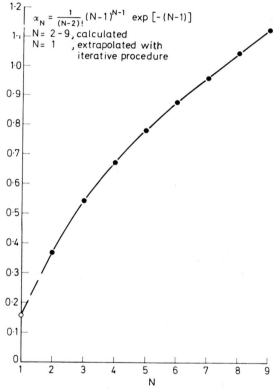

$$\alpha_N = \frac{1}{(N-2)!}(N-1)^{N-1}\,\exp\left[-(N-1)\right]$$

N = 2 - 9, calculated
N = 1 , extrapolated with iterative procedure

Figure 8.5. The relationship between αN and N for the compartmental model of the heart

pulse transducer attached to a thumb or finger. Alternatively, if the recorder is suitable, the patient's ECG should be recorded on the second channel. From a knowledge of the time of occurrence of each contraction of the heart, it is possible to be more precise in defining the volume of the pulmonary circulation rather than just the central blood volume. The CBV includes contributions from both the right and left heart as well as the lungs. With an exponential downslope to the radiocardiogram, a constant proportion of the end-diastolic volume is expelled per stroke. Donato *et al.* (1962) and Lewis *et al.* (1962) have shown how it is possible to calculate from the radiocardiogram the pulmonary blood volume, the right ventricular volume and the right ventricular rate of emptying.

For the patient whose radiocardiogram is shown in *Figure 8.4*, $Q=6\cdot4$ litres per minute, $t_{pR}=5\cdot4$ seconds, $C_{pR}=11\cdot3\times10^5$ and $m=14\cdot3\times10^5$ so that alpha for the right heart peak$=0\cdot45$ corresponding with $N=2\cdot45$ compartments. $t_R=7\cdot2$ seconds and $t_L=14\cdot1$ seconds so that CMTT$=6\cdot9$ seconds. $t_{pL}=11\cdot2$ seconds, and $C_{pL}=8\cdot3\times10^5$ so that alpha for the left heart peak$=0\cdot265$ corresponding to $1\cdot5$ compartments. The central blood volume$=6370\times6\cdot9/60=735$ ml (Hill *et al.*, 1972).

Hobbs (1965) discusses the use of serum albumin labelled with either [121]I or ^{131}I for cardiac output estimations.

Uhrenholdt (1968) has compared the radioactive tracer method with the indocyanine green dye dilution method in 18 patients. He used 45–55 μc of ^{131}I-labelled human serum albumin. The scintillation counter was positioned over the 4th or 5th intercostal space, 3 to 4 cm to the left of the sternal border where the apex beat was most pronounced. The cylindrical sodium iodide crystal 52 mm × 52 mm had a well 22 mm in diameter and 39 mm deep. It was used with a conical collimator (Hallberg and Veall, 1962). Comparisons were made between the two techniques only if the pulse rates agreed within ±4 beats/minute and the mean blood pressures within ±5 mmHg. From 29 simultaneous comparisons it was found that the radio-isotope cardiac output values were always higher than the dye dilution values (mean difference 18·3 per cent, range$+6\cdot6$ to $+35\cdot2$ per cent). The magnitude of the systematic difference between the two methods depends upon the collimator design, counting geometry and the site of the indicator injection. With a conscious patient it is desirable to precede the actual isotope determination with one or two dummy injections of heparinized saline in order to make the patient relax, as lying under the counter may make him feel apprehensive and raise the cardiac output.

Only three to four injections of 50 μc ^{131}I can be made per week without exceeding the permissible dose of 0·3 rads. The number of possible injections can be increased by the use of shorter-lived isotopes such as ^{125}I or [99m]Tc.

With all types of indicator dilution techniques it is difficult to get an answer with patients in shock.

THE THERMAL DILUTION TECHNIQUE FOR THE ESTIMATION OF CARDIAC OUTPUT

It is possible to estimate cardiac output from a dilution curve resulting from the injection of a bolus of 'coolth' (cold indicator). Lowe (1968) shows that when a bolus of cooled indocyanine green dye is injected the area under the dye and thermal dilution curves are not significantly different. The dye was injected into the right atrium and both temperature and dye concentration recorded in the aorta. However, the dye curve reaches its peak earlier and its down-slope is steeper than the thermal dilution curve. These effects arise from the fact that the thermal indicator does leave the circulation and is initially distributed in an unknown proportion to the walls of the heart, blood vessels and lung parenchyma. It is returned from these structures to the blood when the temperature gradient becomes reversed as blood at normal temperatures passes again. Lowe states that an insignificant proportion of the cool indicator is lost outside the body during the first circulation. According to him the major problem in the measurement of cardiac output using coolth arises from the uncertainty of just how much of the injection takes part in the dilution curve. As much as 50 per cent can be lost to the atrial catheter and to the blood outside it. In order to reduce the fraction lost to less than 2 per cent, a high speed injection is made through a catheter which has a low thermal capacity and thermal conductivity and small dead space. Lowe recommends for use in man a concentric tube catheter with an air space separating the two polythene tubes. If the inner tube has a 1-mm internal diameter, 10 ml of cool saline can be injected by hand through the 40-cm catheter in less than 2 seconds.

One advantage of the thermal dilution technique lies in the fact that there is no recirculation peak. This follows since the cool saline warms up to within 0·015°C of the blood temperature while it passes through the peripheral circulation. Five to ten cardiac output measurements are possible, and thirty to forty injections of cold saline can be given to a patient which would be impossible using dye.

In one technique, cooled saline solution is injected via a special catheter into the right ventricle. A thin-walled catheter 80 cm long with a closed tip and six side-openings is suitable for adults, the internal diameter being 2·24 mm and the external diameter 3·33 mm. The side openings ensure almost complete mixing of the cool saline with the blood. With this type of catheter the temperature at the catheter tip is virtually independent of the volume of saline injected.

273

The cool saline is detected by means of a sensitive thermistor placed at the tip of a catheter introduced into the pulmonary artery. In order to warm up that part of the catheter outside the body to body temperature, blood is drawn through the catheter for 4 seconds. The saline at a temperature of 0·5°C is injected as quickly as possible. A volume of 4 ml is usual for normal hearts and 8 ml for greatly dilated hearts. After injection, 4 ml of blood is drawn through the catheter to re-warm it. After the cooled blood has resumed body temperature (5 to 8 seconds) a further injection can be given.

The measuring thermistor would have a resistance of about 1100 Ω at 37°C. Its resistance changes by about 30 ohms/degC. It is used in a Wheatstone bridge arrangement followed by a d.c. amplifier and recorder. The normal chart speed is 10 mm/second. A typical calibration of the recorder would be 0·1degC for 1 cm change in deflection from body temperature.

The cardiac output is given by:

$$\text{Cardiac output} = \frac{V(t_1 - t_2) \cdot \rho_1 s_1 60}{A.K_1.S.\rho_2 s_2}$$

where V is the volume of injected cool saline

t_1 is the temperature of blood in the pulmonary artery measured from the recorder temperature

t_2 is the temperature of saline solution at tip of injection catheter. (7·4°C for Lehman No. 10 catheter and saline volumes of 4–13 ml with a body temperature of 37°C)

ρ_1 is the density of saline solution (1·005 g/ml)

ρ_2 is the density of blood (g/ml)

s_1 is the specific heat of saline solution (0·997 cal/g)

s_2 is the specific heat of blood (cal/g)

A is the area under curve in mm²

K is the temperature calibration of recorder (degC/mm)

S is the chart speed (mm/s)

TABLE 8.1

THE DEPENDENCE OF THE SPECIFIC HEAT AND VISCOSITY OF HUMAN BLOOD UPON THE HAEMATOCRIT

Haematocrit %	Specific heat cal/g	Density of blood g/ml
30	0·89	1·049
35	0·88	1·053
40	0·87	1·058
45	0·865	1·061
50	0·86	1·064
55	0·85	1·068
60	0·84	1·073

Wilson *et al.* (1972) give a critical account of the factors affecting the quantification of the thermal dilution method for cardiac output with particular reference to its use for multiple serial determinations over prolonged periods. Roberts (1969) describes an analogue computer for use with thermal dilution flow measurements.

MEASUREMENT OF CARDIAC OUTPUT BY AN ELECTRICAL IMPEDANCE TECHNIQUE

The indirect measurement of respiratory volumes from observations in the changes of trans-thoracic impedance accompanying respiration is by now well established. The technique has been extended to the indirect measurement of cardiac output by Kubicek *et al* (1966). Four electrodes (2 current and 2 voltage) are applied to the subject as in *Figure 8.6*. The potential changes on the surface of the thorax produced by modifications in the current density distribution

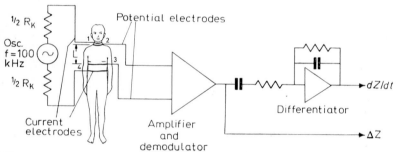

Figure 8.6. *Four-terminal system for indirect measurement by electrical impedance of cardiac output (after L. E. Baker)*

associated with cardiac activity are picked up by electrodes 2 and 3 and recorded as impedance changes. A typical recording is given in *Figure 8.7*. It is apparent that the impedance changes are similar in form to arterial volume changes. They correspond well with the aortic pressure waveform. The method employed by Kubicek to calculate the cardiac output is based upon the formula for resistivity $p = \dfrac{RA}{L}$ or $R = \dfrac{pL}{A}$ where R is the resistance in ohms of a specimen of resistivity p ohm-cm having a length of L cm and cross-section of A cm².

$$R = \frac{pL}{A} = \frac{pl}{L} \cdot \frac{L}{L} = \frac{pL^2}{AL}$$

275

but $AL=V$ the volume of a cylinder if the volume considered is that of a cylindrical conductor of homogeneous material and uniform current density distribution.

Differentiating R with respect to V,

$$\mathrm{d}R/\mathrm{d}V = -pL^2/V^2 \text{ or } \mathrm{d}R = -p(L^2/V^2)\mathrm{d}V$$

Since $R=pL^2/V$, then

$V=pL^2/R$, giving $\mathrm{d}R = -pR^2 = -p(R^2/L^2)dV$ and $\mathrm{d}V = -p(L^2/R^2)\mathrm{d}R$

For a given cylinder of material, $p(L^2/R^2)$ is a constant$=k$, $\mathrm{d}V=k\mathrm{d}R$. Hence the change in volume is directly proportional to the change in resistance. In the general case, the magnitude of the impedance Z is substituted for R, so that $\mathrm{d}V = -p(L^2/Z^2)\mathrm{d}Z$

When this expression is used to calculate the cardiac output, the following substitutions are made:

$\mathrm{d}V$ is the ventricular stroke volume in cc.

p is normally taken as 150 ohm-cm. This is the resistivity of human blood at body temperature and having a normal haematocrit. More detailed values are:

Haematocrit %	Resistivity at 37·5°C
20	110
30	120
35	133
40	148
45	164
50	195
55	230
60	275

Baker *et al.* (1971) found that there was no significant difference between the use of $p=150$ and the values found for the subjects concerned.

L is the length in cm between the two potential electrodes (2 and 3 in *Figure 8.6*).

Z is the value in ohms of the impedance existing between the potential electrodes immediately prior to the rapid decrease of the impedance accompanying ventricular systole.

$\mathrm{d}Z$ is the total change in impedance in ohms associated with the stroke volume.

The specification for $\mathrm{d}Z$ is of importance in this technique. Since the impedance changes have been shown for peripheral arteries (Nyboer 1959) to be similar to blood volume changes, the observed $\mathrm{d}Z$ must reflect a change in blood volume. If the amplitude of $\mathrm{d}Z$

represents blood volume changes in the thorax, these changes correspond to the difference in blood flow into and out of the thorax. It is assumed that upon contraction of the ventricles and the opening of the aortic and pulmonic valves, blood is ejected so rapidly from the heart that the rate of ejection is established before a significant degree of arterial run-off has occurred, that is, loss of blood from the thorax by way of the arterial system, then multiplication of the initial rate of change of impedance by the time

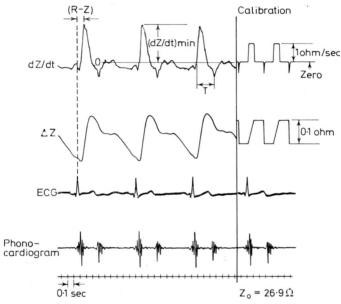

Figure 8.7. The use of the second heart sound to locate the end of ventricular ejection in the calculation of stroke volume by the electrical impedance method

intervals during which the two output valves are open might represent the impedance change which would have been reached had arterial run-off not occurred and would therefore be related to the stroke volume. The maximum rate of impedance change (dZ/dt max) is located by differentiating the impedance waveform and displaying the differential on one channel of the recorder, as in *Figure 8.7*. The maximum rate of change in ohms/second is multiplied by a time interval of 't' seconds derived from the dZ waveform,

(*Figure 8.7*). The formula for the stroke volume now reads $dV = (-pL^2/Z^2).t.\ (dZ/dt)_{max}$. During systole, the thoracic impedance decreases; hence $(dZ/dt)_{max}$ has a negative value, thus making the stroke volume dV positive. The time interval t represents the ejection time. In the original method of Kubicek *et al.* (1966) the start of t is found by projecting a vertical line from the baseline up to the peak of the dZ/dt waveform. At 15 per cent of the height of the peak up from the baseline, a horizontal line is projected to the left to intercept the dZ/dt waveform. The value of 15 per cent was chosen with computer processing in mind for the start of ejection in order to overlook the slow decrease in impedance observed with some individuals at the start of systole. The end of the interval t is determined by the abrupt change in the dZ/dt waveform corresponding with the dichrotic notch in the impedance waveform. This procedure is somewhat arbitrary, but it does provide definite, easy-to-locate, end-points for the time interval.

The dZ waveform can be markedly affected by respiration and it is simpler to use the dZ/dt waveform. The start of t can be taken from when the dZ/dt waveform crosses the $dZ/dt = 0$ baseline to the abrupt change previously described in the dZ/dt waveform. This abrupt change may not always be present. Because of this, it is extremely useful to have available a phonocardiogram. The interval t can then be taken as the interval between the first and second heart sounds (*Figure 8.7*). Using a four channel recorder, the author prefers to record the arterial blood pressure, the ECG (picked up from electrodes 1 and 4), dZ/dt, and the phonocardiogram. From a knowledge of the mean arterial pressure and the cardiac output, the left ventricular stroke work and the total peripheral resistance can be calculated using the nomogram of Mostert *et al.* (1969). Siegal *et al.* (1970) have shown that the inverse of the time interval between the peak of the preceding R-wave of the ECG and $(dZ/dt)_{max}$ gives an estimate of myocardial contractility related to the isometric time-tension index. Changes in myocardial contractility are of interest in assessing the effects of various anaesthetic agents so that recording the ECG together with dZ/dt is valuable.

Because of the shorter time constant involved it is often possible to measure $(dZ/dt)_{max}$ if spontaneous or intermittent positive pressure respiration is not very vigorous. For the best reproducibility it is usual to record $(dZ/dt)_{max}$ close to the end of an expiration. If the patient is conscious and exercising vigorously, as on a treadmill, he should be asked to hold his breath for perhaps five heart beats whilst a cardiac output measurement is taken. If he is unconscious and making excessive respiratory efforts then the anaesthetist can temporarily stop his breathing by vigorously squeezing the re-breathing bag to reduce the patient's arterial carbon dioxide tension and render him apnoeic for a short while. If the patient is connected to an automatic lung ventilator, then this can be turned off for about one minute.

A practical account of the use of the electrical impedance method to measure cardiac output is that of Baker et al. (1971).

Accuracy of cardiac output determinations by the impedance method

Kubicek et al (1966) have carried out a careful evaluation of the impedance method in healthy male volunteers, comparing it with the indocyanine green dye dilution method. Their results showed that, in general, the cardiac output found from the impedance method was higher than that calculated by dye dilution. Based on 115 comparisons, using 10 volunteers, it was found that 63 per cent of the observations lay within a ±20 per cent deviation from the 45 degree perfect correlation line when the impedance cardiac output values were divided by an average factor of $1\cdot19$ to correlate them with the dye dilution values.

Harley and Greenfield (1968) have compared the stroke volumes and cardiac outputs found by the impedance method with the cardiac output found by dye dilution. Thirteen healthy male volunteers and 24 cardiac patients were used. The correlation coefficient between the two methods was $0\cdot68$ for simultaneous values in the volunteers and $0\cdot5$ for the cardiac patients. In 2 patients, the stroke volume measured by impedance was compared with simultaneous deter-minations made by a pressure gradient method. This is a direct measurement of stroke volume based upon the calculation of aortic blood flow from pressure gradients measured by aortic cannulation. For these 2 patients the correlation coefficients were $0\cdot93$ and $0\cdot91$ although the absolute values for the stroke volumes differed considerably for each method. Bache et al. (1969), studying eight patients with cardiomegaly, found that the impedance method did not reliably estimate absolute values for the stroke volumes, the comparison being made with a beat-by-beat pressure gradient technique. In 20 children without shunts or valvular insufficiency, Lababidi et al. (1971) found a $5\cdot5$ per cent mean difference between impedance and dye dilution cardiac output values with the impedance mean being greater than the dye mean.

Baker (1969) compared cardiac outputs from healthy volunteers as found by the impedance and radioisotope dilution methods and obtained a correlation coefficient of only 0·5, although there was a good correlation between the directions of change. It is to be expected that a better correlation would be obtainable between two beat-by-beat methods, rather than a comparison between the impedance method and a dye dilution or Fick method which average over 15 or more beats. This is borne out by the fact that Baker *et al.* (1971)

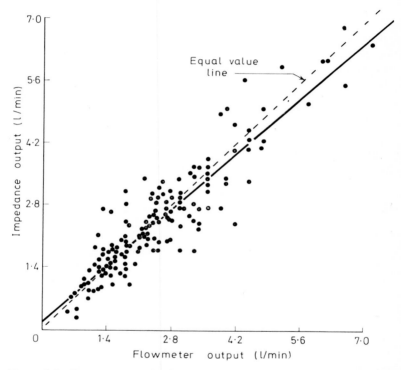

Figure 8.8. Comparison, in the dog, of impedance cardiac output values with those obtained simultaneously by means of an electromagnetic flowmeter arranged to measure blood flow in the ascending aorta (Baker et al., 1971)

found a correlation of 0·68 in normal human male subjects between the impedance and dye dilution methods, whereas the correlation coefficient had a mean value of 0·92 for 214 paired data points taken from 11 dogs in which the impedance stroke volumes were compared with integrated electromagnetic flow probe readings taken from a probe placed around the ascending aorta (*Figure 8.8*).

It is apparent that while the impedance method provides a simple-to-use, non-invasive method for monitoring changes in cardiac output, the problem of deciding on its absolute accuracy in any given patient is by no means easy. Kubicek *et al.* (1966) found that the reproducibility of single impedance observations of cardiac output is greater than for a similar observation obtained by the dye dilution technique. They also found that the ratio of two cardiac output values obtained by the impedance method is more accurate than a similar ratio obtained by the dye dilution technique in predicting true dye cardiac output ratios.

Origins of the impedance changes associated with cardiac activity

The source of the impedance changes accompanying cardiac activity has not, at present, been fully established. Bonjer *et al* (1952) measured the impedance in dogs between the right foreleg to the left hind leg with the heart or lungs being electrically insulated by placing them in rubber bags. Wrapping the heart in a rubber bag did not influence the impedance changes. It appeared that the volume changes of the vascular bed, and not those of the heart, were mainly responsible. When the lungs, but not the heart were insulated, the impedance changes degenerated to small fluctuations. Geddes *et al* (1966) showed that the impedance from base to apex of the heart, which is the probable direction of current flow in the method of Kubicek (1966), increases during systole (emptying) and decreases during diastole (filling). Later experiments, Kubicek *et al* (1967) have shown that it is not the filling and emptying of the heart itself which is causing the impedance changes, but rather the expansion and contraction of the aorta. Karnegis and Kubicek (1970) have correlated the shape of the dZ/dt waveform with a lead 2 ECG and the left ventricular pressure waveform. Lababidi *et al.* (1970) have related specific portions of the dZ/dt waveform with the phono-cardiogram.

Kubicek's equation for stroke volume cannot be expected to apply to all patients, particularly those with pathology of the heart and thorax. It is necessary to postulate a more complicated equation which will take into account redistribution of the blood within the thorax. This point has been well brought out by Cooley (1972).

The use of transthoracic impedance measurements for the early detection of pulmonary oedema

Figure 8.9, taken from a study by D. W. Hill and H. J. Lowe at the University of Chicago Hospitals, shows the variation in Z_0, the transthoracic impedance with chest volume in patients with normal lungs. Patients suffering from the 'shocked lung syndrome' with a substantial amount of fluid in the thorax exhibit a value of thoracic impedance which can be much less than 20 ohms. In one such case, that of a 21-year-old coloured female, Hill and Lowe measured 4·5 ohms. As therapy proceeded and the chest X-ray picture improved, the impedance climbed suddenly to 19 ohms and some

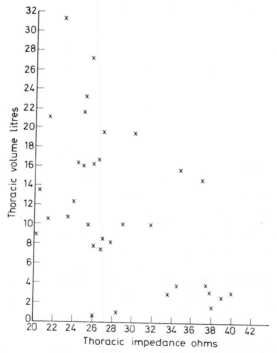

Figure 8.9. The variation of thoracic electrical impedance in ohms with the chest volume in litres for patients with normal lungs

days later stabilized at 33 ohms. Pomerantz *et al.* (1969, 1970) discuss the measurement of the transthoracic electrical impedance as a guide to intrathoracic fluid volumes. In the case of a patient with a pleural effusion, the impedance rose by 1 ohm for each 200 ml of fluid removed. In two cases of respiratory distress syndrome the impedance measured was less than 19–20 ohms. In dogs it was shown that the impedance changed by as much as 45 minutes prior to detectable changes in the central venous pressure, pulmonary compliance arterial pressure or blood-gas values. It was also found that in cardiac by-pass patients, the impedance was lower post-operatively than the pre-operative value. Over the following 7–10 days the impedance rose above the pre-operative levels as the patient's cardio-pulmonary dynamics improved. Similar encouraging reports of the thoracic impedance measurements in the management of thoracic surgery patients have been reported by Van De Water *et al.* (1970, 1971). Van De Water *et al.* (1971) report that the removal of 850 ml of fluid by thoracocentesis from a right pleural effusion increased the thoracic impedance from 17·5 to 19·8 ohms. The measurement of thoracic electrical impedance may well prove to be of considerable value in intensive care units for patients with an accumulation of fluid in the thorax. It should also prove to be a valuable adjunct to blood-gas and pH values for the management of patients having intermittent positive pressure respiration.

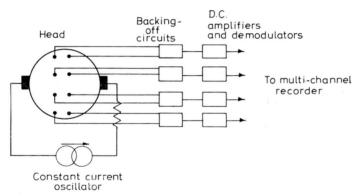

Figure 8.10. Arrangement of typical rheographic recording system

RHEOENCEPHALOGRAPHY

Electrical impedance measurements are also of value in monitoring changes in regional cerebral blood flow. Basically a small constant current, often at a frequency in the range 20–500 kHz, is applied across the head. Pairs of recording electrodes at suitable locations are connected to floating input differential d.c. amplifiers. Provision is made at the input to back off any standing potentials. The output signals are synchronously rectified and fed to a multi-channel recorder. The resulting rheographic curve recorded from each channel is made up from two components. One arises from volume changes synchronous with the pulse occurring in major blood vessels, the other arises from changes in the conductance of the blood dependent upon the blood velocity. The ECG and EEG are normally recorded as well. A computer of average transients triggered from the R-Wave of the ECG is sometimes used to improve the signal-to-noise ratio of the rheographic signal. Rheoencephalography has been shown to be a useful tool in localizing pathology of cerebral blood flow, (Lechner *et al.*, 1969; Allison, 1972). A typical recording system is shown in *Figure 8.10*.

REFERENCES

Cardiac output

Bushman, J. A. (1967). 'Monitoring the ECG waveform.' *Bio-med. Engng.* **2**, 106

Chaplin, H. and Mollison, P. L. (1952). 'Correction for plasma trapped in the red cell column of the haematocrit.' *Blood.* **7**, 1227

Cherrick, G. R., Stein, S. W., Leevy, C. M. and Davidson, C. S. (1960). 'Indocyanine green: observations on its physical properties, plasma decay and hepatic extraction.' *J. clin. Invest.* **39**, 592

Donato, L., Rochester, D. F., Lewis, M. L., Durand, J., Parker, J. O., and Harvey, R. M. (1962). 'Quantitative radiocardiography II. Technic and analysis of curves.' *Circulation* **26**, 183

Dow, P. (1955). 'Dimensional relationships in dye-dilution curves from humans and dogs, with an empirical formula for certain troublesome curves.' *J. appl. Physiol.* **7**, 399

Emanuel, R., Hamer, J., Ching, B., Norman, J. and Manders, J. (1966). 'A dynamic method for the calibration of dye dilution curves in a physiological system.' *Br. Heart J.* **28**, 143

Fox, I. J. and Wood, E. H. (1957). 'Application of dilution curves recorded from the right side of the heart or venous circulation with the aid of a new indicator dye.' *Proc. Staff Meet. Mayo Clin.* **32**, 541

Gott, F. S., Moir, T. W., MacIntyre, W. J., and Pritchard, W. H. (1961). 'A mathematical model of dilution curves for flow study.' *Circ. Res.* **9**, 607

Hallberg, L. and Veall, N. (1962). 'Sodium iodide crystal of well-type for *in vivo* gamma ray measurements.' *Acta radiol.* **58**, 210

Hamilton, W. F., Moore, J. W., Kinsman, J. M., and Spurling, R. G. (1932). 'Studies of the circulation. IV. Further analysis of the injection method and of changes in hemodynamics under physiological and pathological conditions.' *Am. J. Physiol.* **99**, 534

Hamilton, W. F. (1962). 'Measurement of the cardiac output.' In Am. Physiol. Soc. *Handbook of Physiology*. I. *Circulation*. p. 551 Baltimore; Williams and Wilkins

Herd, J. A., Leclair, N. R. and Simon, W. (1966). 'Arterial pressure pulse contours during hemorrhage in anesthetized dogs.' *J. appl. Physiol.* **21**, 1864

Hill, D. W., Valentinuzzi, M. E., Pate, T., and Thompson, F. D. (1972). 'The use of a compartmental hypothesis for the estimation of cardiac output from dye dilution curves and the analysis of radiocardiograms.' *Med. biol. Engng.*, **10,** 43

Hobbs, J. T. (1965). 'Semi-automatic instruments to measure cardiac output and blood volume.' *Wld. med. Electron. Instrum. Lond.* **3,** 324

Horth, T. (1969). 'Arrhythmia monitor.' *Bio-med Engng.* **4,** 308

Johnson, D. E., Liu, C. K., Akcay, M. M., and Taplin, G. V. (1964). 'Radio-pulmonary cardiography for measurement of central mean transit time and its arterial and venous sub-divisions.' In *Dynamic Clinical Studies with Radioisotopes*, Ed. by R. M. Kniseley, W. N. Tauxe and E. B. Anderson, pp. 249–266. U.S. Atomic Energy Commission, Oak Ridge, Tennessee.

Kelman, G. R. (1966). 'Errors in the processing of dye dilution curves.' *Circulation Res.* **18,** 543

Lowe, R. D. (1968). 'Problems in the measurement of blood flow by thermal dilution.' In *Blood Flow Through Organs and Tissues.* p. 6. Ed. by W. H. Bain and A. M. Harper. Edinburgh; Livingstone

Opdyke, D. F. (1952). 'Genesis of the pressure pulse contour method for calculating cardiac stroke index.' *Fed. Proc.* **11,** 733

Payne, J. P. (1960). 'The determination of cardiac output during anaesthesia.' *Ir. J. med. Sci.* **417,** 422

Roberts, V. C. (1969). 'An analogue computer for thermal dilution flow measurement.' *Med. biol. Engng.* **1,** 373

Shipley, R. A., Clark, R. E., Liebowitz, D., and Krohmer, J. S. (1953). 'Analysis of radiocardiogram in heart failure.' *Circ. Res.* **1,** 428

Shubin, H., Weil, M. H. and Rockwell, M. A. jun. (1967). 'Automated measurement of cardiac output in patients by the use of a digital computer.' *Med. Electron. biol. Engng.* **5,** 353

Thorburn, G. D. (1961). 'Estimates of cardiac output from forward part of indicator dilution curves.' *J. appl. Physiol.* **16,** 891

Uhrenholdt, A. (1967). 'A computer as an aid in calculating cardiac output.' *Scand. J. clin. Lab. Invest.* **19,** 38

— (1968). 'Radiocardiography: validity and reproducibility.' In *Blood Flow Through Organs and Tissues.* p. 67. Ed. by W. H. Bain and A. M. Harper. Edinburgh; Livingstone

Valentinuzzi, M. E., Valentinuzzi, M., and Posey, J. A. (1971). 'Dilution curve area; fast estimation by a compartmental procedure.' *Proc. 9th Int. Conf., Med. biol. Engng.*, Melbourne, Paper 30–6

Valentinuzzi, M., Valentinuzzi, M. E., and Posey, J. A. (1972). 'Fast estimation of the dilution curve area by a procedure based on a compartmental hypothesis.' *J. Am. Ass. med. instrum.*

Veall, N. and Vetter, H. (1958). *Radioisotope Techniques in Clinical Research and Diagnosis.* London; Butterworths.

Warner, H. R. and Wood, E. H. (1952). 'Simplified calculation of cardiac output from dye dilution curves recorded by oximeter.' *J. appl. Physiol.* **5,** 111

Warner, H. R., Swan, H. J. C., Connolly, D. C., Tompkins, R. G. and Wood, E. H. (1953). 'Quantitation of beat-to-beat changes in stroke volume from the aortic pulse contour in man.' *J. appl. Physiol.* **5,** 495

Wheeler, H. O., Cranston, W. I. and Meltzer, J. I. (1958). 'Hepatic uptake and biliary excretion of indocyanine green in the dog.' *Proc. Soc. exp. Biol. Med.* **99,** 11

Wilson, E. M., Ranieri, A. J., Updike, O. L., and Damman, J. F. (1972). 'An evaluation of thermal dilution for obtaining serial measurements of cardiac output.' *Med. biol. Engng.*, **10,** 179

Electrical impedance measurements

Allison, R. D. (1972). *Physiological Applications of Impedance Plethysmography*, Pittsburgh; Instrument Society of America.

Bache, R. J., Harley, A., and Greenfield, J. C. (1969). 'Evaluation of Thoracic impedance plethysmography as an indicator of stroke volume in man,' *Am. J. med. Sci.* **258,** 100

Baker, L. E. (1969). 'Biomedical applications of electrical impedance measurements.' In *Progress in Medical Electronics.* Ed. by D. W. Hill and B. Watson. Cambridge; University Press

— Judy, W. V., Geddes, L. E., Langley, F. M., and Hill, D. W. (1971). 'The measurement of cardiac output by means of electrical impedance.' *Cardiovasc. Res. Center Bull.* **9,** 135

Bonjer, F. H., Van den Berg, J. W. and Dirken, M. N. J. (1952). 'The origin of the variations of body impedance occurring during the cardiac cycle.' *Circulation* **6,** 415

Cooley, W. L., (1972). 'The calculation of cardiac stroke volume from variations in transthoracic electrical impedance.' *Bio-med Engng.*, **7,** 316

Geddes, L. A., Hoff, H. E., Mello, A. and Palmer, C. (1966). 'Continuous measurement of ventricular stroke volume by electrical impedance.' *Cardiovasc. Res. Cent. Bull.* **4,** 118

Harley, A. and Greenfield, J. C. (1968). 'Determination of cardiac output in man by means of impedance plethysmography.' *Aerospace Med.* **39,** 248

Karnegis, J. N., and Kubicek, W. F. (1970). 'Physiological correlates of the cardiac impedance waveform.' *Am. Heart J.* **79,** 519

Kubicek, W. G., Karnegis, J. N., Patterson, R. P., Witsoe, D. A. and Mattson, R. H. (1966). 'Development and evaluation of an impedance cardiac output system. *Aerospace Med.* **37,** 1208

— Witsoe, D. A., Patterson, R. P., Mosharrafa, M. A., Marnegis, J. N. and From, A. H. L. (1967). 'Development and evaluation of an impedance cardiographic system to measure cardiac output and development of an oxygen consumption rate computing system utilising a quadrupole mass spectrometer.' *Technical Report No. NAS* 9–4500, NASA Manned Spacecraft Center, Houston, Texas

Lechner, H., Geyer, N., Lugaresi, E., Martin, F., Lifshitz, K. and Markovich, S. (1969) *Rheoencephalography and Plethysmographical Methods.* Amsterdam; Exerpta Medica

Lababidi, Z., Ehmke, D. A., Durnin, R. E., Leaverton, P. E., and Lauer, R. M. (1970). 'The first derivative thoracic impedance cardiogram.' *Circulation*, **61,** 651

— — — — — (1971). 'Evaluation of impedance cardiac output in children.' *Paediatrics*, **47,** 870

Mostert, J. W., Moore, R. H., and Murphy, G. P. (1969). 'Nomograms for estimation of peripheral resistance and work of the Heart.' *Anesthesiology* **30,** 569

Nyboer, J. (1959). *Electrical Impedance Plethysmography.* Springfield, Illinois; Thomas

Pomerantz, M., Baumgartner, R., Laurisdon, J., and Eiseman, B. (1969). 'Transthoracic electrical impedance for the early detection of pulmonary oedema.' *Surgery* **66,** 260

— Delgado, F., and Eiseman, B. (1970). 'Clinical evaluation of transthoracic electrical impedance as a guide to intrathoracic fluid volumes.' *Ann. Surg.* **171,** 686

Siegal, J. H., Fabian, M., Lankau, C., Levine, M., Dove, A., and Nahmad, M. (1970). 'Clinical and experimental use of thoracic impedance plethysmography in quantifying myocardial contractility.' *Surgery* **67,** 907

Van De Water, J. M., Miller, T. D., Milne, E. N. C., Hanson, E. L., Sheldon, G. F., and Kagey, K. S. (1970). 'Impedance plethysmography—a non-invasive method of monitoring the thoracic surgery patient.' *J. thorac. cardiovasc. Surg.* **60,** 641.

— Philips, P. A., Thouin, L. G., Watanabe, L. S., and Lappen, R. S. (1971). 'Bioelectric impedance.' *Archs Surg.* **102,** 541

9–Defibrillators

A.C. DEFIBRILLATORS

In many cases it is possible to restore a sinus rhythm to a heart in ventricular fibrillation by giving a powerful electric shock to the heart. The apparatus for administering the shock is known as a defibrillator. The simplest type of defibrillator is the a.c. defibrillator (Johnson, Kirby and Dripps, 1951). With the chest open, large spoon-shaped electrodes should be used to embrace the heart, the impedance between the electrodes then being of the order of 50 Ω. Basically, an a.c. defibrillator consists of a mains transformer having a number of secondary tappings so that output voltages in the range 85–300 V r.m.s. can be selected by means of a switch (McMillan, Cockett and Styles, 1952), *Figure 9.1.* The current passed through

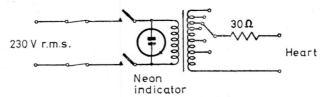

Figure 9.1. Schematic diagram of a simple a.c. defibrillator

the heart will be of the order 4 to 6 A r.m.s. The interelectrode impedance is a pure resistance of approximately 75 Ω. With the chest closed it is necessary to increase the applied voltage to about 500 V, the impedance across the thorax then being about 100 Ω so that a current of some five amperes will flow. It is normally sufficient to pass the current for 0·25 second. This can be done by the operator pressing on a switch, but modern a.c. defibrillators make the foot switch operate a timing circuit that passes five to ten cycles of the mains and then cuts out until the switch is pressed again (Perry and Trotman, 1958). The electrodes are mounted in well-insulated

288

handles, and the use of a foot switch safeguards the operator from an accidental shock.

In a typical commercial a.c. defibrillator two ranges of voltage outputs would be available: 60, 100, 150 and 250 V (for use with internal electrodes placed on the heart) and 250, 400, 600 and 900 V (for use with external electrodes placed on the thorax). A timing circuit allows the current to pass for 5 cycles of the 50 Hz mains (0·1 seconds). Non-interchangeable sockets are provided for the internal and external electrodes so that the higher external range cannot be applied directly to the heart. It is desirable to use electrode jelly with the external defibrillator electrodes which should then be applied with a firm pressure to the thorax in order to avoid burns. Ferris *et al.* (1969) discuss the parameters involved in alternating current defibrillation.

The application of the shock produces a marked convulsion, and in the case of experimental animals, care must be taken to see that this does not damage apparatus connected to the animal, rectal thermometers being a good example. The output secondary winding of the defibrillator should be isolated from earth so that there is no shock risk to anyone touching an earthed object such as the operating table. Modern electrocardiographs are provided with limiting circuits in their input stage and a high degree of isolation from earth so that defibrillation voltages will not permanently damage the recorder. Typically, the protection circuit can be set to operate for input voltages in the range 5 to 60 mV.

A.C. defibrillators have now almost universally been replaced by d.c. defibrillators. This has come about for a number of reasons including:

(1) The fact that d.c. defibrillators can also be used for the conversion of supraventricular arrhythmias such as atrial fibrillation, atrial flutter and paroxysmal atrial tachycardia.

(2) A d.c. discharge is less likely to produce ventricular fibrillation when the pulse is delivered at random during the cardiac cycle than is the case for the passage of an a.c. current; hence the risk of accidentally fibrillating the operator is reduced.

(3) The convulsion of skeletal muscles is less with d.c. defibrillation than with a.c. defibrillation.

(4) D.C. defibrillators have less deleterious affects than a.c. types on parameters such as heart rate, aortic and ventricular pressures and myocardial contractility.

289

D.C. DEFIBRILLATORS

Instead of passing an alternating current through the heart, it is possible to bring about defibrillation by giving the heart one or more single shocks from a capacitor charged to a high voltage. This is the principle of the d.c. defibrillator. Referring to *Figure 9.2*, a variable auto transformer determines the primary voltage of a high-voltage mains transformer. The output voltage from the transformer secondary is applied via the rectifier and vacuum high-voltage switch to charge up the oil-filled 16 µF capacitor via the inductor.

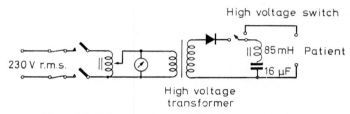

Figure 9.2. Schematic diagram of a basic d.c. defibrillator

When the foot switch is pressed, the high-voltage switch changes over and discharges the capacitor through the inductor across the heart. At the same time a muting circuit shorts out the input to the cardioscope or ECG recorder in order to protect it. The electrode housings contain safety switches so that the capacitor can only be discharged when the electrodes are making firm contact with the heart or chest wall. In this way the risk of burns to the patient and accidental shock to the operator are prevented. Two sets of electrodes are provided, one for internal use and one for external use. The electrode sockets are non-interchangeable and they also select the voltage range available. The higher voltage range is thus only available for use with the external electrodes. An a.c. voltmeter mounted on the front panel of the defibrillator measures the voltage applied to the primary of the high-voltage transformer. The meter is normally scaled in terms of joules or watt-seconds as a measure of the electrical energy stored in the capacitor. This energy is numerically equal to $\frac{1}{2}CV^2$ where C is the capacity of the capacitor in farads and V is the voltage to which it is charged. In order to provide 100 joules a 16 µF capacitor would have to be charged to about 3,500 V. For internal application energies of the order of 50 to 72 J would be used corresponding to voltages of 2,500 and 3,000. For external use energies up to 400 J are available (7,000 V on the capacitor). Power is defined as 'rate of doing work' and the electrical unit of power is the watt. Energy is defined as the 'capacity for doing work' so that energy=power×time. Thus joules and watt-seconds are equivalent and both terms are used in the calibration of defibrillators produced by different manufacturers. The action of the coil (inductor) connected in series with the capacitor is to change the shape of the normal exponential capacitor discharge curve into a pulse which resembles a half sine wave with a duration of about 2·5 milliseconds. Clearly anyone concerned with d.c. defibrillators should be aware of the very high voltages involved. A high standard of workmanship is also required in the apparatus itself. With a charging resistance of 0·25 MΩ the time constant of the 16 μF capacitor is 4 seconds, the peak charging current being 16 mA at 4,000 V. It thus takes 16 seconds to recharge the capacitor. Lown et al (1961) compare the effectiveness of a.c. and d.c. defibrillators.

Whilst the majority of d.c. defibrillators used in hospitals are mains powered, there exists a need for portable, battery powered, versions which can be used anywhere in an emergency. They can, for example, be carried in an ambulance. A typical instrument would be powered by 14 rechargeable nickel–cadmium cells, each of 2 ampere-hours capacity. It would be capable of supplying 40 discharges, each of 400 joules. The time to recharge the capacitor to 400 joules is less than 10 seconds. Switched energy ranges of 15, 30, 45, 60, 100, 150, 200, 250, 300 and 400 joules are available, the output being isolated from earth. The external electrodes of German silver are 96 mm in diameter whilst internal electrodes of 40, 60 or 80 mm diameter are available. The weight of the defibrillator is 20 kg.

Jude et al. (1962) describe an experimental and clinical study of a portable defibrillator. Portable defibrillators are now available which can be powered from either rechargeable cells, a 12 V vehicle battery or a bank of 24 U11 dry cells (each 1·5 V) connected in series. The defibrillator can deliver 50, 100, 200 or 400 joules and weighs 10·5 kg.

Geddes and Tacker (1971) discuss the engineering and physiological considerations of direct capacitor-discharge ventricular defibrillation. In a study on dogs they found an optimum discharge duration of 0·3–4 ms. Cox et al. (1963) describe the successful use of d.c. external defibrillation after the failure of a.c. external defibrillation, whilst Druz (1969) deals with the design rationale of defibrillators.

291

SYNCHRONIZED D.C. DEFIBRILLATORS

In the case of ventricular fibrillation a straight d.c. defibrillator is used, but in order to revert a heart with an atrial arrhythmia to sinus rhythm it is necessary to use a synchronized d.c. defibrillator. The function of the synchronizer unit is to discharge the capacitor of the d.c. defibrillator during the down-stroke of the R-Wave of the patient's electrocardiogram. In this way the discharge occurs before the T-wave, (Lown *et al*, 1962, 1964). There is a risk of producing ventricular fibrillation if the discharge occurs during the T-wave. The patient's electrocardiogram is observed on an electrocardioscope which is fitted with two output terminals. These feed the electrical signal of the ECG into the tuned amplifier of the synchronizer unit.

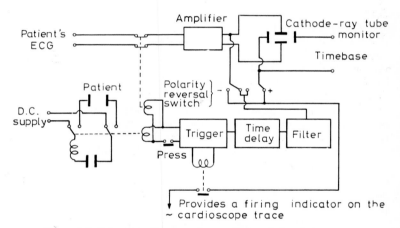

Figure 9.3. Schematic diagram of a synchronized d.c. defibrillator

This picks up the R-wave of the ECG and uses this to trigger a delay circuit (*Figure 9.3*). After an interval of about 30 milliseconds the capacitor is discharged across the electrodes. A synchronized d.c. defibrillator suitable for trolley mounting is illustrated in *Figure 9.4*. The associated cardioscope is fitted with bradycardia and tachycardia alarms and a heart rate meter so that it can be used for monitoring the patient. D.C. defibrillators are now available in many hospitals. Gilston, Fordham and Resnekov (1965) discuss the technique from the viewpoint of the anaesthetist.

292

DOUBLE SQUARE PULSE DEFIBRILLATORS

Conventional a.c. and d.c. defibrillators are quoted by Kugelberg (1968) as producing myocardial injury with a diminished ventricular function for a period of approximately 30 minutes following the delivery of the shock. As a result, if the chest can be opened, there is a need to work with lower energy shocks applied to the heart. These facts led Kugelberg to develop a double-pulse system using voltages in the range 8–60 V compared with the 800–1500 V

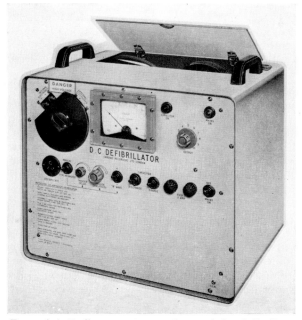

Figure 9.4. Trolley mounting synchronized d.c. defibrillator.
(Reproduced by courtesy of Cardiac Recorders Ltd.)

employed in d.c. capacitor discharge defibrillators. The rationale of the double-pulse approach is based upon the hypothesis that at the moment of passing the current some of the fibrillating cells will be excitable. They will be depolarized. However, cells which are refractory will continue to fibrillate. In order to obtain a total defibrillation, the second pulse operates on this later group of cells. The pulse amplitude and width together with the interval should be such that the cells defibrillated by the first pulse will be refractory

293

to the second. The timing of the second pulse should be such that it defibrillates those cells which were refractory to the first pulse but which have now become excitable. For human use the duration of each pulse is set at 30 ms with an interval between pulses of 100 ms. The pulse amplitude can be set within the range 50–300 V. Kugelberg reports that out of 41 patients, in 40 cases ventricular fibrillation was terminated by the use of the double-pulse defibrillator. The shocks were given directly to the heart after open-heart surgery. On average, successful defibrillation was achieved at the third attempt with a mean energy of 2·4 watt-seconds, and a mean amplitude of 50 V. Kugelberg (1967) states that in dogs both a.c. defibrillation (280 V r.m.s. at 840 watt-seconds) and d.c. defibrillation (40 watt-seconds) reduced ventricular function by 50 per cent for 30 minutes, whereas there was no diminution with the double-square-pulse system.

CHECKING D.C. DEFIBRILLATOR PERFORMANCE

In the course of visiting a number of intensive care units, the author has been struck by the forcibly expressed opinion that it is necessary to check the operation of d.c. defibrillators at least daily in order to be sure that they will function correctly when an emergency arises. The tester should present a resistive load of 50 ohms to the defibrillator so that the current drawn is realistic. At any instant the power dissipated in a resistance of R ohms is V^2/R in watts where V is the voltage drop appearing across the resistor. To take the simplest case, suppose that a square pulse of 50 joules energy and 2·5 ms duration is applied to a 50 ohm resistor. The power dissipated is $V^2/50$ which equals 50 joules over a period of 2·5/1000 seconds. Thus $(V^2/50)(2·5/1000)=50$ so that $V=1000$ volts. In the case of a practical d.c. defibrillator, the pulse is not flat-topped, but is likely to look like that shown in *Figure 9.5*. Since the voltage across the load now varies with time, the power dissipated is given by $P=(1/R)\int_{t_1}^{t_2} V^2 dt$.

In *Figure 9.5* it can be seen that the pulse is biphasic having an initial positive portion followed by a negative portion. The total power is the sum of that produced in each portion. Good versions of defibrillator testers square the voltage developed across the 50 ohm load and integrate it over the pulse duration. Typical energy ranges provided would be 0–40, 0–100 and 0–400 joules. In theory, it is also possible to determine the energy dissipated by measuring the temperature rise produced in the 50 ohm load. A thermocouple should be used rather than a mercury-in-glass thermometer since the time response of the latter is slow.

294

The concept of delivered energy

The energy stored in the capacitor of a conventional capacitor discharge type of d.c. defibrillator is given by $\frac{1}{2}cv^2$ joules where C is in farads and V is in volts. Such defibrillators are also known as RLC defibrillators since the simplest versions consist of a d.c. power supply, a storage capacitor and a series inductor. The winding of the inductor has a windings resistance. Hagan (1972) discusses the case of a 40 μF capacitor charged to 5000 V and discharged through a 50Ω patient via 0·1 Henry inductor having a 50Ω windings resistance. The stored energy $\frac{1}{2}cv^2 = 500$ joules. For this situation, Hagan calculates the energy delivered to the patient to be 250 joules.

In comparing the performance of various models of d.c. defibrillator, especially ones with different waveforms (e.g. RLC and square wave) delivered and not stored energies should be quoted. (Sutton *et al.*, 1970; Stratbucker *et al.*, 1971). The delivered energy can be measured with a defibrillator tester which solves the energy equation $W = \int_{o}^{t} \frac{V^2}{R} \, dt$ where R is the patient load resistance and V is the instantaneous voltage developed across it.

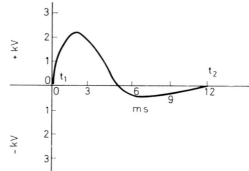

Figure 9.5. The waveform of a typical 200 joule Lown-type d.c. difibrillator pulse

Routine inspection of d.c. defibrillators

For ventricular defibrillation purposes, d.c. defibrillators are usually required in a hurry. Hence, they should be subjected to routine inspections to check for breaks in the insulation of the electrode cables, a good condition of the mains lead and plug, clean electrodes, intact fuses, battery condition if applicable and operation of indicator lights and controls. The power delivered should be checked and the leakage current from the chassis to earth when the case is not earthed and also the leakage current from the electrodes to earth. Excessive leakage current could produce ventricular fibrillation in a patient with a cardiac catheter when the defibrillator is to be used for the conversion of atrial arrhythmias.

REFERENCES

Cox, A. R., Dodds, W. A., and Trapp, W. G. (1963). 'Successful use of d.c. external defibrillation after failure of an a.c. external defibrillator.' *Can. med. Ass. J.* **89**, 1193

Druz, W. S. (1969). 'The design rational of defibrillators.' *J. Am. Ass. med. Instrum.*, **3**, 65

Ferris, C. D., Moore, T. W., Khazei, A. H., and Cowley, R. A. (1969). 'A study of parameters involved in alternating-current defibrillation.' *Med. biol. Engng.*, **9**, 185

Geddes, L. A., and Tacker, W. A. (1971). 'Engineering and physiological considerations of direct capacitor-discharge ventricular defibrillation.' *Med. biol. Engng.*, **9**, 185

— (1971). 'Electrical ventricular defibrillation.' *Cardiovasc. res. Center Bull.* **10**, 3

Gilston, A., Fordham, R. and Resnekov, L. (1965). 'Anaesthesia for direct current shock in the treatment of cardiac arrhythmias.' *Br. J. Anaesth.* **37**, 533

Hagan, W. (1972). 'Defibrillation techniques.' *Med. Electron. Data*, **3**, 33

Johnson, J., Kirby, C. K. and Dripps, R. D. (1951). 'Defibrillation of the ventricles by electric shock with complete recovery.' *Ann. Surg.* **134**, 116

Jude, J. R., Kouwenhoven, W. B., and Knickerbocker, G. G. (1962). 'An experimental and clinical study of a portable external cardiac defibrillator.' *Surg. Forum* **13**, 185

Kugelberg, J. E. W. B. (1967). 'Ventricular defibrillation. A new aspect.' *Acta. chir. scand.* Suppl. 372.

— (1968). 'Ventricular defibrillation with double square pulse.' *Med. Electron. biol. Engng.* **6**, 167

Lown, B., Amarasingham, R. and Neuman, J. (1962). 'A new method for terminating cardiac arrhythmias; use of a synchronized capacitor discharge.' *J. Amer. med. Ass.* **182**, 548

— Kleiger, R. and Wolff, G. (1964). 'The technique of cardioversion.' *Am. Heart J.* **67**, 282

— Neuman, J., Amarasingham, R. and Berkovits, B. V. (1961). 'Comparison of alternating current with direct current electroshock across the closed chest.' *Am. J. Cardiol.* **10**, 223

McMillan, I. K. R., Cockett, F. B. and Styles, P. (1952). 'Cardiac arrest and ventricular fibrillation.' *Thorax* **7**, 205

Perry, B. J. and Trotman, R. E. (1958). 'An internal defibrillator with current measuring facilities.' *Electron. Engng.* **30**, 24

Stratbucker, R., Chambers, W. and Hagan, W. (1971). 'Defibrillation performance characteristics.' *J. Ass. advancem. med. Instrum.* **5**, 2

Sutton, W., Galysh, F. and Hagan, W. (1970). 'Significant determinants of successful reversions of fibrillation by a new d.c. defibrillator.' *Am. Heart J.*, **79**, 630

10–Cardiac Pacemakers and Bladder and Anal Stimulators

IMPLANTED CIRCUITS

One branch of medical electronics that is of particular interest to surgeons and anaesthetists is the application of electronic circuits that can be implanted within the body for extended periods. For use with human patients the two most useful systems are the cardiac pacemaker and the electronic stimulator for the control of urinary incontinence. For use during experiments with animals, implanted electromagnetic and ultrasonic blood flow probes and miniature solid-state blood pressure transducers are enabling comprehensive monitoring of physiological variables to be carried out from free-ranging animals. Apart from the obvious need to use highly reliable miniature circuit components, there are the requirements of providing the circuit with sufficient power and ensuring that the body does not reject the implant. The first requirement has led to the development of reliable miniature mercury batteries, the evolution of methods of bringing leads out through the skin from an implanted circuit without introducing infection, and radio-frequency links for coupling power from an external source into an implant. The second requirement has only been met by the development of epoxy resin 'potting' techniques and the use of an outer covering of a biologically inert silicone material.

According to Braley (1967) the carbon-silicon bond does not occur in the animal or vegetable kingdoms, the various silicones having to be produced artificially. If the body is able to metabolize silicones this is an extremely slow process, and for this reason silicones appear to be virtually inert when implanted. There is no exudation of plasticizer material from silicones, and this fact prevents the occurrence of irritant reactions.

ELECTRODE ARRANGEMENTS FOR USE WITH CARDIAC PACEMAKERS

Both bipolar and unipolar systems are in use. Myocardial stimulation can be performed with two electrodes placed on the heart (bipolar leads) or with a single electrode on the heart and another electrode situated elsewhere in the body (unipolar leads). This second or 'indifferent' electrode should be connected to the positive terminal of the pacemaker, since the normal depolarization of the heart is mimicked by negative stimulation. Davies and Sowton (1966) report that in their patients a comparison of the stimulus amplitudes required to pace the heart with different polarities revealed that up to 16 times more energy was needed to initiate ventricular contraction when an initial stimulus of positive polarity was used rather than one of negative polarity. A mathematical model for the polarization impedance of cardiac pacemaker electrodes is given by Jaron, Schwann and Gesolowitz (1968).

A typical bedside pacemaker for use with a catheter electrode would provide an output voltage range from 0·2 to 8 V in 0·2 V steps, from 0·2 to 3 V in 0·5 V steps from 6 to 8 V and 1 V steps from 6 to 8 V. The rate range might be 30 to 150 beats per minute and the pulse width is usually 2 ms. Power sufficient for about six months pacing can be provided by four dry batteries. When used in the demand, as opposed to the fixed rate, mode, each output pulse is inhibited if a spontaneous R–wave from the heart has been detected having an amplitude in the range 1–1·5 mV. If the expected beat is not found then the unit delivers a pacing pulse. If the spontaneous heart rate drops below a pre-set stand-by value then the unit will pace continuously at this stand-by rate.

PACEMAKER SYSTEMS FOR SHORT-TERM PACING

The use of an external pacemaker coupled to the heart by means of an electrode catheter with the electrode tip situated in the apex of the right ventricle was developed by Furman and Schwedel (1959) and is the method of choice for emergency pacing of Siddons and Sowton (1967), provided suitable X-ray apparatus is available for positioning the electrode. Both unipolar and bipolar catheters have been used. The catheter is passed via an arm vein in most cases. This arrangement requires the passage of only small currents which are painless and do not give rise to muscle twitching.

Bedside pacemaker units powered from rechargeable batteries are available with facilities for both internal and external pacing. For internal pacing with a catheter electrode, the output voltage is limited to a maximum of 15 V, whilst for use with external electrodes the maximum is 150 V. The repetition rate is typically 20 to 120 per minute with a 3 ms pulse width.

For short-term use in emergency it is possible to pace the heart from electrodes placed on the chest wall. Two-inch square metal plate electrodes covered with electrode jelly are placed over the manubrium and the left axilla just lateral to the apex beat. Pulse amplitudes in the range 50 to 200 V are required with a pulse width usually of 2 ms but not greater than 3 ms. The pulse generator should have controllable rates within the range 30–120 beats per minute. Conscious patients may have to be anaesthetized to overcome the pain from muscular contractions and the electrode sites changed to prevent the formation of burns (Zoll, Linenthal and Zarsky 1960).

Pulses of 10 V or less will pace the heart when applied directly to the myocardium by means of a percutaneous myocardial needle. The use of such a needle inserted through the fourth or fifth left interspace is described by Thevenet, Hodges and Lillehei (1958), and insertion using another procedure by Lillehei *et al* (1964).

PACEMAKER SYSTEMS FOR LONG-TERM PACING

As with systems for short-term pacing, the electrodes can make contact either from within the heart or on its surface. In conjunction with these two basic arrangements of electrodes the pacemaker circuit can be either entirely implanted, entirely external, or consisting of a passive implant coupled via a radiofrequency link to an external pulser.

External pacemakers

An external pacemaker offers the advantage of an easy change of battery and heart rate, but is more liable to trouble from wire breakages than a totally implanted system and makes the patient aware that he is dependent upon the correct functioning of an external unit. External pacemakers are not now much used in conjunction with a wire running to an electrode situated on the surface of the heart. This is because sepsis tends to track along the wire and leads to an inflammatory reaction around the electrode thus increasing the pulse amplitude threshold for pacing (Davies and Sowton 1966). Sepsis may be delayed and Senning (1964) has used this technique for up to 3 years.

The use of an endocardial electrode in conjunction with an external pacemaker is feasible for long-term pacing, the external jugular vein being used as the site of entry for the electrode catheter. If pacing is performed for more than three or four weeks by this method, the incidence of bacteraemia is high. Siddons (1963) reports 3 bacteraemias out of 27 patients paced in this way for more than four weeks. Lagergren et al (1965) found only 3 non-fatal septicaemias in 100 patients paced by this method, but with the wire now running a long subcutaneous course from the site of the neck vein entry before traversing the skin in the groin.

Implanted pacemakers

An implanted pacemaker with electrodes placed on the surface of the heart has been the most extensively used. Both bipolar and monopolar lead arrangements are used. Stainless steel is a good electrode material for use when a negative electrode is placed on the heart because of its satisfactory mechanical properties. Because of the deterioration of positive electrodes arising from electrolysis it is desirable to make the indifferent tissue electrode from platinum-iridium alloy and not subject to the continual movement of the heart (Davies and Siddons 1965).

The use of a transvenous endocardial electrode with an implanted pacemaker avoids the necessity of exposing the heart during surgery. The electrode is passed via a jugular vein and the pacemaker implanted in the abdomen, the connecting wire running a long subcutaneous course. Alternatively, the pacemaker can be implanted in the axilla or beneath the breast (Chardack, Frederico and Gage (1965); Senning (1964); Bluestone et al (1965).

It is possible to couple power through the thoracic wall into a passive implant from an external unit either by simple inductive coupling or by a radiofrequency transformer system. In the first case, the external unit is placed on the chest wall accurately positioned in respect of the implant. This consists of a coil, which may be iron-cored, whose leads are run to the surface of the heart. The external unit pulses a coil which by mutual induction induces a pulse into the implant coil. The implant consists simply of a coil, but as it picks up only a small proportion of the available energy, care must be taken in the design of the external unit to prevent its being cumbersome. Induction type pacemakers have been described by Abrahms, Hudson and Lightwood (1960) and Abrahms and Norman (1964). Although the implant associated with induction systems is as simple as possible, it does not allow complete control of the impulse waveform. For this reason the radiofrequency system employs pulse modulation of a radiofrequency carrier which is picked up by a tuned coil in the implant and demodulated by a diode-capacitor combination. Radiofrequency systems have been described by Cammilli *et al* (1964) and by Glenn *et al* (1964). Both inductive and radio-frequency pacemakers have been modified to work with an endocardial electrode. To obviate trouble with wire breakages, Schuder and Stoeckle (1962) used a miniature receiver mounted on the heart.

Two useful review papers dealing with the technical and clinical aspects respectively of cardiac pacemakers are those of Kahn and Mavens (1972) and Bleese *et al*. (1972).

EXTERNAL RATE CONTROL FOR IMPLANTED PACEMAKERS

The simpler types of implanted pacemaker operate at a fixed rate, but in some models provision is made to vary the rate from outside the body. Possible methods for doing this are: (1) the use of a switch operated by an external magnet, Berg (1964); (2) electrical induction, Davies (1962); or (3) the insertion of a needle screw through the skin into a socket in the pacemaker.

ATRIAL-TRIGGERED PACEMAKERS

This type of pacemaker is triggered by the natural pacemaker of the heart and delivers an impulse to the ventricle after a suitable P-R interval. The system allows for the alteration of cardiac output by variation of rate as well as stroke volume and ensures that ventricular contraction is timed at a sufficient interval to allow for atrial filling. Triggering can be obtained from an additional electrode. Center *et al* (1963) placed this electrode on the left atrium, while Rudewald *et al* (1964) placed its tip within the right atrium. The use of an atrial-triggered pacemaker is also described by Carlens *et al* (1963).

'ON-DEMAND' PACEMAKERS

Most 'on-demand' pacemakers detect spontaneous ventricular activity and are inhibited unless the R-R interval exceeds a preset limit (Goetz, Dormandy and Berkovits, 1966). Neville *et al* (1966) have used a different principle. The stimulus is triggered by the spontaneous R-wave so that it falls in the absolute refractory period of the heart. If the R-R interval should exceed the preset limit the unit functions as a fixed-rate pacemaker. With some types of on-demand unit the application of an external magnet will temporarily convert the unit to fixed rate pacing.

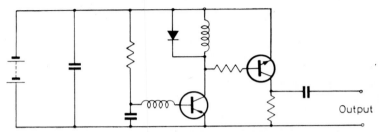

Figure 10.1. Blocking oscillator, St. George's Hospital circuit, for a cardiac pacemaker. (Reproduced by courtesy of Devices Implants Ltd.)

CARDIAC PACEMAKER CIRCUITS

Blocking oscillator circuits are commonly used for cardiac pace-makers, and an outline circuit for the St. George's Hospital type pacemakers produced by Devices Ltd is shown in *Figure 10.1*. The

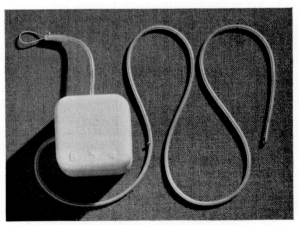

Figure 10.2. St. George's Hospital pacemaker designed for implantation in the axilla

version designed to be implanted in the axilla is illustrated in *Figure 10.2*. It is a fixed rate unit powered at 4 V from three mercury cells. The rate is normally set by the manufacturer at 70 per minute, but rates in the range 40–120 per minute can be provided. The pulse output is passed through a blocking capacitor to give an initial short negative portion followed by a long positive portion so that there are equal areas above and below the baseline (*Figure 10.3*). There is now no mean d.c. voltage across the electrodes which would produce a rapid polarization. The pulse width is 0·5–0·8 ms, and the

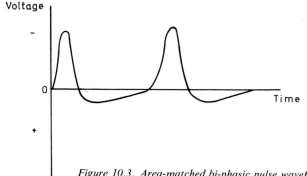

Figure 10.3. Area-matched bi-phasic pulse waveform

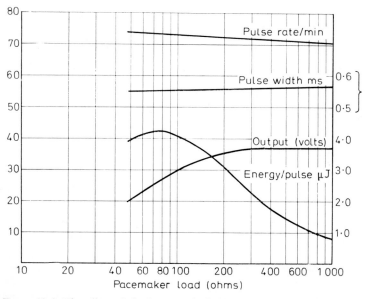

Figure 10.4. The effect of alteration in the load on a St. George's Hospital type pacemaker. (Reproduced by courtesy of Devices Implants Ltd.)

303

pulse amplitude is 2·5 V minimum into a 150-ohm load, approximately 25 µJ of energy being delivered into a 300-ohm load. From *Figure 10.4* it is seen that the impulse duration, stimulation rate and output voltage remain virtually constant with loads in the range 200–1000 Ω. The energy delivered by each impulse is markedly dependent upon the circuit loading. The anticipated life of the batteries is three years and the stimulation frequency decreases as the batteries near exhaustion.

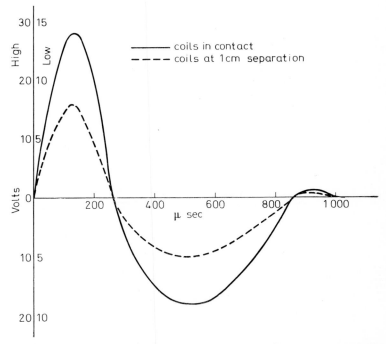

Figure 10.7. Pulse waveform generated by the Lucas inductive pacemaker. (Reproduced by courtesy of Joseph Lucas Ltd.)

Another widely used pacemaker circuit is the complementary pair transistor multivibrator. The circuit of the Model FM139 implantable pacemaker by Elema–Schonander is shown in *Figure 10.5*. The supply voltage is 6·7 V from five mercury cells. The rate is normally fixed at 70 per minute, with an impulse width of 2–2·5 ms, and the leading edge of the negative pulse being at least 6 V. The impulse energy is approximately 100 µJ into a 300-ohm load.

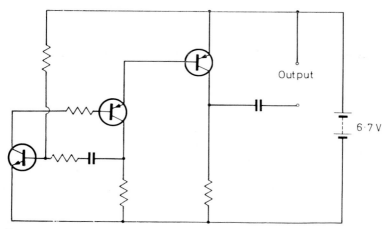

Figure 10.5. Complementary pair cardiac pacemaker circuit. (Reproduced by courtesy of Elema-Schonander)

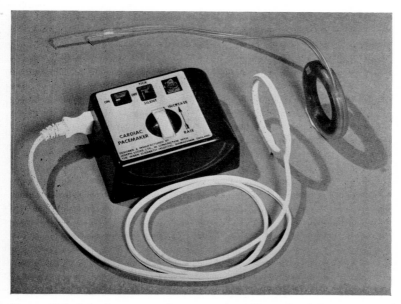

Figure 10.6. Inductive-type cardiac pacemaker. (Reproduced by courtesy of Joseph Lucas Ltd.)

The Lucas induction pacemaker is depicted in *Figure 10.6* together with the external primary coil, internal secondary coil and bipolar myocardial electrodes. The box contains a voltage-converter unit which steps up the 1·5 V battery supply voltage to approximately 100 V which charges a capacitor. This is discharged into the external primary coil via a silicon-controlled rectifier. The pulse width does not vary with load impedance and can be altered by changing the primary coil. Alternative 'high' and 'low' power outputs are provided. The impulse waveform appearing across a 180-ohm load is shown in *Figure 10.7*. The rate is variable over the range 30 to 100 pulses per minute.

ELECTROLYTIC DISINTEGRATION OF PACEMAKER ELECTRODES

In order to prevent placing a mean d.c. voltage across pacemaker electrodes these are normally fed from a good quality capacitor to give an 'area-matched' waveform. Compared with pessary stimulators for the treatment of urinary incontinence, the current density at pacemaker electrodes is high and cases of the electrolytic destruction of the positive stainless steel indifferent electrode have been reported, Siddons and Sowton (1967) report three cases of electrolytic failure of stainless steel positive electrodes in their first 60 cases, even though area-matched biphasic pulses were used. The reaction will proceed more rapidly with monophasic pulses. Rowley (1963) implanted stainless steel electrodes into the leg muscles of dogs and planned to pass a d.c. current of 10 mA for 5 days which would be equivalent to pacing for 10 years with monophasic pulses. He found that stainless steel failed after only 6 hours, whereas platinum-iridium electrodes were unaffected after the 5 days. Platinum is now commonly used for the indifferent electrode, with a stainless steel wire cathode attached to the myocardium.

ELECTRICAL HAZARDS WITH CARDIAC PACEMAKERS

Since the use of cardiac pacemakers involves the attachment of one or more electrodes directly to the heart, particular care must be taken to see that currents capable of causing ventricular fibrillation are not passed through it. An obvious source of such current lies in leakage from mains powered apparatus. For this reason pacemaking equipment should be battery powered. Another hazard can arise from implanted coils and leads acting as an aerial and picking up signals from surgical diathermy during surgery, or other apparatus situated close to the patient during his work.

Although some workers, Kohler and Mackinney (1965), have reported that the use of surgical diathermy for example during prostatectomy, did not affect the pacemaker implanted in the patient, care must be exercised in the use of surgical diathermy under these circumstances. It would be best to avoid the use of diathermy altogether in patients with pacemakers, since Lichter, Borrie and Miller (1965) report the onset of ventricular fibrillation in 2 pacemaker patients induced by the use of surgical diathermy.

Carleton, Sessions and Graettinger (1964) tested 3 pacemakers and found that electrical interference was obtained only when the pacemakers were within 6 cm of the distributor of a car or within 30 cm of a therapeutic diathermy set (13·5 to 27 MHz). Kraft *et al* (1967) have carried out a detailed study of possible electrical influences on implanted pacemakers. Trouble arises from the induction currents from high-frequency electromagnetic fields which are rectified by transistor diodes. These can result in a shift of the transistor working points and a change in the pacing rate. Kraft *et al* make the following recommendations:

(1) At least 15 cm must be allowed between short-wave diathermy electrodes and the pacemaker and its electrodes, thus only the extremities should be irradiated.

(2) It is safe to be within the aerial area and in the transmitter room of medium- and short-wave radio stations and television stations if the distance from the output amplifier is not less than 50 cm. It is not safe to work on the transmitter.

(3) It is safe to work in a power station.

(4) It is safe to work in a radar station if the distance from the working set is not less than 1 m.

(5) It is safe to occupy a seat in the passenger cabin of an aircraft.

(6) It is safe to ride in a car, but not to adjust the engine while it is running.

(7) It is not safe to ride motor scooters.

(8) No effect was experienced from electric shavers, TV sets or X-ray machines.

The evidence as to the effect on implanted pacemakers of defibrillator currents is not conclusive. Norman (1964) mentions that a Lucas induction pacemaker had not been damaged when the patient concerned was defibrillated. Norman (1965) also found that the General Electric pacemaker would usually withstand the use of both a.c. and d.c. defibrillators. Kantrowitz (1964) and Cole and Yarrow (1964) respectively found that a General Electric and a Medtronic type 5860 implanted pacemaker withstood the use of a d.c. defibrillator.

RELIABILITY OF PACEMAKERS

Reliability figures for a complementary pair multivibrator pacemaker have been quoted by Glass (1965) as 0·01 per cent failure per 1,000 hours for each of 2 transistors, 2 capacitors and 5 batteries; as 0·001 per cent per 1,000 hours for each of 4 resistors, and as 0·0001 per cent per 1,000 hours for each of 30 soldered joints. The over-all reliability of the complete pacemaker as regards its electronic components alone is the sum of the separate reliabilities, that is, 0·097 per cent per 1,000 hours. On this basis, only one of 100 such pacemakers put into use should fail within one year. Blocking oscillator circuits differ in that they make use of a transformer. Greatbatch of Buffalo has determined the failure rate of a miniature transformer to be 0·16 per cent per 1,000 hours, and that of the batteries to be 0·025 per cent per 1,000 hours. He found the over-all electronic failure rate (excluding electrodes) to be 1·2 per cent per 1,000 hours. Rembert and Cooley (1967) discuss the radiologic appearance of satisfactory implanted pacemakers and those complications which can be detected by radiology, including malposition of the electrodes, fracture of the leads and battery exhaustion. Furman et al (1967) describe a pulse method for measuring the impedance of the myocardial electrode circuit in the patient. Van den Berg et al (1967) have developed a method of 'photo-analysis' to check the condition of implanted pacemakers and electrode circuits. It is based upon the fact that the voltage of the pacemaker signals across Einthoven leads is proportional to the current through the heart electrode circuit. Knuckey, Mcdonald and Sloman (1965) describe a method of evaluating the performance of a pacemaker in vivo by analysing the stimulus artefact produced by the generator. Green (1971) has developed a pacemaker frontal plane vector technique for following the condition of implanted pacemakers.

A greater reliability can be expected from the use of a 'thin film' construction. With this the electronic circuit is enclosed in a hermetically sealed unit and is safe from corrosion by leaking batteries or the ingress of body fluids. It also protects the components from mechanical stresses generated by the epoxy resin encapsulation.

The type TF thin film pacemaker by Devices Implants Ltd is illustrated in *Figure 10.8.*

BIO-ELECTRIC ENERGY SOURCES FOR CARDIAC PACEMAKERS

Implanted pacemakers, other than induction and radiofrequency types, require surgery for the replacement of their mercury batteries. This would not be necessary if the body itself could supply the power requirements of the pacemaker. Possible sources of this power are electro-chemical generators based on metabolic processes, and piezo-electric or electro-mechanical systems utilizing the motion of the ventricles.

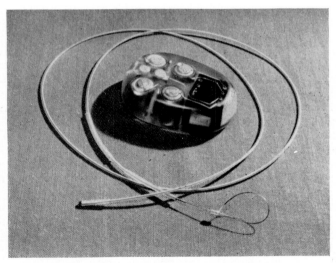

Figure 10.8. Thin film cardiac pacemaker. (Reproduced by courtesy of Devices Implants Ltd.)

Enger (1967) describes a three-gram batteryless pacemaker which is small enough to be placed on the surface of the left ventricle of a dog. The electrical output of the pacemaker is directed to the myocardium by 2 platinum electrodes which penetrate the ventricle to a depth of approximately 9 mm. The power is produced by the mechanical flexing of a piezo-electric bimorph. The internal impedance of such a generator is as high as 10 MΩ and it is not easy to insulate it from the conducting fluids of the body. Enger has found beeswax to be a suitable insulant, and that the motion of the right ventricle can produce enough power. Schaldach, Nasseri and Bucherl (1967) report on long-term experiments with an electro-chemical generator. Racine and Massie (1966) employ a pair of electrodes (one of platinum black, the other of high-speed steel) to supply 0·5–0·6 V d.c. to a capacitor. The electrode pair was buried in the myocardium of a patient. A pulser circuit connected the capacitor to a current amplifier, the output pulse of which was fed to a step-up transformer to provide a 1·5 to 3 V pulse which was applied to the heart. The pulse frequency was continuously adjustable in the range 60–200 per minute and the pulse width could be varied from 1 to 5 ms.

DEVELOPMENTS IN POWER SOURCES FOR CARDIAC PACEMAKERS

With conventional mercury cells the life of an implanted pacemaker is usually in the region of 24–30 months. Improvements in reducing the ingress of body fluids into the device have to be matched with power sources having a longer life expectancy. Greatbatch (1971) mentions two new types of primary cells having lithium anodes. The first uses a nickel sulphide cathode and an organic (propylene carbonate) electrolyte. The open-circuit voltage is 1·8 V. No gas is evolved during life so that the cell can be hermetically sealed. Preliminary tests have indicated an energy density which is greater than that of the conventional zinc–mercury cells normally used. The second cell is a lithium–iodine cell which is all solid-state in construction. The electrolyte is crystalline lithium iodide and the open circuit voltage is 2·8 V for a single cell. Both cells have a higher source impedance than the 6 ohms of a zinc–mercury cell. The lithium-nickel cell has a value of about 100 ohms whilst the lithium–iodine cell has about 1 kΩ at the start and 16 kΩ at the finish of life. Greatbatch (1971) gives the circuit of a pacemaker designed to work with a lithium–iodide cell. It is hoped to obtain a five-year life with these cells. The chemical capacity of conventional zinc–mercury cells used in pacemakers should be sufficient for three years or more. The average pacemaker life of 24 months is usually related to the corrosive liquid electrolyte (NaOH) since the cells cannot be hermetically sealed due to the evolution of hydrogen.

Other promising approaches are in the use of radioactive sources. One approach is based on the heat developed by the radioactive decay of a sealed 0·2g uranium-238 source. This is applied to a thermo-pile based on semiconductor bismuth telluride material. The thermo-

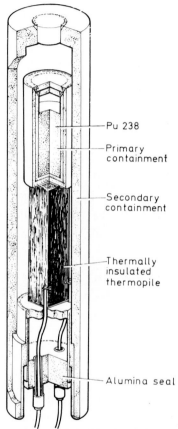

Pu 238

Primary containment

Secondary containment

Thermally insulated thermopile

Alumina seal

Figure 10.9. Isotope battery. (Reproduced by courtesy of the United Kingdom Atomic Energy Authority)

pile output voltage of about 0·4 is stepped up to 6 V to drive the pacemaker circuit by means of a d.c.-to-d.c. converter. The half-life of the isotope is 87 years and the expected life of the power unit is

311

10 years. The limitation arises because of the build-up of helium gas emanating from the source, and its sealed container has to be strong enough to contain the high pressure which is built up over a 10 year period. The container also provides shielding for the source. The use of a semiconductor thermopile offers the greatest efficiency at present, the power available being about 400 microwatts at 0·4 V into a 100Ω load. The ^{238}Pu is virtually a pure alpha emitter. It is housed as shown in *Figure 10.9.*

Another approach uses tritium (the radioactive isotope of hydrogen) which has a toxicity of approximately one five hundredth of plutonium-238, a low maximum energy of 18·1 ke V, and a half-life of 12·3 years. Beta particles emitted by the tritium are absorbed in a semiconductor diode. There, they lose energy liberating electron-hole pairs which induce a voltage and current flow across the junction. A practical device consists of several cells in series made by laminating tritiated zirconium foil with silicon diodes. Gatt (1971) mentions that a 200 micro-watt, 10-year life battery could be made to give 40 μA at 5 V with 0·5g of tritium chemically combined in a stable form and with a 4500 cm^2 diode junction area. The battery volume would be 15 cm^3 and its mass 100 g. Such betavoltaic devices are non-thermal in nature, but with the tritium source a pressure of 70 atmospheres is possible due to the evolution of helium.

IMPLANTED ELECTRONIC STIMULATORS FOR THE TREATMENT OF URINARY INCONTINENCE

By applying a continuous train of pulses to electrodes situated in the region of the bladder neck, Caldwell (1967) has shown that it is possible to restore continence in many cases both to male and female patients. It is preferable that electrical leads to the electrodes should not pass through the skin since this can lead to sepsis and therefore fibrosis, or the development of further fibrosis in an already damaged muscle which is working imperfectly. In order to overcome the problem of periodic battery replacement the complete stimulator is not implanted. As will be explained later a 'passive implant' system is employed, a radio frequency link being employed to provide stimuli from a generator external to the body.

Caldwell (1967) reports the treatment of 36 cases, 29 women and 7 men. Of the women, 28 suffered from stress incontinence and 1 was a multiple sclerotic. Of the men 4 were post-operative prostatectomy cases, 1 suffered from a spinal injury, 1 was incontinent following a proctocolectomy, and 1 was a senile incontinent. Of the 36 cases, 24 had a good result, one showed some improvement and 11 did not improve. Other accounts are those of Caldwell (1963 and 1965) and Caldwell, Flack and Broad (1965).

In women, Caldwell uses an operative approach which is retropubically down to the bladder neck. This is done through a vertical or transverse skin incision separating the recti muscles and approaching the retropubic space. A subcutaneous cave is fashioned to hold the implant. A small balloon attached to a water-filled catheter and pressure transducer is inserted into the urethra (James, 1968). The implant electrodes are placed on the bladder neck or the region of the anterior fibres of the levator. When the stimulus is applied the transducer will normally indicate a marked rise in pressure of the order of several tens of centimetres of water pressure. A single stitch may be used to fix the electrodes in position. The leads are then brought out through the rectus sheath, the muscles are sewn together and the implant placed in its cave. The stimulator box in its sterile towel is placed on the skin over the implant and the system tested once more. Ten days later when the wound has healed sufficiently, the stimulator box is gently approximated to the implant and held in place with adhesive plaster or placed in a pocket of a belt. In men, Caldwell places the electrodes either in the perineum or retropublically at the apex of the prostate. Technically, Caldwell finds the perineum to be the easier site. Good contraction of the water-filled balloon placed in the urethra in the sphincter region can usually be seen. The operative procedure and testing follows the same pattern as in women.

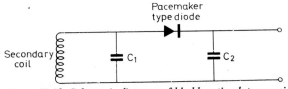

Figure 10.10. Schematic diagram of bladder stimulator passive implant

Commercially available stimulators for this type of work use a complementary pair multivibrator feeding a 1 MHz radiofrequency oscillator. The output circuit consists of a primary coil close to the skin. The circuit is powered by a PP3 9-V dry battery or by its rechargeable equivalent. The implant consists of a secondary pick-up coil tuned to 1 MHz by a capacitor C_1 in parallel (*Figure 10.10*). The resulting radiofrequency output is demodulated by the silicon diode, which is of the quality used in cardiac pacemakers, capacitor C_2 removing the bulk of the residual radiofrequency. The whole of this circuit is potted first in an epoxy resin and then covered with a biologically inert silicone rubber (Braley, 1967). The leads are made from a multi-start spiral of platinum-iridium wire wound on a Nylon core. When the implant feeds a load resistance of 150 Ω the output consists of 4-V pulses one millisecond wide at a repetition frequency of 20 Hz.

The pulser circuit and primary coil are encapsulated in epoxy resin and mounted in a single box together with the battery and an on-off switch. The battery thickness determines the depth of the box to be about 0·75 inch which many women patients find too prominent when it is placed on the centre of the abdomen. Some patients require a more powerful stimulus, so that the latest commercial design has the batteries and pulser circuit mounted in a separate box which can be worn by the patient in a more inconspicuous position, the primary coil being relatively flat and connected to the box by a flexible lead.

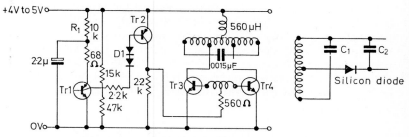

Figure 10.11. Circuit diagram of a pulser and radio frequency stages for exciting a passive bladder stimulator implant

An alternative circuit is that of Hill and Griffiths (1968) (*Figure 10.11*). The pulse repetition frequency of 20 per second is derived from a relaxation oscillator based upon the silicon controlled switch Tr_1. The 2·2 μF capacitor charges via R_1 until Tr_1 fires. This process takes about 50 ms. The capacitor discharges via the 68-ohm resistor and Tr_1 taking about 1 ms. Only during a pulse does Tr_2 draw current. Tr_3 and Tr_4 constitute a Baxandall Class D oscillator (Baxandall, 1959), base drive being applied from Tr_2. The 0·0015 μF capacitor tunes the over-winding of the transformer to approximately 900 kHz. Positive feedback is applied from the secondary winding

314

to the bases of Tr_3 and Tr_4. This circuit uses no high-value resistors so that thin film construction is a possibility. With a 4·5-V supply and a spacing of $\frac{3}{8}$ inch between the pulser primary coil and the implant, the implant delivered 4·5-V pulses into a 450-ohm load, or 3·5-V pulses into a 150-ohm load. The variation of output pulse amplitude with the separation between the pulser and implant is shown in *Figure 10.12(a)* and *Figure 10.12(b)* shows the variation

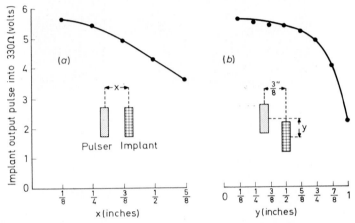

Figure 10.12.(a) The variation of the output pulse amplitude from a silicon switch type bladder stimulator with separation between pulser and implant

Figure 10.12(b) The variation in pulse amplitude at a constant spacing as the distance between centres of the pulser and implant is altered

in pulse amplitude at a constant spacing as the distance between centres of the pulser and implant is altered. The alignment of the pulser over the implant is seen not to be critical. The circuit will run for 30 hours from a 150-mAh rechargeable accumulator. If desired the circuit can be potted inside a rubber colostomy flange. *Figure 10.13* shows a commercial pulser unit and implant by Devices Implants Ltd, together with the silicon switch circuit constructed inside a plastic box and also inside a colostomy ring. For both these latter cases the separate battery box is not shown. A later commercial system in which the energizing coil is connected to the pulser box via a flying lead is shown in *Figure 10.14*.

During the pre-operative testing of patients it is usual to employ an external adjustable stimulator having a low output impedance

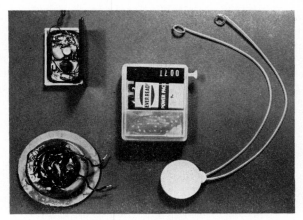

Figure 10.13. A commercial bladder stimulator by Devices Implants Ltd. together with a silicon switch circuit mounted in a plastic box and also inside a colostomy ring

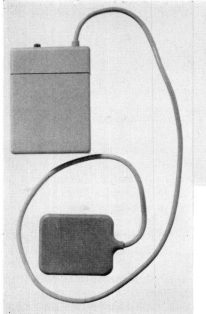

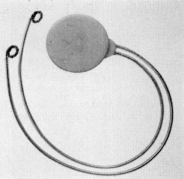

Figure 10.14. Bladder stimulator unit connected to its energizing coil via a flying lead. (Reproduced by courtesy of Devices Implants Ltd.)

316

and connected to a pair of needle electrodes placed in the perineum. In women, ball pointed electrodes may also be used mounted at the tips of a pair of tongs for use in the vagina. Lale (1966) describes the design of a suitable stimulator. This is also fitted with a radio-frequency output stage and plug-in coil for energizing bladder stimulator implants. A current meter is fitted, the current increasing as the implant draws power. It is useful to use this fact to check that there is no electronic failure when an implant is actually in a patient.

A detailed account of 14 cases fitted with radiofrequency type implants for the treatment of urinary incontinence is that of Alexander and Rowan (1968a). There were 10 women and 4 men the youngest being 23 years old and the oldest 77 years. Of the women, 8 suffered from 'stress incontinence' the remaining 2 women and 4 men suffered from 'neurogenic incontinence' (5 from upper motor and 1 from lower motor neurone disease). Alexander and Rowan first make two small incisions in the perineum over the inner aspect of each ischiopubic ramus and the periosteum is identified without attempting to visualize the pudendal nerves. A pair of probe electrodes connected to a stimulator are applied to locate the area of maximum perineal contraction and the loop electrodes of the implant are attached to the periosteum at this point by two un-absorbable sutures. The implant is energized by bringing up the pulser box and, if the resultant contraction is less than before, the electrodes are re-sited. The stimulator used by Alexander and Rowan (1968a) has two selectable output powers. At 'low' power, with a coupling distance of 0·5 inch a pulse amplitude of 4 V is developed across a load of 300 Ω. Under the same conditions but at the 'high' power setting the pulse amplitude is 7 V, in each case the pulse width is 1 ms and the repetition rate 20 per second. The aerial coil is taped to the skin over the implant, and the pulser box which measures $4\frac{1}{2} \times 3 \times 1$ inches is carried under the axilla in a holster. Of the 14 implants, 9 were judged to be successful. Four of the 8 stress incontinence patients were successfully treated. Five of the 6 neurogenic incontinent patients were successfully treated, the failure being the case of lower motor neurone disease in a man with in-complete traumatic paraplegia and completely flaccid perineal sphincter muscles.

In one of the patients of Alexander and Rowan (1968a), radiated interference from two household electrical appliances (a vacuum cleaner and a washing machine) was picked up by the implant and gave rise to a skin sensation similar to stimulation. The longest period for which an implant had been *in situ* in this series was 16 months.

Use of implanted stimulators to induce micturition in cases of neurogenic bladder

A much harder problem lies in the use of stimulators to evacuate the bladder in patients having a neurogenic bladder. The design of a radiofrequency stimulator for the treatment of urinary incontinence has much in common with that needed to induce micturition. References to the technique to be used with neurogenic bladders are Bradley *et al* (1962), Bradley, Chou and French (1963), Schamaun and Kantrowitz (1963), Glenn *et al* (1964), Boyce, Lathem and Hunt (1964), Hageman *et al* (1966), Stenberg, Burnet and Bunts (1967) and Talibi *et al* (1970).

Use of electronic pessary to control stress incontinence and urgency in women

An alternative approach in women to the use of a radiofrequency-powered implanted bladder sphincter stimulator is the use of an external stimulator connected to a pair of pessary-mounted electrodes (Alexander and Rowan 1968b; Hill *et al* 1968). Although the positioning of the pessary electrodes is not as precise as that possible with implanted electrodes, the pessary system offers the advantage of not requiring surgical intervention. For this reason it is well suited to out-patient control. Because the stimulus is applied directly to the electrodes via a flexible lead the cost of a transmitter-receiver unit is avoided. Since the entire unit is easily removeable, repairs or modifications can quickly be performed. If control of the incontinence can be achieved, the apparatus can be made available for another patient.

Hill *et al* (1968) used a correctly fitting pessary of either a Portex polythene ring type, or more usually a Hodge, Perspex type. The pessary is modified to hold two electrodes (*Figure 10.15*) each consisting of 4 turns of 0·020 inch diameter silver wire spaced over a distance of 7 mm. The spacing between the electrodes varies between 15 and 25 mm depending upon the size of the pessary. The electrodes are connected to a flexible double plastic covered wire of the type used in hearing aids. The distal end of the wire terminates in a miniature socket which mates with a corresponding plug on the stimulator. This comprises a complementary-pair multivibrator circuit powered from either a pair of mercury cells or a rechargeable miniature accumulator. The life of the mercury cells is at least 14 days. The output pulses from the stimulator have the following characteristics when measured across a 200-ohm load: repetition rate 20 per second, amplitude 5 to 6 V, width 5 ms. A switch is provided for use when the stimulator is not used at night, otherwise it is left switched on permanently. Patients are able to micturate as desired without difficulty when the device is operational. The stimulator box can be worn inconspicuously by carrying it in a pocket provided in a pair of briefs. A pessary of the correct

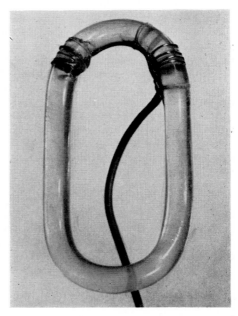

Figure 10.15 Polythene Hodge pessary carrying two silver wire electrodes

size for the patient concerned is first selected and the electrodes subsequently attached. The pessary is then inserted so that the electrodes lie anteriorly against the region of the bladder-urethral junction. The patients can be trained in douching and to be able to remove and re-inert the pessary so that it occupies the same position. Normally no difficulty is experienced in wearing the pessary throughout menstruation. When the pessary is first used the patient may be conscious of a slight sensation of 'vibration'. The siting of the electrodes is important, and some degree of experiment may be required in order to determine the most effective type of pessary and electrode placing. When tried on patients who have undergone

319

much surgery in the region of the bladder neck, it may be found that the electronic pessary is rendered ineffective due to the stimulus now being directed towards fibrous tissue. Alexander and Rowan (1968b) employed a stimulus of 12 V, 1 ms at 20 pulses per second.

Vincent (1972) describes an interesting technique in the form of, a 'demand' stimulation of the sphincter mechanism. Sensing electrodes, mounted on a vaginal pessary or anal plug, detect or sense EMG activity due to pelvic floor potentials. The circuit stimulates for 2 seconds and then looks for EMG potentials in excess of 100 μV. If these are detected the sensing mode lasts for only 150 ms and the stimulus is again applied. If the potentials have fallen below 100 μV then the unit continues waiting in the sense mode. Thus, coughing or straining can automatically apply the stimulus to the anal canal or vaginal wall via the same electrodes which were used for sensing. Spread of the stimulus affects the voluntary urethral sphincter mechanism. Patients with urgency and frequency due to certain causes can be taught to actuate the stimulator as they require it by voluntary effort.

Edwards *et al.* (1971) describe the operation of a clinic for the investigation and treatment of resistant urinary incontinence. They state that a patient's incontinence must be clearly defined as being primarily due to either sphincter disturbance or detrusor dysfunction. The following investigations are undertaken: (1) physical examination, including a careful neurological examination; (2) electromyographic studies of the legs and perineum; (3) cystometrogram; (4) urethral pressure profile (Brown and Wickham, 1969; Harrison and Constable, 1970); (5) pressure flow study; (6) examination under anaesthesia—which includes urethral pressure profile and a cystometrogram—both of these investigations being undertaken in conjunction with perineal stimulation of the pelvic floor; (7) intravenous pyelogram; and (8) micturating cystometrogram.

One of the problems encountered in the assessment of the degree of incontinence present in a given patient is the amount of urine which has leaked away James *et al.* (1971) describe an ingenious 'nappy' which is fitted with electrodes between which is passed a low voltage alternating current. The deposition of urine into the nappy reduces the electrical conductivity between the electrodes which can be related to the urine volume.

Choice of material for pessary electrodes

Alexander and Rowan (1968b) employed stainless steel for their electrode material, while Hill *et al* (1968) used silver wire. Electron microscope studies of these materials pulsed in saline reveal that both metals are electrolytically attacked. In the case of silver wire the attack occurs preferentially along the lines formed during the drawing down of the wire. The deposit is silver chloride. With stainless steel the attack occurs at the grain boundaries, a brown deposit forming on the negative electrode and a suspension of rust forming close to this electrode. Platinum is not affected by the pulsing and is the electrode material of choice. This is confirmed from the reported experiences of workers with cardiac pacemakers (Siddons and Sowton 1967).

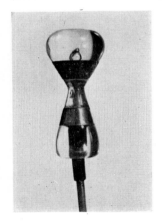

Figure 10.16. Anal plug and control box. (Reproduced by courtesy of Cardiac Recorders Ltd.)

THE USE OF AN ANAL PLUG

Another useful approach, particularly in men, is to apply stimulus pulses to the anus by means of a so-called anal plug. This consists of a dumb-bell shaped plastic moulding carrying a pair of cylindrical metal strip electrodes (*Figure 10.16*). One manufacturer supplies 3 sizes of plug. A flexible cable leads from the plug to the control box which can be placed in a pocket or clipped to a belt. The box is powered from a 9-V battery or rechargeable cell and delivers 1 ms-wide pulses of up to about 7 V in amplitude. A variable amplitude control is provided so that the patient can adjust the strength of the stimulus. The pulse repetition rate provided by one commercial system is 100 per second.

The use of an anal plug stimulator was recommended by Hopkinson and Lightwood (1967) for the treatment of anal incontinence with a pulse repetition frequency of 80 per second. However, it has also

321

proved to be effective in the treatment of urinary incontinence in cases of post-prostatectomy incontinence and urinary diversion (Riddle, Hill and Wallace 1969). While some patients find it convenient to wear the plug continuously, in many cases it is sufficient to wear the plug for only a few hours per day. This reduces the possibility of fatiguing the rectal muscles. The stainless steel electrodes should be cleaned regularly with a metal polish.

SOME OTHER CLINICAL APPLICATIONS OF IMPLANTED CIRCUITS

Currently interest is widening in the therapeutic applications of implanted stimulator circuits. This is consequent upon the availability of reliable power supplies and microcircuitry. Dunning (1972) has described the use of an implanted circuit to stimulate the carotid sinus nerves in man in order to produce a fall in arterial blood pressure and a decrease in peripheral vascular tone to relieve angina pectoris even in cases which cannot be managed by drug therapy. The stimulator provided a pulse rate variable between 20 and 200 per second with a pulse amplitude of between 1 and 6 V and a pulse width of 350 μs. The implant was passive in nature with a radio frequency transmitter external to the body.

Nashold, Somjen and Friedman (1972) have been making use of a passive implant and radio frequency transmitter to stimulate the spinal cord dorsal columns in order to relieve certain patients of otherwise uncontrollable pain. The stimulus frequency could be varied from 9 to 55 V per second with a pulse width of 300 μs and an amplitude variable from 0·3 to 30 V.

REFERENCES

Pacemakers

Abrahms, L. D. and Norman, J. C. (1964). 'Experience with inductive coupled cardiac pacemakers.' *Ann. N.Y. Acad. Sci.* **111**, 1030
— Hudson, W. A. and Lightwood, R. (1960). 'A surgical approach to the management of heart block using an inductive coupled artificial pacemaker.' *Lancet* **1**, 1372
Berg, J. V. van den (1964). 'Techniek van Pacemakers.' *Ned. Tijdschr. geneesk.* **108**, 2003
— Rodrigo, F. A., Thalen, H. J. T. and Koops, J. (1967). 'Photoanalysis of the condition of implanted pacemakers and electrode circuits.' *Proc. K. ned. Akad. Wet. Sec. C.* **70**, 419
Bleese, N., Kalmar, P., Harms, H., Rodewald, G., and Westermann, K. W. (1972). 'Implanted cardiac pacemakers; clinical experience and evaluation.' *Med. Prog. through technol.* **1**, 69

Bluestone, R., Davies, G., Harris, A., Leatham, A and Siddons, H. (1965). 'Long-term endocardial pacing for heart block.' *Lancet* **2**, 307

Braley, S. (1967). 'The silicones in clinically-orientated bio-engineering.' In *Engineering in the Practice of Medicine*. p. 159. Ed. by B. L. Segal and D. C. Kilpatrick. Baltimore; Williams and Wilkins

Cammilli, L., Pozzi, R., Drago, G., Pizzichi, G. and de Saint-Pierre, G. (1964). 'Radio-frequency pacemaker with receiver coil implanted on the heart.' *Ann. N.Y. Acad. Sci.* **111**, 1007

Carlens, E., Johansson, L., Karlof, I. and Lagergren, H. (1965). 'New method for atrial-triggered pacemaker treatment without thoracotomy.' *J. thorac. cardiovasc. Surg.* **50**, 229

Carleton, R. A., Sessions, R. W. and Graettinger, J. S. (1964). 'Environmental influence on implantable cardiac pacemakers.' *J. Am. med. Ass.* **190**, 938

Center, S., Nathan, D., Wu, C-Y, Samet, P. and Keller, W. (1963). 'The implantable synchronous pacer in the treatment of complete heart block.' *J. thorac. cardiovasc. Surg.* **46**, 744

Chardack, W., Frederico, A. and Gage, A. (1965). 'Pacemaker leads routed down jugular.' *Wld. med. J.* **1**, 46

Cole, D. W. and Yarrow, S. (1964). 'Artificial electrical pacing for heart block: A review based on 24 cases treated with implanted pacemakers.' *N.Z. med. J.* **63**, 126

Davies, J. G. (1962). 'Artificial cardiac pacemakers for the long-term treatment of heart block.' *J. Br. Instr. Radio. Engng.* **24,** 453

— Siddons, H. (1965). 'Experience with implanted pacemakers: technical considerations.' *Thorax* **20**, 128

— Sowton, G. E. (1966). 'Electrical threshold of the human heart.' *Br. Heart J.* **28**, 231

Enger, C. C. (1967). 'A piezoelectrically powered three gram pacemaker.' *Digest of 7th Int. Conf. Med. and Biol. Engng. Stockholm.* p. 79.

Furman, S., and Schwedel, J. B. (1959). 'An intracardiac pacemaker for Stokes-Adams seizures.' *New Engl. J. Med.* **261**, 943

— Parker, B., Escher, D. J. W. and Schweidel, J. B. (1967). 'Instruments for evaluating function of cardiac pacemakers.' *Med. Res. Engng.* **6**, 29

Gatt, F. C. (1971). 'A tritium pacemaker battery design.' *Digest, 9th Int. Conf. Med. biol. Engng.*, Melbourne, 278

Glass, H. I. (1965). 'Problems associated with the design of implantable electronic devices.' In *Resuscitation and Cardiac Pacing*. Proc. Conf. Glasgow, March 1964. p. 207

Glenn, W. W. L., Hageman, J. H., Mauro, A., Eisenberg, L., Flanigan, S, and Harvard, M. (1964). 'Electrical stimulation of excitable tissue by radio frequency transmission.' *Ann. Surg.* **160,** 338

Goetz, R. H. (1963). 'Bipolar catheter electrode as temporary pacemaker in Stokes–Adams syndrome.' *Surgery Gynec. Obstet.* **116**, 712

— Dormandy, J. A. and Berkovits, B. (1966). 'Pacing on demand in the treatment of atrioventricular conduction disturbances of the Heart.' *Lancet* **2**, 599

Greatbatch, W. (1971). 'A new pacemaking system utilizing a long-life lithium cell.' *Digest of 9th Int. Conf. Med. and Biol. Engng. Melbourne.* p. 79.

Green, G. D. (1971). 'Assessment of cardiac pacemakers: pacemaker frontal plane vectors.' *Am. Heart. J.* **81,** 1

Jaron, D., Schwann, H. P. and Gesolowitz, D. B. (1968). 'A mathematical model for the polarization impedance of cardiac pacemaker electrodes.' *Med. Electron. biol. Engng.* **6,** 579

Kahn, A. R., and Mavens, T. C. (1972). 'Technical Aspects of Electrical Stimulation Devices.' *Med. Prog. through technol.* **1,** 58

Kantrowitz, A. (1964). 'Problems in the clinical use of implantable pacemakers.' *J. cardiovasc. Surg.* **5,** 668

Knuckey, L., Mcdonald, R., and Sloman, G. (1965). 'A method of testing implanted cardiac pacemakers.' *Br. Heart J.* **27,** 483

Kohler, F. P. and Mackinney, C. C. (1965). 'Cardiac pacemakers in electro-surgery.' *J. Am. med. Ass.* **193,** 855

Kraft, D., Emmrich, K., Gunther, K. and Ursinus, K. (1967). 'Physical influences on heart pacemakers.' *Digest 7th Int. Conf. Med. and Biol. Engng. Stockholm. p.* 70

Lagergren, H., Johansson, L., Landegren, J. and Edhag, O. (1965). 'One hundred cases of treatment for Adams–Stokes syndrome with permanent intravenous pacemaker.' *J. thorac. cardiovasc. Surg.* **50,** 710

Lichter, I., Borrie, J. and Miller, W. M. (1965). 'Radio-frequency hazards with cardiac pacemakers.' *Br. med. J.* **1,** 1513

Lillehei, C. W., Levy, M. J., Bonnabeau, R. C., Long, D. M. and Sellers, R. D. (1964). 'The use of a myocardial electrode and pacemaker in the management of acute postoperative and postinfarction complete heart block.' *Surgery* **56,** 463

Neville, J., Millar, K., Keller, W. and Abidskov, J. A., (1966). 'An implantable demand pacemaker.' *Clin. Res.* **14,** 256

Norman, J. C. (1964). *Ann. N.Y. Acad. Sci.* **111,** 1044 (Discussion)

— (1965). *J. thorac. cardiovasc. Surg.* **50,** 866 (Discussion)

Racine, P. and Massie, H. L. (1966). 'An experimental internally powered cardiac pacemaker.' *Med. Res. Engng.* **5,** 24

Rembert, F. M. and Cooley, R. N. (1967). 'Implantable cardiac pacemakers: radiologic appearance.' *Tex. Med.* **63,** 72

Rowley, B. A. (1963). 'Electrolysis—a factor in cardiac pacemaker electrode failure.' *I.E.E.E. Trans. biomed. Engng.* **10,** 176

Rodewald, G., Giebel, O., Harms, H. and Scheppakat, K. T. (1964). 'Intravenös-Intakardiale Applikation von vorhofgesteurten elektrischen Schrittmachern.' *Z. Kreislaufforsch.* **53,** 860

Schaldach, M., Nasseri, M., and Bucherl, E. S. (1967). 'Bioelectric energy sources for cardiac pacemakers.' *Thoraxchirurgie,* **15,** 608

Schuder, J. C. and Stoeckle, H. (1962). 'A micromodule pacemaker receiver for direct attachment to the ventricle.' *Trans. Am. Soc. artif. internal Organs* **10,** 366

Senning, A. (1964). 'Problems in the use of pacemakers.' *J. cardiovasc. Surg.* **46,** 259

Siddons, A. H. M. (1963). 'Long-term artificial cardiac pacing: experience in adults with heart block.' *Ann. R. Coll. Surg.* **32,** 22

— Sowton, E. (1967). *Cardiac Pacemakers.* Springfield; Thomas

Thevenet, A., Hodges, P. C. and Lillehei, C. W. (1958). 'The use of a myocardial electrode inserted percutaneously for control of complete atrio-ventricular block by an artificial pacemaker.' *Dis. Chest* **34,** 621

Zoll, P. M., Linenthal, A. J. and Zarsky, L. R. N. (1960). 'Ventricular fibrillation—treatment and prevention by external electric currents.' *New Eng. med. J.* **262**, 105

Bladder, anal and other stimulators

Alexander, S. and Rowan D. (1968a). 'Electrical control of urinary incontinence by radio implant.' *Br. J. Surg.* **55**, 358

— — (1968b). 'An electronic pessary for stress incontinence.' *Lancet* **1**, 728

Baxandall, P. J. (1959). 'Transistor sine-wave c.c. oscillators.' *Proc. Instn. elect. Engrs.* **106**, 748

Boyce, W. H., Lathem, J. E. and Hunt, L. D. (1964). 'Research related to the development of an artificial electrical stimulator for the paralyzed human bladder: review.' *J. Urol.* **91**, 41

Bradley, W. E., Chou, S. N. and French, L. A. (1963). 'Further experience with the radio transmitter receiver unit for the neurogenic bladder.' *J. Neurosurg.* **20**, 953

— Wittmers, L. E., Chou, S. N. and French, L. A. (1962). 'Use of a radio transmitter receiver unit for the treatment neurogenic bladder'. *J. Neurosurg.* **19**, 782

Braley, S. (1967). 'The silicones in clinically-orientated bioengineering.' In *Engineering in the Practice of Medicine.* p. 159. Ed. by B. L. Segal and D. G. Kilpatrick. Baltimore; Williams and Wilkins.

Brown, M., and Wickham, J. E. A. (1969). 'The urethral pressure profile.' *Br. J. Urol.*, **41**, 211

Caldwell, K. P. S. (1963). 'The electrical control of sphincter incompetence.' *Lancet* **2**, 174

— (1965). 'A new treatment for rectal prolapse.' *Proc. R. Soc. Med.* **58**, 792

— (1967). 'The treatment of incontinence by electronic implants.' *Ann. R. Coll. Surg.* **40**, 447

— Flack, F. C. and Broad, A. F. (1965). 'Urinary incontinence following spinal injury treated by electronic implant.' *Lancet* **1**, 846

Edwards, L., Harrison, N. W., and Williams, J. P. (1971). 'Investigation and treatment of resistant urinary incontinence.' *Br. med. J.*, **1**, 543

Dunning, A. J. (1972). 'Electrical Stimulation of the Carotid Sinus Nerves.' *Med. Prog. through technol.* **1**, 75

Glenn, W. W. L., Hageman, J. H., Mauro, A., Eisenberg, L., Flanagan, S. and Harvard, M. (1964). 'Electrical stimulation of excitable tissue by radio-frequency transmission.' *Ann. Surg.* **160**, 338

Hageman, J., Flanigan, S., Harvard, B. M. and Glenn, W. W. L. (1966). 'Electromicturition by radiofrequency stimulation.' *Surgery Gynec. Obstet.* **123**, 807

Harrison, N. W., and Constable, A. R. (1970). 'Urethral pressure measurement: a modified technique.' *Br. J. Urol.* **42**, 229

Hill, D. W., and Griffiths, C. A. (1968). 'An electronic stimulator for the treatment of urinary incontinence.' *Br. J. Urol.* **40**, 187

— Mable, S. E. R., Wallace, D. M. and Dewhurst, C. J. (1968). 'Electronic pessary for incontinence.' *Lancet* **2**, 112

Hopkinson, B. R. and Lightwood, R., (1967). 'Electrical treatment of incontinence.' *Br. J. Surg.* **54**, 802

James, E. D. (1968). 'Equipment and methods involved in the treatment of urinary incontinence by electronic stimulation.' *Med. Electron. biol. Engng.* **6**, 595

— Flack, F. C., Caldwell, K. P. S., and Martin, M. R. (1971). 'Continuous measurement of urine loss and frequency in incontinence patients.' *Br. J. Urol.* **43,** 233

Lale, P. G. (1966). 'Muscular contraction by implanted stimulators.' *Med. Electron. biol. Engng.* **4,** 319

Nashold, B. S., Jnr., Somjen, G., and Friedman, M. (1972). 'The Effects of Stimulating the Dorsal Columns of Man.' *Med. Prog. through Technol.* **1,** 89

Riddle, P. R., Hill, D. W. and Wallace, D. M. (1969). 'Electronic techniques for the control of adult urinary incontinence.' *Br. J. Urol.* **41,** 205

Schamaun, M. and Kantrowitz, A. (1963). 'Evacuation of the chronic cord bladder by a radio-linked stimulator.' *Surg. Forum* **14,** 491

Siddons, H. and Sowton, E. (1967). *Cardiac Pacemakers.* Springfield; Thomas

Stenberg, C. C., Burnette, H. W. and Bunts, R. C. (1967). 'Electrical stimulation of human neurogenic bladders: experience with 4 patients.' *J. Urol.* **97,** 79

Talibi, M. A., Drolet, R., Kunov, H., and Robson, C. J. (1970). 'A model for studying the electrical stimulation of the urinary bladder of dogs.' *Br. J. Urol.* **42,** 56

Vincent, S. A. (1972). 'The engineering approach to the study of bladder control.' In *Biomedical Technology in Hospital Diagnosis,* Ed. by A. T. Elder and D. W. Neill, p. 453. Oxford; Pergamon

11 –Surgical Diathermy Apparatus and Electrical Safety Precautions in the Operating Room

Apart from the patient-monitoring equipment, the most commonly encountered electrical apparatus in the operating room is the surgical diathermy unit. If routine safety precautions are not observed it is possible for the patient to suffer a diathermy burn, and there is always the possibility of the diathermy igniting an explosive anaesthetic agent. Finally, it is quite likely that the operation of the diathermy will upset the performance of any patient-monitoring units that may be connected to the patient. For all these reasons, it is necessary that surgeons and anaesthetists should be familiar with the operating principles of surgical diathermy units and of the safety precautions required when electrical apparatus (particularly if it is mains powered) is connected to a patient.

SURGICAL DIATHERMY UNITS

In essence, a surgical diathermy unit consists of a radiofrequency power oscillator. Current practice uses valve oscillators, but older diathermy sets consisted of spark gap oscillators. Although spark-gap sets are being steadily replaced by valve units, they are very robust and many are still giving good service.

Spark-gap surgical diathermy units

In a typical spark-gap set, *Figure 11.1*, the 1500 V r.m.s. secondary winding of the mains power transformer is applied across two spark-gaps in series. The metal rods forming the gaps are fitted with fins in order to dissipate heat. The spark-gaps are in parallel with a series-tuned circuit consisting of two mica capacitors and a· tapped

327

inductor. During each half cycle of the mains the voltage from the 1500 V winding steadily rises, charging the capacitors. When the voltage becomes sufficiently high to break down the gaps, sparking occurs, and the capacitors discharge through the coil. As the current dies away the back e.m.f. produced in the inductance drives current in the reverse direction back into the capacitors. Hence while the gaps are conducting, radiofrequency oscillations are generated by the tuned circuit. The power drawn from this radiofrequency 'tank' circuit can be varied by altering the tapping point on the inductor.

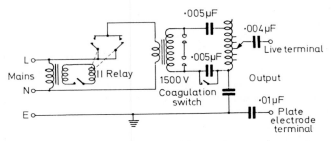

Figure 11.1. Circuit diagram of a typical spark-gap surgical diathermy set

The mica coupling capacitor connected to the tapping point prevents any d.c. voltage from getting to the patient. The voltage across the gaps rises to a peak twice per cycle of the a.c. mains, so the output waveform of this type of diathermy apparatus consists of trains of damped radiofrequency oscillations produced at 10 millisecond intervals. The capacitors in the tuned circuits are each of 0·005 μF capacity. When they are both in series in the circuit the effective capacity becomes 0·0025 μF. This is the condition when the diathermy set is used for cutting and the frequency is basically about 450 kHz. For coagulation, one capacitor is shorted out and the frequency falls to about 350 kHz. Power is applied from the mains to the transformer primary by means of a relay operated via a 6-V secondary winding from the surgeon's foot switch. This arrangement keeps the mains voltage away from the foot switch which is likely to be situated on a wet floor. The maximum output power available is of the order of 150 W into a load of 150 Ω. The complete diathermy unit is mounted inside a sealed cabinet to prevent the ingress of explosive agents such as cyclopropane.

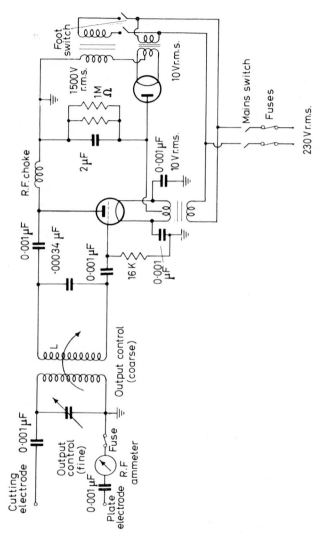

Figure 11.2. Circuit diagram of a low-power valve surgical diathermy set

329

Thermionic valve diathermy sets

The simplest type of valve diathermy set consists of a power oscillator such as the circuit of *Figure 11.2*. The power output can be varied by altering the spacing and hence the mutual inductance between the coil L of the anode tuned circuit and the coupling coil feeding the output circuit. The frequency of oscillation for valve sets lies in the range 1–3 MHz. In the majority of valve diathermy sets, in order to save cost, a separate rectifier valve is not provided for the oscillator H.T. supply. Instead, the valve is fed from the raw high voltage secondary winding of the mains power transformer. The valve can only pass current when its anode is positive to its cathode so that it acts as its own rectifier. Thus the output waveform from this type of unit consists of bursts of radiofrequency oscillation at a repetition rate of 50 Hz. The fact that the output is modulated 100 per cent at 50 Hz makes this type of set, and spark-gap sets, liable to cause a great deal of interference to monitoring equipment such as electroencephalographs and electrocardiographs. This will be mentioned in more detail in a later paragraph.

With the simpler types of valve circuit just described, provision is made to use a lower impedance tapping point from the tuned circuit during coagulation. This results in a better power transfer to the larger electrodes now used.

More sophisticated diathermy units consist of a main power oscillator generating up to 500 watts at 1·75 MHz with a sine waveform into a 150-ohm load. A separate rectifier and smoothing is provided for the h.t. supply to the oscillator. The radio frequency output can be modulated at either 60 kHz or 20 kHz to give bursts of current.

The straight sine wave output is used for the smooth cutting of tissues in air or under water without fulguration. Sufficient power is available to cut even heavy layers of fatty or muscle tissue. When the 60 kHz modulation is used, different effects are obtained depending upon the type of electrode used. For cutting and coagulation, cutting electrodes produce a fulgurized cut which bleeds very little. The coagulation action prevents contamination with cellular material or bacteria and the ingress of toxic substances by closing the capillaries and lymph channels. When special coagulation electrodes such as plates or balls are employed, the 60 kHz modulation can be used in tumour surgery to seal larger blood vessels or to fulgurate tissue sections. The 20 kHz modulation gives a very good coagulating action, similar to that found with spark-gap generators. It is used for coagulation without cutting and is good for closing up areas of small seeping blood vessels, in conjunction with cutting electrodes such as resection loops and needles. The small cutting action of the 20 kHz modulated signal prevents any undesirable penetration of the electrodes into the tissue to be coagulated. For cutting under water, the modulation frequency is still further reduced to 50 Hz. In some units, two independent outputs are provided; both the waveform and intensity can be set separately for each. Eight steps of

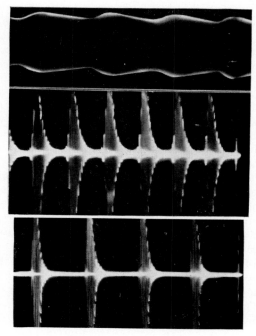

Figure 11.3. Output waveforms from a valve diathermy unit. Upper: continuous sine wave, middle and lower: pulsed waveforms for cutting with coagulation. (Reproduced by courtesy of the Transformatoren und Röntgenwerk, Dresden)

intensity can be provided for each channel and provision may be made to reduce automatically the current when working with small electrodes. Dobbie (1969) gives a detailed account of the output waveforms produced by both valve and spark-gap diathermy sets. *Figure 11.3* shows typical output waveforms for a modulated valve generator.

331

BURNS FROM DIATHERMY SETS

The main causes of patients receiving burns from the surgical diathermy set arise from a fault in the indifferent plate electrode or in the cable to this electrode. It will be recalled that the high potential terminal of the radiofrequency output leads, via a cable, to the surgeon's cutting needle which is mounted in an insulated handle. When the arc is struck, the high current density at the tip of the needle gives rise to intense local heating and the cutting action. The low potential terminal of the diathermy unit is connected to the patient usually via a cable connected to a lead plate electrode. The plate is wrapped in a cloth bag soaked in saline solution and strapped on to the patient's thigh. Although the same current passes through the plate electrode as goes through the needle, the current density at the plate is much less, so that no heating occurs here if the contact impedance between the plate and the patient's body is low. This is so when the plate is flat and the covering wet. However if the lead plate has become ridged due to bending or the cloth covering has been allowed to dry out, then the contact impedance may become sufficiently high for enough heat to be generated to give rise to a burn. It is important that the condition of the plate and its covering be checked regularly. An alternative is to use a 0·008-inch thick stainless steel flexible plate without any covering. The plate is springy and can be placed under the patient easily. No covering is necessary since a film of perspiration forms between the plate and the patient's body. For work with infants, a sheet of 0·005-inch thick aluminium foil can be used. This is not sufficiently opaque to prevent a radiograph being taken through it.

Apart from a faulty contact with the plate electrode, another fault can arise due to a broken lead connecting the set to the plate electrode. When this happens the patient's body may attain a radiofrequency potential of 100–150 V r.m.s. If, say, the patient's hand or foot makes a loose contact with an earthed object, sufficient current may pass to cause a burn. There is the possibility of a capacitive current flowing without a direct contact to an earthed body, and the possibility of any member of the operating room staff getting a shock if he happens to touch the patient under these conditions while touching an earthed object. Many diathermy sets incorporate a simple system for monitoring the continuity of the plate electrode lead. Two leads may be connected to the plate and a low d.c. current passed through the leads. If an open circuit occurs an audible and visible alarm is activated. Some manufacturers are now producing a disposable metal foil plate electrode with two metal foil leads connected to it. This electrode can be used with a separate alarm unit for fitting to older diathermy sets which do not have built-in plate electrode monitoring facilities. This simple continuity arrangement will not sound an alarm if the plate electrode has not been attached to the patient, or has accidentally fallen from under the patient. It is better to use two entirely separate plate electrodes and cables, one under the back and the other under the buttocks of the patient. The chances of both electrodes being forgotten or falling off, or of both cables breaking are obviously small.

In current (1973) practice, the plate electrode is no longer connected directly to earth, but is connected via a capacitor situated inside the diathermy set to the earth terminal of the set. This capacitor is an 0·01 μF mica type having a high working voltage and a good insulation resistance. Its impedance is 0·3 MΩ at 50 Hz and 30 Ω at 400 kHz. Thus the plate is effectively returned to earth at radio-frequencies but not at d.c., so that the risk to the patient of receiving a dangerous shock as a result of a fault arising in the earthing of any apparatus connected to him is minimized.

Dobbie (1968) reports that of 13 cases of diathermy burns coming to his attention during 1966/67, six appeared to be due to the use of a dry saline pad on the plate electrode. In 5 cases the burns appeared to be due to the surgeon's diathermy needle being placed on the patient while the foot switch was accidently activated. One case of a burn on the patient's thigh was reported by the surgeon concerned as arising from a broken plate lead. A case of a burn at the external meatus of the penis was also reported by the surgeons as being due to a broken plate electrode lead. However, investigation revealed that the cause of this burn was faulty insulation of the resectoscope. The 6 cases of burns due to the dry saline pad could have been eliminated by the use of a bright-metal plate electrode, and the 5 cases of burns arising from accidental activation of the foot switch would not have occurred if the surgeon's electrode holder had been fitted with a finger switch.

Another source of burns to patients can arise from the action of the diathermy arc in setting on fire drapes and towels lying on the patient's skin. The risk is, of course, increased if surgical spirit has fallen on the material. In this case it is possible for the spirit to catch fire beneath a loose drape.

ELECTRICAL INTERFERENCE FROM DIATHERMY SETS

Radiated interference from surgical diathermy sets to apparatus at a distance is not normally a problem as the length of the radio-frequency leads attached to a set is but a small fraction of the wavelength (150 m for a frequency of 2 MHz). When it is necessary to operate sensitive recording apparatus such as an electroencephalo-graph close to the operating room then the level of interference can usually be reduced to an acceptable level by simple R-C filters attached to each electrode and also at the input to each amplifier. The filter arrangement is illustrated in *Figure 11.4* where the series resistors have a value of 1 kΩ each and the shunt capacitors are each 330 pF (Dobbie 1965).

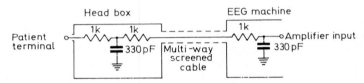

Figure 11.4. R-C filter network for use with an EEG machine in the presence of radiated interference from a surgical diathermy unit (after Dobbie, 1965)

The problems involved in recording signals continuously, such as the ECG from a patient undergoing surgery, while the diathermy is in use are more severe since the diathermy signal will be several thousand times greater than the wanted signal in amplitude. In the case of those older sets which use the oscillator valve also as the rectifier for the power supply, the output is 100 per cent modulated at the mains frequency. The galvanometers of the recording system are unable to respond to the radio frequency, but can be overloaded and damaged by the 50 Hz modulation signal. It may prove to be impracticable to obtain a sufficiently high degree of filtering of the radio frequency for this type of set as in the case of spark-gap sets. In order to prevent possible damage to the recording pens, Mapleson (1961) has used a simple radio receiver to pick up the diathermy set's radiation. The signal from the receiver is caused to actuate a relay which substitutes dummy-load resistors in place of the recording pens.

With a diathermy set having a sine-wave output the problems are eased, and the leads to the ECG apparatus can be run into a screened filter box which connects via a screened multi-way cable to the recorder. Each lead passes through an L-C filter, the radiofrequency chokes wound on ferrite cores giving a better rejection than the resistors previously used. A considerable radiofrequency signal is often passed back from the diathermy set along the mains cable and thus gets into recording equipment which is also connected to the mains. An efficient radiofrequency filter unit should be fitted to the mains outlet socket for the diathermy equipment.

The author recently encountered an interesting case of severe 50 Hz interference blotting out the ECG recording from a patient during surgery as soon as the plate electrode was connected to the patient's thigh. This happened even when the diathermy set was switched off but plugged into the mains. The trouble was traced to the fact that the mains plug had been wired incorrectly, the earth and neutral being interchanged. On another unit two cables connected the diathermy set to the plate electrode. Interference was experienced from the low-voltage 50 Hz current passed through them continuously to check for a break in the cable.

When making measurements of radiofrequency currents and voltages in connection with studies on surgical diathermy sets, Dobbie (1968) advocates the use of low-impedance radiofrequency thermocouple type meters. This avoids the pick-up of unwanted signals with high-impedance devices such as cathode-ray tube oscilloscopes. Typical radiofrequency currents into the patient during cutting will be in the range 100–400 mA r.m.s. It is very difficult to measure the power delivered into tissue while cutting as the charring producd rapidly alters the contact impedance with the needle electrode and thus the current.

Although a pure radiofrequency would not directly affect the recording pens it could cause a severe overloading of the signal amplifiers. As a result of working in a non-linear portion of their characteristics, rectification of the radiofrequency wave can occur, the resulting d.c. signal deflecting the pens off scale.

THE USE OF SCREENED ROOMS

When high-gain amplifiers are to be used, particularly with cathode-ray tube displays, in the presence of strong radiated interference signals, the only satisfactory solution may be to conduct the work in a screened room. This should be made from a fine mesh wire-netting mounted on a wooden frame and earthed at only one point to a plate buried in the ground. Particular care should be paid to the bonding of the mesh sheets and to ensuring that flexible metal strips at the edges of the door make good contact with similar strips on the frame when the door is shut. The mains supply to the room should be well filtered from radiofrequency signals and fluorescent lamps should not be used inside the mesh. The design of screened rooms is described by Leadbitter (1963), and by Thompson and Yarborough (1967). In the author's experience, a screened room proved to be most useful in a laboratory which was in direct line-of-sight with a powerful television transmitter. It prevented the appearance of the line-sync pulses on oscilloscopes.

ELECTRICAL SAFETY PRECAUTIONS WITH PATIENT MONITORING APPARATUS

The use of an earth-free mains supply

Whenever electrical apparatus is connected to a patient, particular care must be exercised to ensure that there is no possibility of the patient receiving a dangerous shock, the risk is obviously greater when the equipment is mains powered. When a substantial amount of monitoring apparatus is to be employed a good additional safety precaution is to have the room fed from an earth-free mains supply. Should a fault condition develop in any of the monitor units so that a part in contact with the patient rises to the line voltage of the mains there is now no return path for current should the patient be earthed. For locations such as cardiac and neurosurgical operating rooms and hyperbaric chambers the mains supply should be derived from a one-to-one ratio mains transformer having a suitable load

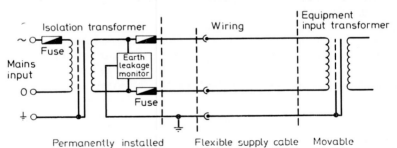

Figure 11.5. The use of a symmetrical isolation transformer feeding the symmetrical mains transformer of an equipment in order to minimize earth leakage currents (Klomp and Lucas, 1972)

capacity. *Figure 11.7* gives an outline of an earth-free mains power distribution arrangement for feeding a number of beds in an intensive care area. The mains earth is only attached to the shield of the 1 : 1 isolating transformer and to the earth leakage detector. A cluster of electrical sockets is provided for each patient and these are fed via individual circuit breakers for each cluster. All exposed metal pipes and metal surface near to each bed are bonded to a good earth (not the mains earth). In order to avoid the pick-up of excessive mains hum from the action of earth loops it is desirable that all equipment which may be used together should work to the same earth 'bus-bar'. This is particularly important when signals from patient monitors are to be interrogated by a digital computer.

Normally, the isolated mains supply should not come into contact with an earthed object. If it does, then a small leakage current will flow. An earth leakage current detector should be fitted to give warning of leakage currents down to 5 mA r.m.s. If this current is exceeded a warning is given of a fault condition existing and this should be corrected as soon as possible. Meanwhile no danger will arise of the patient being connected between the live lead of the mains and earth. The mains leads inside any piece of monitoring apparatus should be doubly insulated from earth so that two faults must occur before the mains voltage can get on to the chassis. Full details of the manufacturing standards required for electro-medical equipment used in the United Kingdom are set out in the *Hospital Technical Memorandum No. 8.* 'Safety code for electro-medical apparatus', available from Her Majesty's Stationery Office. A useful American paper on safety precautions is that of Bruner (1967).

A stringent requirement occurs for the safety performance of electrical equipment which may come into contact with a patient having a saline filled catheter connected to an electrical pressure transducer and introduced into the heart (Mody and Richings, 1962) or when electrodes have been implanted into the myocardium. The greatest risk occurs with the catheter in either the right or left ventricle. In man, currents in either of the ventricles of the order of 150 to 200 µA can produce ventricular fibrillation, whereas more than 3 mA may be required into either atrium. From an extrapolation of animal experiments, Geddes *et al.* (1969) deduce that a current of 310 µA at 60 Hz flowing between right arm and left leg would be adequate to produce ventricular fibrillation, whilst Dalziel (1956) estimates between 100 and 275 µA at 60 Hz. Current thinking in the United Kingdom (1972) suggests that a maximum permissible leakage current into a patient of 100 µA would be satisfactory. American practice is favouring a limit of 5 µA. This is substantially more expensive to achieve than the 100 µA. Possible approaches include

337

the use of a low-voltage battery-powered input stage, for example, to an ECG monitor, followed by a photo-isolator and then the main amplification circuitry. In the photo-isolator, the output signal from the first stage modulates the light output from a light-emitting diode; this modulated light can then be detected by means of a photo-cell. Other approaches make use of audio-frequency modulation anp transformers to couple power into the input stage and extract the signal from it.

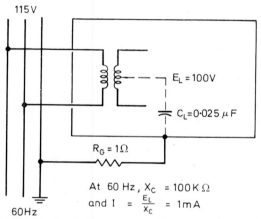

$$\text{At } 60 \text{ Hz}, X_C = 100 \text{ K}\Omega$$
$$\text{and } I = \frac{E_L}{X_C} = 1 \text{ mA}$$

Figure 11.6. The dotted line indicates a capacitive leakage current path from the mains transformer to the chassis of an electrocardiograph. If the case is well earthed, the leakage current is safely bypassed to earth (Hopps, 1969)

Klomp and Lucas (1972) discuss in detail the performance of isolation transformers for medical electronic equipment. They found the results shown in Table 11.1.

TABLE 11.1

Mains supply	Equipment mains transformer	Earth leakage current (μA)
Ordinary mains	Normal transformer	42
Isolation transformer	Normal transformer	25
Isolation transformer	Symmetrical transformer	21
Symmetrical transformer	Normal transformer	5
Symmetrical transformer	Symmetrical transformer	21

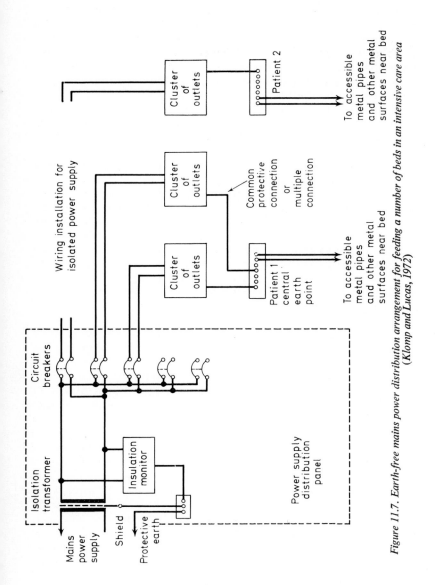

Figure 11.7. Earth-free mains power distribution arrangement for feeding a number of beds in an intensive care area (Klomp and Lucas, 1972)

In order to achieve leakage currents less than 5μA with this technique, it is necessary to use an isolation transformer which has a centre tapped secondary winding which is symmetrical about earth and supplies power to the equipment mains transformer which has primary windings centre tapped and symmetrical about earth. Both sets of symmetrical windings have a screen which is connected to the centre tap and the value of the capacitance from both ends of the windings to earth is arranged to be almost equal (*Figure 11.5*). Thus transformer techniques can minimize leakage currents from the mains to earth. They cannot guard against hazards arising from the breakdown of insulation inside the apparatus allowing a dangerous voltage to be applied to the heart. The use of a low-voltage, isolated, input circuit is required for this.

Hopps (1969) indicates that a leakage voltage of 100 V from a mains transformer with a leakage capacitance to earth of 0·025 μF will send a 1 mA leakage current at 60 Hz though a patient whose resistance might be 5,000 ohms (*Figure 11.6*). If the patient had an earthed cardiac pacemaker electrode connected to a ventricle, then fibrillation might result. Hopps also makes the point that a patient with a cardiac catheter or electrode in one bed may be fibrillated by a short circuit occurring elsewhere. The resulting surge current flowing in the mains earth conductor may raise the right leg potential of the patient to a voltage level sufficient to cause fibrillation if the heart is earthed independently. The current required to produce ventricular fibrillation rises markedly with increasing frequency, so that frequencies of the order of 100 kHz are used for thoracic impedance measurements (Geddes *et al.*, 1969).

Noordijk, Oey and Tebra (1961) describe the pathways of current from an incorrectly earthed electrocardiograph through the heart to a mains-powered cardiac pacemaker which resulted in ventricular fibrillation. Starmer, Whalen and McIntosh (1964) describe the measurement of leakage currents to earth in medical equipment. Hopps and Roy (1963) discuss the electrical hazards which may arise during cardiac investigations and treatment. Said and El-Shiribiny (1962) report the case of a patient who, while anaesthetized, received 11 shocks from an accidental electrical connection and went into ventricular fibrillation. Starmer, Whalen and McIntosh (1964) review the hazards of electric shock in cardiology. They cover hazards of pacing, defibrillating and cardiac catheterization.

Bracale and Marsico (1970) and Van Der Weide and Van Bemmel (1968) describe amplifiers for use with ECG's and other physiological signals and incorporating a photo-isolator stage. The use of isolator stages is now becoming commonplace in order to eliminate hazards arising from leakage currents to earth.

THE USE OF MONITORING APPARATUS AND SURGICAL DIATHERMY IN THE PRESENCE OF EXPLOSIVE ANAESTHETIC AGENTS

In the United Kingdom, the agents likely to be encountered which can give rise to explosions or fires are cyclopropane and diethyl ether. Both on the grounds of economy and safety, cyclopropane is nearly always used in a closed circuit arrangement. Explosions have resulted from sparks from the surgical diathermy unit igniting a mixture of oxygen and cylopropane when the lungs were punctured during a thoracotomy. Barrkman (1965) reports a case of intestinal explosion after a caecostomy with diathermy. This was due to an explosion of hydrogen or methane in the gut together with air let in from the surgical incision. The most dangerous region in the operating room itself will be immediately adjacent to the anaesthetic machine, anaesthetic circuit tubing, the relief valve and the patient, particularly his head (Bulgin, 1953). The high-risk zone for explosions extends out about three feet farther horizontally and downwards to the floor. Beyond this, with a good ventilation system, the concentrations of the agents will generally be less than the limit for ignition. Thus if there is any doubt about the sparking-risk of a piece of apparatus, it should be placed more than four feet from the patient and anaesthetic equipment. Ether vapour and cyclopropane are heavier than air and so will gravitate towards the floor. For this reason, electrical wall outlets if not of a sparkless type should be mounted well above floor level. In American operating rooms, apparatus which is not certified as explosion-proof must be mounted at least five feet above the floor. In the United Kingdom the level is four feet six inches. This requirement applies to permanently installed switches and to switches on portable apparatus if the apparatus is closer than four feet to the anaesthesic apparatus. It is obvious that an efficient ventilation system in the operating room will greatly reduce the chance of a dangerous concentration of anaesthetic building up. From 5 to 10 changes per hour of air are recommended (Report, 1956). The air extraction points should be situated near floor level, and the inlet points as high in the walls as possible, certainly not less than six feet above the floor. Any apparatus used in the operating room should be designed in such a way as to prevent the build-up on it of static charges of electricity. These could give rise to a spark leading to an explosion. Further details are covered by Hill (1967).

Clearly, the use of a surgical diathermy in the presence of explosive anaesthetic agents such as ether and cyclopropane must be approached with great caution. Some manufacturers of surgical diathermy units

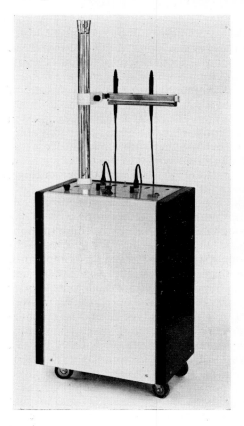

Figure 11.8. Air purged surgical diathermy unit (Reproduced by courtesy of Transformatoren und Röntgenwerk, Dresden)

provide that the generator can be located outside the operating room, or, if it is inside, it is purged with room air taken in at a height of 1·5 metres above floor level in order to avoid the ingress of explosive agents. The average pressure inside the unit is kept about

0·4 mm Hg above atmospheric and the unit cannot be activated until purging has taken place for one minute. Arrangements can also be made to purge the region surrounding the cutting electrodes with nitrogen. This is particularly important when working in the vicinity of the face and neck of the patient. *Figure 11.8* shows a surgical diathermy unit produced in the German Democratic Republic. The tall column functions both as an inlet for the purging air stream and also as a support for the electrode holder.

THE USE OF SURGICAL DIATHERMY ON PATIENTS USING CARDIAC PACEMAKERS

The use of surgical diathermy on patients using a cardiac pacemaker should be avoided, since pick-up of unwanted signals from the diathermy set may cause false triggering of the pacemaker. Lichter, Borrie and Miller (1965) observed ventricular fibrillation in 2 patients when an American Cystoscope Company diathermy unit was used. The pacemaker in question was the I.M.E. Model C.V. 2371. On the other hand, Kohler and Mackinney (1965) report patients having implanted pacemakers by Medtronic and General Electric undergoing transurethral prostatectomy without any interference to their pacing. The surgical diathermy unit employed is quoted as having a frequency in the range 1–3·5 MHz with modulation at 120 Hz. It is clear that care must be exercised when using surgical diathermy apparatus on patients who are being paced. This statement is underlined by the paper of Titel and el-Etr (1968). These authors report the case of a man aged 51 years undergoing surgery for an aortic valve replacement and open mitral commissuratomy. Myocardial electrodes were implanted and connected to an external Medtronic demand pacemaker using extension wires and alligator clamps. The clamp on one wire was inadvertently placed on a wet drape near the incision. Surgical diathermy was then performed, the plate electrode being placed beneath the patient's buttocks. Each time the diathermy electrode was operated the heart was observed to fibrillate, reversion to the paced rhythm returning on stopping the diathermy. Removal of the clamp from the wet drapes allowed the diathermy to proceed without the occurrence of fibrillation.

When electrodes are connected to the myocardium, particular care must be taken to avoid their receiving leakage currents arising from other apparatus connected to the patient. Whalen and Starmer (1967) state that a current as low as 180 μA will fibrillate a human

343

heart when applied to the myocardium. The findings of Kohler and Mackinney are substantiated by Fein (1967) again in prostatectomy patients where a well-insulated, battery-powered pacemaker was used during surgical diathermy.

REFERENCES

Barrkman, M. F. (1965). 'Intestinal explosion after opening a caecostomy with diathermy.' *Br. med. J.* **1,** 1594

Bracale, M., and Marsico, M. (1970). 'A photon-coupled amplifier for measuring and recording physiological signals.' *Med. biol. Engng.*, **8,** 103

Bruner, J. M. R. (1967). 'Hazards of electrical apparatus.' *Anesthesiology*, **28,** 396

Bulgin, D. (1953). 'Factors in the design of an operating theatre free from electrostatic risks.' *Br. J. appl. Phys.* **4,** S87

Dalziel, C. F. (1956). 'Effects of electric shock on man.' *I.R.E. Trans. Med. Electron.*, **PGME-5,** 44

Dobbie, A. K. (1965). 'Why screened rooms in hospitals?' *Wld. med. Electron. Instrum. Lond.* **3,** 157

— (1966). 'Electrical safety of patient monitoring equipment.' *Br. Hosp. J.*

— (1968). 'Personal communication'.

— (1969). 'The electrical aspects of surgical diathermy.' *Bio-med Engng.* **4,** 206

Fein, R. L. (1967). 'Transurethral electrocautery procedures in patients with cardiac pacemakers.' *J. Am. med. Ass.* **202,** 101

Geddes, L. A., Baker, L. E., Moore, A. G., and Coulter, T. W. (1969). 'Hazards in the use of low frequencies for the measurement of physiological events by impedance.' *Med. biol. Engng.*, **7,** 289

Hill, D. W. (1967). *Physics Applied to Anaesthesia*, p. 166 London; Butterworths

Hopps, J. A. and Roy, O. Z. (1963). 'Electrical hazards in cardiac diagnosis and treatment.' *Med. Electron. biol. Engng.* **1,** 135

Hopps, J. A. (1969). 'Shock hazards in operating rooms and patient-care areas.' *Anesthesiology*, **31,** 142

Klomp, A. M., and Lucas, J. H. M. (1972). 'Advantages of symmetrical isolation transformers in the reduction of patient hazards.' *Med. biol. Engng.*, **10**

Kohler, F. P. and Mackinney, C. C. (1965). 'Cardiac pacemakers in electro-surgery.' *J. Am. med. Ass.* **193,** 855

Leadbitter, A. F. C. (1963). 'Screening against electrical interference.' *World med. Electron. Instrum. Lond.* **2,** 17

Lichter, I., Borrie, J. and Miller, W. M. (1965). 'Radio-frequency hazards with cardiac pacemakers.' *Br. med. J.* **1,** 1513

Mapleson, W. W. (1961). 'Device for protecting recording pens from interference from surgical diathermy.' *J. Scient. Instrum.* **38,** 260

Mody, S. M., and Richings, M. (1962). 'Ventricular fibrillation resulting from electrocution during cardiac catheterisation.' *Lancet*, **2,** 698

REFERENCES

Noordijk, J. A., Oey, F. T. I. and Tebra, W. (1961). 'Myocardial electrodes and the dangers of ventricular fibrillation.' *Lancet* **1**, 975

Report of a Working Party on Anaesthetic Explosions (1956). London; H.M.S.O.

Said, K. and El-Shiribiny, A. (1962). 'Accidental repeated electric shocks during anaesthesia.' *Acta anaesth. scand.* Suppl. **12**, 111

Starmer, C. F., Whalen, R. E. and McIntosh, H. D. (1964). 'Hazards of electric shock in cardiology.' *Am. J. Cardiol.*, **14**, 537

— — —(1966). 'Determination of leakage currents in medical equipment.' *Am. J. Cardiol.* **17**, 437

Thompson, N. P. and Yarnbrough, R. B. (1967). 'The shielding of electro-encephalographic laboratories.' *Psychophysiology* **4**, 244

Titel, J. H., and el-Etr. (1968). 'Fibrillation resulting from pacemaker electrodes and electrocautery during surgery.' *Anesthesiology* **29**, 845

Van Der Weide, H., and Van Bemmel, J. H. (1968). 'A photon-coupled amplifier for the transmission of physiological signals.' *Med. biol. Engng.*, **6**, 447

Whalen, R. E., and Starmer, C. F. (1967). 'Electric shock hazards in clinical cardiology.' *Mod. Concepts cardiovasc. Dis.* **36**, 7

12–Oximeters, Densitometers and Colorimeters

PRINCIPLES OF OPTICAL ABSORPTION

If I_0 is the intensity of a definite monochromatic wavelength of light passing into a layer of a substance limited by two parallel planes and of thickness d and I is the intensity emerging from the layer, then the Lambert–Beer Law states that $I = I_0 \exp(-e.c.d.)$ where c is the concentration of the substance concerned, and e is called the extinction coefficient. Its dimensions depend upon the units selected for the concentration. If c is in moles/litre, then e is called the molecular extinction coefficient. The optical density of the solution is given by $D = e.c.d.$ so that $I = I_0 \exp(-D)$. Since $D = e.d.c$, if the liquid obeys Beer's Law a plot of the optical density against concentration for a particular wavelength and cell thickness will yield a straight line. Instruments such as oximeters, densitometers and spectrophotometers basically measure optical densities. Modern spectrophotometers are usually calibrated directly in terms of both the optical density and the percentage transmission of light by the sample.

The optical density must be dimensionless, since it is simply the index of a power; $e.c$ is the reciprocal of the thickness required to reduce the intensity of the incident light to 37 per cent of its original value (by analogy with the definition of the time constant). Beer's Law states that the optical density is a linear function of the concentration c. This fact is used in colorimeters for estimating the concentration of a solution.

THE USE OF A MONOCHROMATIC DENSITOMETER IN COLORIMETRY

As has just been shown for a liquid which obeys Beer's Law, $I = I_0 \exp(-D)$ where D is the optical density. Thus $-D = \log_e(I/I_0)$

or $+D=\log_e(I_0/I)$. Simple colorimeters are widely used to measure the optical density of solutions at a known wavelength. A typical application occurs in a haemoglobinometer (Burn 1968). The cuvette is 0·5 cm deep, and the blood is diluted 1 in 100 with saline solution. Haemolysis is brought about and the ghosts dissolved with ammonia. Light from an incandescent bulb is passed through a 540 nm optical interference filter and then through the measuring cuvette and an identical air-filled reference cell. The output of a photomultiplier situated behind the reference cell is proportional to I_0, while that from the same photomultiplier situated behind the cuvette is proportional to I. Since the optical density of the solution is proportional to the haemoglobin concentration, it is necessary to evaluate $\log_e(I_0/I)$. The method used by Burn (1968) is shown in *Figure 12.1*. A voltage proportional to I_0 controls the frequency of a

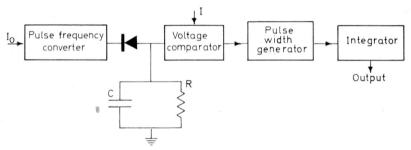

Figure 12.1. Logarithmic circuit for the estimation of optical density (after Burn 1968)

pulse generator. Each pulse charges capacitor C which discharges through R so that it is completely discharged before the arrival of the next pulse. The voltage on C is compared with a voltage proportional to I and a pulse is generated by the comparator when the voltage on C is greater than I. The charging voltage for C is also proportional to I_0, that is the voltage that would be given by I when the optical density is zero. Under these conditions the width of the generated pulse would be zero. If the pulse width is t seconds when the voltage on the capacitor is proportional to I then $I = I_0 \exp(-kt)$, so that t is proportional to $\log_e(I_0/I)$, that is, to D. A rotating shutter allows the light to pass alternately through the reference cell and the measuring cuvette. The output pulses from the pulse-width generator are integrated and fed to a recorder to give an output proportional to the haemoglobin concentration.

THE BASIC THEORY OF OXIMETRY

Measurements of the degree of oxygen saturation of the blood by spectrophotometric means are usually based upon the assumption that blood behaves as an ideal absorber of light and obeys Beer's Law. Haemolysed blood obeys Beer's Law so that $I_d = I_o \exp(-ecd)$ where

I_d is the intensity of the transmitted light of wavelength λ and at depth d.

I_o is the intensity of the incident light of wavelength λ.

d is the depth of the blood.

c is the concentration of the haemoglobin.

e is the extinction coefficient of haemoglobin at an oxygen saturation S and wavelength λ.

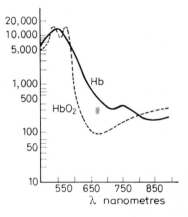

Figure 12.2. The absorption of light expressed in terms of the molecular extinction coefficient for haemoglobin and oxyhaemoglobin plotted against the incident light wavelength

In *Figure 12.2* is shown a plot of the molecular extinction coefficient for haemoglobin and oxyhaemoglobin against wavelength in the visible and near infra-red regions of the spectrum. It can be seen that at 805 nm (8,050 Å) there is an isobestic point, that is to say, that the molecular extinction coefficients for fully saturated ($S=1$) and fully reduced ($S=0$) blood are equal at this wavelength. The fact that an isobestic point exists is vital to the principle of operation of oximeters.

In practice, the transmission of light through thin layers of non-haemolysed whole blood does not obey Beer's Law exactly. These deviations are thought to arise from the scattering of light by the cells. To account for the deviations the Beer's Law equation can be

348

modified to become $I_d = I_0 \exp(-ecdf)$ where f is a function expressing the variation of the extinction coefficient for whole blood for a given wavelength in respect of the sample depth, haemoglobin concentration and degree of oxygen saturation. For haemolysed blood $f = 1$.

Consider the measurement of the transmitted light intensity through a sample of haemolysed blood at two separate wavelengths, 650 nm in the red and 805 nm in the infra-red. In the red the extinction coefficient for reduced haemoglobin is e_{Hb}^r while that for oxyhaemoglobin is $e_{HbO_2}^r$. In the infra-red $e_{Hb}^{ir} = e_{HbO_2}^{ir} = e^{ir}$

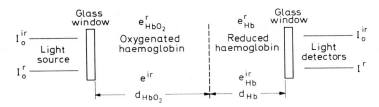

Figure 12.3. The use of light of two wavelengths (red and infra-red) to measure the oxygen saturation of blood in a cuvette

Referring to *Figure 12.3* the relative oxygen saturation by volume is $S = d_{HbO_2}/(d_{HbO_2} + d_{Hb}) = d_{HbO_2}/d$, where

d_{HbO_2} is the effective depth of sample occupied by oxyhaemoglobin;

d_{Hb} is the effective depth of sample occupied by reduced haemoglobin;

$d = d_{HbO_2} + d_{Hb}$ is the depth of the sample cuvette.

For the infra-red $I^{ir} = I_o^{ir} \exp(-e^{ir} cd)$

For the red, the two exponents are additive, so that:

$$I^r = I_o^r \exp\left[(-(e_{HbO_2}^r . d_{HbO_2} + e_{Hb}^r . d_{Hb})c)\right]$$

A solution for S can be obtained by eliminating the product cd to give:

$$S = \left\{ \frac{e_{\mathrm{Hb}}^{\mathrm{r}}}{e_{\mathrm{Hb}}^{\mathrm{r}} - e_{\mathrm{HbO2}}^{\mathrm{r}}} - \frac{e^{\mathrm{ir}}}{e_{\mathrm{Hb}}^{\mathrm{r}} - e_{\mathrm{HbO2}}^{\mathrm{r}}} \right\} \cdot \left\{ \frac{\log_e I^{\mathrm{r}} - \log_e I_o^{\mathrm{r}}}{\log_e I^{\mathrm{ir}} - \log_e I_o^{\mathrm{ir}}} \right\}$$

The expression for S is independent of the cuvette depth d and the haemoglobin concentration c; S is linearly related to $(\log_e I^{\mathrm{r}} - \log_e I_o^{\mathrm{r}})/(\log_e I^{\mathrm{ir}} - \log_e I_o^{\mathrm{ir}})$. The constant of proportionality is generally determined for a particular instrument by measuring the saturation of blood samples with the oximeter and also with a gasiometric technique (Van Slyke and Neill, 1924). This expression derived from the ideal behaviour of haemolysed blood has generally been applied to whole blood oximetry, but this leads to some uncertainty in the measurements. Although the effects of scattering are not included, an analysis of a number of errors which can occur in oximetry is given by Tait, Sekelj and D'Ombrain (1966), particularly in regard to the use of ear oximeters.

THE EFFECT OF SCATTERING UPON THE TRANSMISSION OF LIGHT THROUGH BLOOD

Oximeters are basically instruments used to measure the degree of saturation of the blood with oxygen and they operate on a photo-electric basis by measuring the light transmitted through or reflected from a layer of blood at known wavelengths. Each millilitre of blood contains about 5 million cells, the cells being approximately 7 micrometres in diameter by 2 micrometres thick ($1 \ \mu\mathrm{m} = 1,000$ nm). Because of the presence of the cells, as has been mentioned, a simple Beer's Law transmission will not apply exactly. Light incident upon the blood will not only be absorbed, but will be scattered in both the forwards and backwards directions by the processes of reflection, refraction and diffraction.

Following Reichert (1966) consider a beam of light of intensity I_o and wavelength λ incident upon a layer of blood of thickness d, with reference to the transmission and reflection which occurs in a layer of blood of thickness dx situated at a distance x from the incident surface measured in the forward direction, *Figure 12.4*. In passing through this layer of blood some of the light will be absorbed, some will be diffusely reflected backwards, and some will be scattered forwards by the blood cells. A fraction of the light scattered backwards will be re-scattered in the forward direction.

I is the intensity of light incident on the front surface of the blood $(x = O)$.

a is the extinction coefficient of blood for light in the forward direction.

s is the scattering coefficient of blood for light in the forward direction.

s' is the scattering coefficient of blood for light in the backward direction.

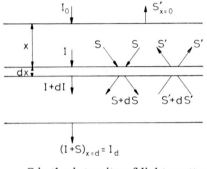

Figure 12.4. The transmission of light through blood, with scattering in the forwards and backwards directions

S is the intensity of light scattered in the forward direction.

S' is the intensity of light scattered in the backward direction.

x is the distance from the front surface of the thin layer of blood of thickness dx

d is the thickness of the layer of blood contained in a cuvette

c is the concentration of haemoglobin

e_0 is the extinction coefficient per unit concentration of haemoglobin when there is no scattering.

e is the extinction coefficient per unit concentration of haemoglobin when there is both absorption and scattering.

Then the change in intensity dI occurring over a distance dx is given by

$$dI = -I(a + s + s')dx \qquad (1)$$

In particular, the change in intensity of the light scattered in the forward direction with distance is

$$dS/dx = \underset{\substack{\text{scattered} \\ \text{in forward} \\ \text{direction}}}{sI} - \underset{\text{absorbed}}{aS} - \underset{\substack{\text{scattered} \\ \text{in backward} \\ \text{direction}}}{s'S} + \underset{\substack{\text{scattered in} \\ \text{forward direction} \\ \text{from the light flux} \\ \text{in the backward} \\ \text{direction}}}{s'S'} \qquad (2)$$

351

The change in intensity of the light scattered in the backward direction with distance is

$$-dS'/dx = s'I \quad - \quad aS' \quad - \quad s'S' \quad + \quad s'S \qquad (3)$$

<table>
<tr><td>scattered in backward direction</td><td>absorbed</td><td>scattered in forward direction from the light flux in the backward direction</td><td>scattered in backward direction</td></tr>
</table>

From equations (1), (2) and (3) it is possible to obtain I, S and S'

Re-arranging (1) gives $dI/I = -(a+s+s')dx$ (4)

Integrating (4), if $I = I_0 \exp-(a+s+s')x$ (5)

From (2), $dS/dx = sI-(a+s')S+s'S'$ (6)

From (3), $-ds'/dx = s'I-(a+s')S'+s'S'$ (7)

From (6) $S' = (I/s')[(dS/dx)+(a+s')S'-sI)]$ (8)

Substituting in (7) from (8) and (5),

$$d^2S/dx^2 = (a+2as')S-[2as+(s+s')^2]I_0 \exp-(a+s+s')x \qquad (9)$$

From (7), $S = (I/s')(dS'/dx)-I+[(a+s')/s']S'$ (10)

Substituting in (6) $d^2S'/dx^2 = (a^2+2as')S'$ (11)

Since (11) is simpler than (10) the boundary conditions that $S=0$ at $x=0$ and $S'=0$ at $x=d$ are applied to (11). The solution of this second-order differential equation will be of the form $S' = A\exp(\alpha x)+B\exp(-\alpha x)$, where A and B are constants

Substituting for dS^1/dx and S^1 in (7) from (12) and (8),

$$s'(I+S) = [A.\exp(\alpha x)](a+s'-\alpha)+[B.\exp(-\alpha x)](a+s'+\alpha) \qquad (12)$$

Since $S=0$ at $x=0$,

$$s'I_0 = A(a+s'-\alpha)+B(a+s'+\alpha) \qquad (13)$$

Since $S'=0$ at $x=d$,

$$0 = [A\exp(\alpha d)](a+s'-\alpha)+[B\exp(-\alpha d)](a+s'+\alpha) \qquad (14)$$

From (13), (14) and (5),

$$A = [s'I_0\exp(-\alpha d)]/[(a+s'+\alpha)\exp(\alpha d)-(a+s'-\alpha)\exp(-\alpha d)] \qquad (15)$$

$$B = [s'I_0\exp(\alpha d)]/[(a+s'+\alpha)\exp(\alpha d)-(a+s'-\alpha)\exp(\alpha d)] \qquad (16)$$

From (12), (10), (5) and (6),

$$S' = s'I_0 \{\exp[\alpha(d-x)]-\exp[-\alpha(d-x)]\}/[(a+s'+\alpha)\exp(\alpha d) \\ -(a+s'-\alpha)\exp(-\alpha d)] \qquad (17)$$

When $x=0$, from (17),

$$S' = s'I_0[\exp(\alpha d)-\exp(-\alpha d)]/[(a+s'+\alpha)\exp(\alpha d)-(a+s'-\alpha) \\ \exp(-\alpha d)] \qquad (18)$$

when the cuvette thickness d is large enough so that light incident upon the back of the cuvette can be neglected, then $\exp(-\alpha d)$ is approximately equal to zero.

$$\text{Thus } S'=s'I_0\exp(\alpha d)/(a+s'+\alpha)\exp(\alpha d) \tag{19}$$

Since $\alpha=\sqrt{a^2+2as'}$,

$$S'=s'I_0/[(a+s')+\sqrt{(a^2+2as')}] \tag{20}$$

This is the equation governing the intensity of the light scattered from the blood in the cuvette in the backward direction. It can be compared with the Lambert–Beer Law governing the total transmission of light through the blood in the forward direction, that is,

$$I_d=I_0\exp(-ecd) \tag{21}$$

From (7),

$$s'(I+S)=(dS'/dx)+(a+s')S' \tag{22}$$

From (5) and (16),

$$s'(I+S)=\frac{S'I_0[(a+s'+\alpha)\exp\alpha(d-x)-(a+s'-d)\exp-\alpha(d-x)]}{(a+s'+\alpha)\exp(\alpha d)-(a+s'-\alpha)\exp(-\alpha d)} \tag{23}$$

When $x=d$

$$I_d=I_0\exp[-d\sqrt{(a^2+2as')}]\times$$

$$\left\{\frac{2\sqrt{(a^2+2as')}}{[a+s'+\sqrt{(a^2+2as')}]-[a+s'-\sqrt{(a^2+2as')}]\exp[-2d\sqrt{(a^2+2as')}]}\right\} \quad 24$$

When the values for a and s' are substituted into (24), the term in the braces { } has a value which is approximately unity. This fact can be verified by putting $(a+s')\simeq\sqrt{(a^2+2as')}$. This makes the numerator and denominator equal, giving

$$I_d=I_0\exp[-d\sqrt{(a^2+2as')}] \tag{25}$$

This is the equation governing the transmission of light through blood, taking into account the effect of the cells in scattering light.

All types of oximeter contain the following basic components:

Light source, generally an incandescent lamp.

Cuvette to hold the blood sample. It may have a rectangular or cylindrical cross-section and be made of glass or plastic. Some cuvettes are designed for flow-through operation.

Optical filters to select appropriate wavebands in the visible or near infra-red spectral regions.

Radiation detector. Currently, cadmium sulphide or selenide photocells are usually employed.

Optical arrangement. Basically the transmitted or reflected light is measured at either a single wavelength (650 nm in the red) or at two wavelengths (650 nm and 805 nm in the near infra-red) or (550 nm in the green and 650 nm in the red).

Electrical systems

Five different electrical arrangements have been used in oximeters, as follows. Direct deflection at 650 nm only, a double-scale meter using red and infra-red, a ratio system operating upon the ratio of red to infra-red intensities, a single-scale meter showing the difference between red and infra-red, and a single-scale meter showing the difference between red and infra-red with the infra-red now held constant.

DICHROMATIC TRANSMISSION OXIMETERS

The high optical density of whole blood arises mainly from the scattering and reflection of light by the red cells. The optical density of a sample of blood will therefore vary with conditions affecting the size, shape and aggregation of the cells. Factors which may be important are variations in the rate of blood flow through the cuvette, the addition of non-isotonic solutions to the blood and variations in the blood carbon dioxide tension. All single wavelength (monochromatic) oximeters will suffer from artefacts such as these, since the instruments cannot distinguish between variations in optical density at the chosen wavelength due to changes in the blood saturation, and non-specific optical density variations arising from changes in the red cells.

By measuring at 650 nm in the red and 805 nm in the near infra-red it is possible to achieve a high degree of compensation for non-specific optical density changes. At 650 nm the absorption of red light by oxyhaemoglobin is much greater than that for reduced haemoglobin. The red photocell thus monitors changes in blood oxygen saturation. At the isobestic wavelength, the infra-red photocell is insensitive to changes in oxygen saturation, but monitors non-specific changes in optical density. By using it in a compensating circuit the dichromatic oximeter can be made insensitive to changes in haemoglobin concentration, blood flow and so on.

Dichromatic densitometers for dye dilution curve recording

A requirement for measuring the optical density of blood also arises with the dye dilution method for the measurement of cardiac output. Indocyanine green dye is now widely used in this technique, the dye absorbing light heavily at around 800 nm. This is a desirable property, since the optical density is now independent of the degree of saturation of the blood. However, since there is no other isobestic wavelength for blood it is not possible to make use of a second photocell in the normal way to compensate for non-specific changes in blood optical density. The matter was resolved in an ingenious fashion by Sutterer and Wood (1962). A special dichroic mirror is employed to reflect light in the region of 800 nm to one photocell, while simultaneously transmitting light of wavelengths shorter and longer than this to a second photocell. Since the transmission by blood of wavelengths longer and shorter than 800 nm is affected in opposite directions by changes in oxygen saturation it is possible

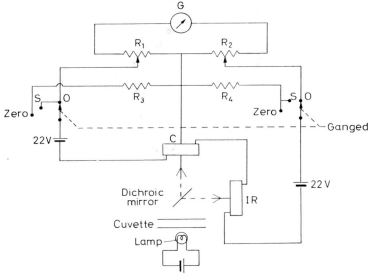

Figure 12.5(a). Schematic diagram of a compensated dichromatic densitometer (after Sutterer and Wood, 1962)

by correctly choosing optical filters and the spectral sensitivity of the photocell to ensure that the responses to the longer and shorter wavelengths cancel. Thus the output of the second photocell is unaffected by saturation changes and can be used to monitor non-specific optical density changes. The optical arrangement is shown in *Figure 12.5a* and the spectral sensitivities of the two photocells in *Figure 12.6*. Light from the filament lamp transmitted through the cuvette L is split by the dichroic mirror and falls on the compensating (C) and dye detecting (IR) photocells. Each photocell is situated behind an optical filter. The sensitivity is set by R_1 and R_2

355

situated in the galvanometer circuit; these are 10-turn helical potentiometers. The load resistors R_3 and R_4 are chosen to keep the load on the photocells constant and hence minimize drift in the cells. A dichromatic densitometer of the compensated type is shown in *Figure 12.5b* together with its catheter cuvette and earpiece cuvette.

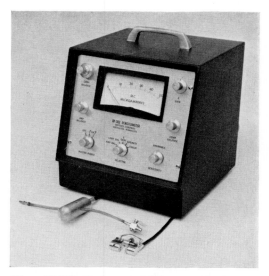

Figure 12.5(b). Compensated dichromatic densitometer with catheter and earpiece cuvettes. (Reproduced by courtesy of Waters Co.)

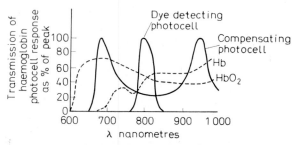

Figure 12.6. The spectral sensitivities of the two photo-cells used in a compensated dichromatic densitometer (after Sutterer and Wood, 1962)

Another version of a compensated dye curve densitometer for use with indocyanine green is that of Sekelj *et al* (1967).

When a dye dilution curve is to be recorded, the control switch is first set to position 0 and the zero reading of the galvanometer set to a predetermined position near to the bottom of the scale of the associated recorder. With blood being drawn through the cuvette and the switch in position S, the sensitivity of the compensating photocell is adjusted by R_1 to bring the recorder reading back to the previously arranged zero or baseline. Finally with the switch in the 0 (operate) position, the sensitivity of the detecting photocell is adjusted by R_2 to return the recorder to the baseline. The outputs of the two photocells are then nearly equal and opposite. The sensitivity of the densitometer is proportional to the difference in the galvanometer readings with the switch in the S and 0 positions. The photocells, the filament lamp and the cuvette are all mounted in a cylindrical housing 2·5 cm in diameter by 7 cm long. The volume of the cuvette and its inlet connection is only 0·05 ml in total so that the densitometer has a good dynamic response.

THEORY OF THE REFLECTION OXIMETER

The oxygen saturation of the blood is defined by

$$\overline{S} = \frac{(HbO_2)}{(Hb)+(HbO_2)} = \frac{(HbO_2)}{c} \qquad (26)$$

where c is the concentration of haemoglobin.

When the blood is fully reduced, $\overline{S}=0$, and $e^r = e_{Hb}^r$ where e^r is the absorption coefficient for blood in the red when there is both absorption and scattering, and e_{Hb}^r is the corresponding figure for haemoglobin. When the blood is fully oxygenated, $\overline{S}=1$ and $e^r = e_{HbO2}^r$

$$e^r = e_{Hb}^r - \overline{S}\left(e_{Hb}^r - e_{HbO2}^r\right)$$

From (26), since $e = e_0.c$,

$$\frac{S'}{I_o} = \frac{s'}{2\left[e_{Hb}^r - \overline{S}\left(e_{Hb}^r - e_{HbO2}^r\right)\right]c + s'}$$

It can be shown (Rodrigo, 1953) that a plot of the logarithm of the reciprocal of the oximeter deflection for reflected light against oxygen saturation will yield a straight line.

357

Reichert (1966) describes a reflection-type oximeter using cuvettes made of Tygon tubing designed for flow-through use during an extra-corporeal circulation. The light diffusely reflected from the blood is measured in the red and infra-red, and the ratio of the two intensities measured with a self-balancing bridge circuit. Zijlstra (1958) covers the principles of reflection oximetry in detail.

EAR OXIMETERS

A transmission oximeter can be employed to measure the arterial oxygen saturation using the pinna of the ear as a cuvette (Sekelj, 1954), since the oxygen content of the blood in the capillaries of the vasodilated ear is very nearly the same as that of arterial blood. Making the usual assumptions that (1) the light used is sufficiently monochromatic; (2) Beer's Law of optical absorption holds for non-haemolysed blood and (3) that the ear is a good cuvette, if I_o^r is the red photocell output current for the compressed 'bloodless' ear, I_o^{ir} the corresponding value for the infra-red photocell, I^r the red photocell output for the flushed ear, d_1 the apparent depth of fully oxygenated blood, d_0 the apparent depth of fully reduced blood, d the apparent total depth of blood in the ear, then

$$I^r = I_o^r \exp[-(d_1 e_{HbO_2}^r + d_0 e_{Hb}^r)]$$

If I^{rs} is the red photocell output current for the fully saturated flushed ear, I^{irs} is the corresponding value for the infra-red photocell, the values for the flushed ear give $I^{rs} = I_o^r \exp(-d.e_{HbO_2}^r)$ and $I^{irs} = I_o^{ir} \exp(-d.e^{ir})$ where $d = d_1 + d_0$ and $\bar{S} = d_1/d$.

Anderson, Sekelj and McGregor (1961) have shown that a constant relationship exists between the transmitted intensities of the red and infra-red light through the 'bloodless' compressed ear, that is, $k = I_o^r / I_o^{ir}$. An empirical relationship has also been found to exist between the transmitted red and infra-red intensities for the flushed ear such that $I^{rs} = a(I^{irs} - b) \log_{10} H$ where a and b are constants for a particular earpiece and H is the haemoglobin concentration of blood in g/100 ml determined from a venous blood sample.

$$S = 1 - d_0/d = 1 - (e^{ir} - e^r_{HbO2}) . \frac{(\log_e I^{rs} - \log_e I^r)}{(e^r_{Hb} - e^r_{HbO2})(\log_e I^{rs} - \log_e I^r - \log_e K)}$$

Let $C = \dfrac{e^{ir} - e^{rs}}{e^r_{Hb} - e^r_{HbO2}}$

$$\overline{S} = 1 - C + \frac{C}{\log_e \left[\dfrac{a.\log_{10} H}{K} \dfrac{(1-b)}{I^{ir}} \right]} . (\log_e I^r - \log_e I^{ir} - \log_e K)$$

b is usually small enough to be neglected so that

$$\overline{S} = 1 - C + \left[\frac{C}{\log_e \left(\dfrac{a.\log_{10} H}{K} \right)} \right] . (\log_e I^r - \log_e I^{ir} - \log_e K)$$

If the output voltages from the red and infra-red photocells are E^r and E^{ir} then $E_r = k_1 . I^r$ and $E_{ir} = k_2 . I^{ir}$

Then $$\overline{S} = 1 - C + \left(\frac{C}{\log_e \dfrac{a.\log_{10} H}{K}} \right) . (\log_e E^r - \log_e E^{ir} - \log_e (K.k_1/k_2))$$

Changing the base of the logarithms from e to b gives

$$\overline{S} = 1 - C + \frac{C \log_{10} b}{\log_{10} \dfrac{a.\log_b H}{K}} . [\log_b E^r - \log_b E^{ir} - \log_b (K.k_1/k_2)]$$

Hence $\overline{S} = 1 - C + A(D + \log_b E^r - \log_b E^{ir})$ where $A = C.\log_{10} b /$
$\log_{10} \dfrac{(a.\log_{10} H)}{K}$ and $D = -\log_b (K.k_1/k_2)$

This equation can be solved by means of an on-line analogue computer to give a direct read-out in terms of percentage oxygen saturation. The system described by Tait and Sekelj (1967) employs three operational amplifiers and two logarithmic function generators. Paul and Woolf (1967) describe an ear oximeter using operational amplifiers.

TRANSMISSION OXIMETERS

Neglecting the absorption of light by water, let the intensity of red light passing through the cuvette be I^r_0 when the cuvette is filled with water, and I^r when it is filled with blood. The optical density of the blood is $D^r = \log I^r_0 / I^r = e^r . c . d$

The saturation $\bar{S} = HbO_2/c$ and $e^r = e^r_{Hb} - \bar{S}(e^r_{Hb} - e^r_{HbO2})$.

By measuring at a constant concentration c, and different known saturations, $\bar{S}$, e^r_{Hb} and e^r_{Hb} can all be determined. In a similar manner e^{ir}_{Hb} is found.

$$D^r = [e^r_{Hb} - \bar{S}(e^r_{Hb} - e^r_{HbO2})].c.d.$$

$$D^{ir} = [e^{ir}_{Hb} - \bar{S}(e^{ir}_{Hb} - e^{ir}_{HbO2})].c.d.$$

$$= e^{ir}_{Hb}.c.d. \text{ since } e^{ir}_{Hb} = e^{ir}_{HbO2}$$

$$\frac{D^r}{D^{ir}} = \frac{e^r_{Hb} - \bar{S}(e^r_{Hb} - e^r_{HbO2})}{e^{ir}_{Hb}}$$

so that the ratio of the optical densities of the blood in the red and infra-red is linearly related to the oxygen saturation.

THE USE OF AN OXIMETER AS A DENSITOMETER IN DYE DILUTION STUDIES

In many oximeters by replacing the red photocell with a fixed resistor it is possible to use the cuvette as a densitometer for recording cardiac output curves with the dye Cardio Green. If a blue dye is to be used, then the red photocell is used, the infra-red photocell now being replaced with a fixed resistor.

FIBRE OPTIC OXIMETERS AND DENSITOMETERS

The development of flexible fibre optics which can be the length of a cardiac catheter has made it possible to have the light source and the photocells all mounted outside the body (Fromer 1967). The most commonly used type is a reflection oximeter, the catheter containing two fibre bundles one to transmit the usual red and infra-red wavelengths, the other to transmit back the reflected light at these wavelengths to the photocells. By this means it is possible to correlate oxygen saturation variations within the heart with intracardiac, ECG and blood pressure measurements (Kapany *et al*, 1967). It is also possible to carry out dye curve measurements.

Fibre optics work on the principle of total internal reflection. Each fibre consists of a central core of glass surrounded by a cladding of glass having a lower refractive index than that of the core. Light incident upon the interface at angles of incidence greater than the critical angle suffers total internal reflection and is efficiently transmitted down the fibre, *Figure 12.7*

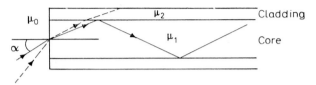

Figure 12.7. Principle of operation of a fibre optic

Let μ_0 be the refractive index of the external medium, μ_1 the refractive index of the core and μ_2 the refractive index of the cladding. A ray of light making an angle of incidence greater than α, the critical angle, is refracted at each interface, as shown by the dotted line, but escapes from the core. A ray having an angle of incidence of α or less suffers total internal reflection and is transmitted. The numerical aperture of a fibre is given by $N.A. = \mu_0 \sin\alpha = \sqrt{(\mu_1^2 - \mu_2^2)}$. Typically $N.A. = 0.55$ so that $\alpha = 33$ degrees, if $\mu_0 = 1$ (air). When the fibre optic is only required to transmit light then the fibre diameters can be of the order 50 to 100 μm and the individual fibres do not need to be accurately aligned with respect to each other. When a coherent system is needed for viewing an image, smaller fibres, typically 10 μm in diameter, are used and they are carefully aligned so that their relative positions are the same at each end of the fibre. Obviously great care is needed in the manufacture of fibre-optic gastroscopes and cystoscopes in order that a clear image is available.

In one version of a fibre optics oximeter, Gamble *et al* (1965), light from a tungsten filament lamp is focused by means of two lenses on to the transmitting bundle of fibre optics in the cardiac catheter. Light reflected back from blood at the catheter tip passes through a rotating glass disc, *Figure 12.8*, having alternate clear and mirror segments near its periphery. By this means the reflected light is divided into 550 pulses per second. The clear glass segments allow light to fall on to the 650-nm filter, while the reflecting segments direct it on to the 805-nm filter. Light from both filters falls on to the same photomultiplier. The output from the photomultiplier is amplified and then synchronously rectified. The phase reference signal for the synchronous rectifier is obtained from the chopper disc segments by means of an auxilliary lamp and phototransistor. The signals corresponding to the reflected light intensities at 650 and 805 nm are then compared and their ratio displayed on a meter calibrated in percentage oxygen saturation. An optical wedge placed in the path of the 805-nm light acts as a ratio adjustment. The

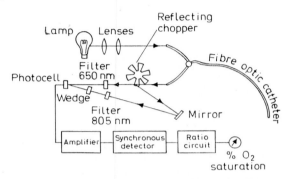

Figure 12.8. Schematic diagram of a high-speed fibre optic reflection oximeter (after Gamble et al, *1965)*

response time of the instrument is only 0·1 second and it can be used *in vivo* for up to 3 hours. It has been used to monitor mixed venous oxygen saturation changes in the pulmonary artery during treadmill exercises, and the effects of respiration and the Valsalva manoeuvre upon pulmonary oxygen saturation in patients with valvular heart disease, and in patients with atrial septal defects and left-to-right shunts.

FIBRE OPTIC DENSITOMETER

The dye, indocyanine green, widely used in cardiac output measurements by the indicator dilution technique, has its peak optical absorption in the region of 800 nm. Since this is an isobestic point for blood, the absorption reading is not affected by the state of oxygenation of the blood. The fibre optic oximeter can be changed to a densitometer for indocyanine green dye by leaving the 805 nm filter in place and replacing the 650 nm filter with a 900 nm filter. The ratio of the reflected light intensities at these wavelengths is linearly related to the dye concentration. The output signal corresponding to reflection at 805 nm only is markedly affected by cardiac pulsations, but the ratio is relatively unaffected. With the tip of the fibre optic catheter placed in the left ventricle, there is no re-circulation peak on the dye dilution curve. Thus, the area under the curve, which is required for a cardiac output determination, can be obtained by the use of a simple integrator circuit fed from the output of the densitometer.

The instrument is calibrated by placing the catheter tip in samples of blood containing known concentrations of dye and stirred by a magnetic stirrer (Hugenholtz *et al.*, 1965).

COMBINED FIBRE OPTIC OXIMETER AND PRESSURE TRANSDUCER

It is possible to mount a small reflecting diaphragm at the end of a fibre optic cardiac catheter. White light is directed down the catheter and, after reflection from the proximal side of the diaphragm returns via the remaining fibres. The shape of the diaphragm is affected by the pulsations of the blood pressure which is in contact with the distal side of the diaphragm. The modulated light beam is led to a photo-transistor and, after amplification, is fed to a recorder. The frequency response of the device is sufficiently high for it to record heart sounds as well. Such an arrangement has been described by Lindstrom (1970). Ohno *et al.* (1971) have extended the technique by arranging with a cardiac catheter containing 300 fibres each of 50 μm diameter to measure both oxygen saturation and intracardiac pressure. The frequency response for the pressure system is linear out to 100 Hz and 9 dB down at 1200 Hz. The catheter size is No. 7 French.

REFERENCES

Anderson, N. M., Sekelj, P. and McGregor, M. (1961). 'The transmission of red and infra-red light through the human ear.' *I.R.E. Trans. biomed. Electron.* **8,** 133
Burn, G. (1968). 'An automatic haemoglobinometer and haemocyto-meter.' In *Proc. 2nd European Symposium Med. Electron.* p. 62. London; Hanover Press
Fromer, P. L. (1967). 'The principles of fibre optics and their clinical applications.' In *Engineering in the Practice of Medicine.* p. 422. Baltimore; Williams and Wilkins
Gamble, W. J., Hugenholtz, P. G., Monroe, R. G., Polanyi, M. and Nadas, A. S. (1965). 'The use of fiberoptics in clinical cardiac catheterisation.' *Circulation.* **31,** 328
Hugenholtz, P. G., Gamble, W. J., Monroe, R. G., and Polyani, M. L. (1965). 'The use of fibre optics in clinical cardiac catheterization. 2. *In vivo* dye-dilution curves.' *Circulation,* **31,** 344

Kapany, N. S., Harrison, D. C., Silbertrust, N., Drake, R. P., McLaughlin, T. and Miller, H. A. (1967). 'Fibre optics oximeter—densitometer for cardiovascular studies.' *Appl. Opt.* **6**, 565

Lindstrom, L. H. (1970). 'Miniaturized pressure transducer intended for intravascular use.' *I.E.E.E. Trans. Biomedical Engng.*, **BME-17**

Ohno, H., Kameya, S., Mizoi, K., Oshima, M., Kustakabe, M., Iwai, Y., Nakashika, M., and Saito, K. (1971). 'A study in fiberoptic oximetry—measurement of oxygen saturation and pressure of intracardiac blood.' *Digest 9th. Int. Conf. med. biol. Engng.*, Melbourne, 106

Paul, W. and Woolf, C. R. (1967). 'An ear oximeter using d.c. operational amplifiers.' *Can. J. Physiol.* **45**, 1001

Reichert, W. J. (1966). 'Theory and construction of oximeters.' In *Oxygen Measurements in Blood and Tissues.* p. 81. Ed. by J. P. Payne and D. W. Hill. London; Churchill

Rodrigo, F. A. (1953). 'The determination of the oxygenation of blood *in vitro* by using reflected light.' *Am. Heart J.* **45**, 809

Sekelj, P. (1954). 'Further studies on oximetry.' *Am. Heart J.* **48**, 746

— Oriol, A., Anderson, N. M., Morch, J. and McGregor, M. (1967). 'Measurement of indocyanine green dye with a cuvette oximeter.' *J. appl. Physiol.* **23**, 114

Stephen, C. R., Slater, H. M., Johnson, A. L. and Sekelj, P. (1951). 'The oximeter—a technical aid for the anesthetist.' *Anesthesiology* **12**, 541

Sutterer, W. F. and Wood, E. H. (1962). 'A compensated dichromatic densitometer for indocyanine green.' *I.R.E. Trans. biomed. Electron.* **BME-9**, 133

Tait, G. R., Sekelj, P. and D'Ombrain, G. L. (1966). 'A theoretical analysis of some errors in oximetry.' *I.E.E.E. Trans. biomed. Electron.* **BME-13**,' 200

— and Sekelj, P. (1967). 'An analog computer for ear oximetry.' *Med. Electron. biol. Engng.* **5**, 463

Van Slyke, D. D. and Neill, J. M. (1924). 'Determination of gases in blood and other solutions by vacuum extraction and manometric measurements.' *J. biol. Chem.* **61**, 523

Zijlstra, W. G. (1958). '*A Manual of Reflection Oximetry and some other Applications of Reflection Photometry*.' Assen, Holland; Van Gorcum

13–The Measurement of Body Temperature

For the routine measurement of body temperature, even when patient-monitoring systems are in use in an intensive care unit, many medical and nursing staff prefer to use the traditional clinical thermometer. The method is inexpensive and causes little trouble since the staff will be spending a good deal of time at the bedside in any case. A mercury-in-glass clinical thermometer gives its indication at the site where the temperature is being measured. The advantage offered by electrical thermometers is that their output indication can be remote from the site of measurement. This requirement can arise when the temperatures of a number of patients have to be recorded at a central location, or during surgery when the patient is covered in drapes, or during the technique of hypothermia when it may be necessary to know the temperature of the patient at several sites in the body. As with most measurements several possible techniques exist and it is best to have more than one available.

RESISTANCE THERMOMETERS

Whereas a metal will show a slight increase in resistance when its temperature is raised, a suitable semiconducting material will show a large decrease in resistance. The wire coil or semiconductor is placed in a bridge circuit and the change in resistance expressed in terms of temperature.

Although use has been made of compact wire coils to measure temperature in the axilla, the technique has not proved to be attractive because of the difficulties of winding the fine diameter wire to give a reliable construction. The small change in resistance occurring with changes in body temperature requires stable high-gain amplification. In some arrangements, the coil forms one arm of an a.c.

bridge energized at about 2 kHz and followed by an amplifier tuned to this frequency.

THERMISTORS

Nearly all commercially available patient-monitoring systems use well-aged semiconductor elements which are temperature sensitive. These are known as thermistors since they are thermally-sensitive resistors. The resistance of the thermistor decreases with temperature according to a relationship of the form $R = A.\exp(b/T)$ where R is the resistance of the thermistor in ohms and T is the absolute temperature and A and B are constants (Scarr and Setterington, 1960). A typical thermistor resistance would be 2,000 Ω at 20°C falling to 1,400Ω at 40°C. The active portion of the thermistor consists of a bead, made from a mixture of nickel, cobalt and manganese oxides, about the size of a pin-head. It is suspended from a pair of lead wires and mounted inside the tip of a glass envelope so that only a thin layer of glass separates it from the surroundings. This protects the element but allows the speed of response to be fast enough for the thermistor to be able to sense respiratory gas flows. The bridge current flowing through the thermistor is set to a value where self heating will keep the bead temperature above ambient so that it is affected by the cooling produced when it is placed in a gas stream. The maximum power dissipation in a bead of this type is about 10 mW. The normal tolerance on resistance is ±20 per cent at 20°C, but matching down to ±1 per cent is available at a higher price. In order to improve their stability thermistors should be aged, according to Trolander and Sterling (1962) for 3 eight-hour periods at 95°C when they are to be used in the region of 40°C.

Taking natural logarithms of both sides of the thermistor equation, $\log_e R = (b/T) + \log_e A$. It can be seen that the relationship between R and T is non-linear. It is desirable that the scale of a clinical temperature monitor should be linear, and that it should be possible to either interchange thermistor probes or to switch the recording instrument to more than one probe. Differentiating the thermistor equation gives the change in thermistor resistance with temperature $dR/dT = (-b/T^2).R$ and so this depends upon the actual value of the temperature giving a curved relationship. However, by shunting a thermistor with a fixed resistor, one can almost obtain a linear temperature-resistance characteristic over a limited temperature range (Norden and Bainbridge, 1962). If a thermistor with a resistance of

2,000 Ω at 20°C is shunted with a 2,000-ohm resistor, the resistance-temperature characteristic of the combination will be almost linear from 0–50degC and is linear from 0–30degC. When the resistances of the thermistor and its shunt are equal, the temperature sensitivity of the combination will be about one half that of the thermistor alone. One can make two similar thermistors the equivalent of two nearly identical thermistors by the use of shunt and series resistors with each thermistor (Godin, 1962). This arrangement is adopted in commercial multi-probe instruments. The attainment of a linear output from a thermistor bridge is also discussed by Scott (1964). Richards (1967) uses a closely specified thermistor in an a.c. bridge circuit to make a direct reading thermometer with a nearly linear scale. Without calibration, typical errors are plus or minus 0·5degC over a range of 20degC. A typical transistorized physiological temperature-monitoring system using up to 10 interchangeable thermistor probes has three ranges. Two are conventional and cover 20–32°C and 30–42degC with an accuracy of $\pm$0·2degC. The third range is a sensitive one covering only $-$2degC to $+$2degC about any temperature set in the range 34–42degC. This is used to monitor changes occurring in a patient's temperature with time. An electrical output of 1 V d.c. for full scale is provided for tape recording or to operate an alarm system.

The use of a data logger in conjunction with thermistor probes to measure the oral temperature of several hundred women patients in the Juntendo Women's Hospital, Tokyo, provides an interesting example of this technique.

Several times each day the patients are instructed over the public address system to put the probes in their mouths. The patients lie still while music is played, and the data logger scans the probes, printing out the temperature and bed number for each patient. Unoccupied beds are distinguished by the printing of the ambient temperature.

METAL RESISTANCE THERMOMETERS

Metal resistance thermometers constructed from a coil of nickel or platinum wire have been used for the measurement of skin, rectal, oesophageal and oral temperatures. The coil and its connecting leads are placed in one arm of a bridge circuit, with a dummy pair of leads in an opposite arm, *Figure 13.1*. The ends of the dummy leads are shorted out, and the coil and dummy leads are run together. In this way any changes occurring in the resistance of the coil leads with ambient temperature changes are cancelled by corresponding changes in the dummy leads. Resistance coils tend to be a little bulky and are not suitable for mounting in needles. A typical resistance thermometer unit would be scaled 25–42degC with an accuracy of 1 per cent of the scale span.

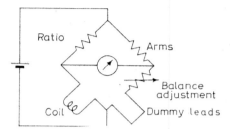

Figure 13.1. A simplified electrical resistance thermometer circuit

The increase in coil resistance with temperature is linear over the range 0–100degC. If R_0 is the resistance of the coil at 0°C and R_t is the resistance at t°C, then $R_t = R_0(1 + \alpha t)$ where α is the temperature coefficient of resistance of the wire. For platinum $\alpha = 0.004$/degC. Hence a 100-ohm platinum coil would increase its resistance by 0.4degC for each 1degC change. If R_0 and α are known, a measurement of R_t will give a value for t°. Platinum and nickel are chosen because they are stable and easily obtainable.

THERMISTOR ENDORADIOSONDES

Temperature sensitive endoradiosondes or 'radio pills' are of great value in transmitting the deep body temperature of mobile patients

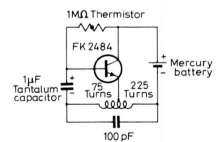

Figure 13.2. Circuit of a temperature sensitive endoradiosonde (after Mackay, 1967)

or free-ranging animals. In *Figure 13.2* is illustrated a simple transmitter which can be assembled into the volume of a sphere approximately 1 cm in diameter (Mackay, 1967). This is basically a Hartley oscillator. As a result of the circuit's oscillating, a voltage builds up on the 1 μF capacitor sufficient to cut off the transistor. The charge leaks away, the time constant being determined by the resistance of the thermistor. Thus the frequency of squegging (the rate of interruption of the oscillator frequency) is dependent upon the thermistor resistance and hence of the temperature of the gut in which the radio pill is placed. The transmission from the pill can be received on an ordinary pocket transistor receiver as a series of clicks which can be timed with a stop watch. The click rate is linearly related to temperature.

THERMOCOUPLES

A thermocouple consists of a circuit made from two dissimilar metals, and having the two junctions maintained at different temperatures, *Figure 13.3*. The temperature difference gives rise to a thermal electromotive force which drives a current around the circuit.

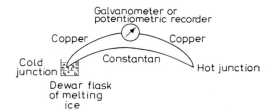

Figure 13.3. A simple thermocouple circuit

Over a limited temperature range the thermal e.m.f. and hence the current, is proportional to the temperature difference. One junction, the reference junction, is maintained at a constant temperature, and the other junction used to sense the temperature to be measured. The reference junction is often held at 0°C inside a Dewar flask containing melting ice, or in an ice-point apparatus controlled by a thermo-electric cooler. In some cases it may be sufficient to mount the thermocouple reference junction inside a large block of metal, to give thermal inertia, at room temperature.

Convenient combinations of metals for sensing clinical tempera-tures are iron-constantan or copper-constantan (constantan is an alloy of 60 per cent copper, 40 per cent nickel). Copper-constantan develops a thermal e.m.f. of 40 μV per degC temperature difference between the junctions. With the reference junction at 0°C and the other at 38°C, the output from the thermocouple is about 1·5 mV.

369

This can be readily measured with a precision d.c. potentiometer using a Weston cadmium-mercury cell as a voltage reference, or with a good quality digital voltmeter. With a 0°C reference temperature the output is too great to be indicated on the usual 1 mV full-scale potentiometric recorder, and a recorder having a full-scale deflection of 2 or 5 mV will be needed. The use of a multi-channel printing-type potentiometric recorder is helpful when up to 12 different temperatures have to be recorded.

Clinical thermocouple instruments often make use of a galvano-meter display to indicate rectal or axillary temperatures. For ward or operating room use it is usually not convenient to have a cold junction at 0°C, so that these instruments employ an automatic cold junction compensation device. In one system, the thermocouple cold junction is mounted close to the galvanometer which has one of its coil suspension springs made from a bimetal. Changes in the ambient temperature affect the cold junction, but cause the bimetal spring to twist in such a direction as to offset the deflection of the galvanometer produced by the ambient temperature change.

The e.m.f. produced by thermocouples is small and requires care for its measurement; however, thermocouples possess the advantage of reproducibility, since a number can be made from a batch of each of the two wires. Constantan will not soft solder, and the thermo-couple junctions are best made by twisting the ends of wires together and spot welding them with a dental spot welder. As an alternative, hard solder may be used. Thermocouples can be robust since the strength is largely set by that of the wires. The temperature-sensing junction can be mounted at the tip of a hypodermic needle for the measurement of tissue temperatures (Krog, 1954). Thermo-couples are particularly useful when temperatures have to be measured under difficult circumstances. Bracken, Broughton and Hill (1968) mounted three thermocouples (one at the top, middle and bottom) of a steel cylinder filled with Entonox nitrous oxide-oxygen mixture to 2,000 lbf/in².

Laws of thermocouples

The production of the thermoelectric e.m.f. in a thermocouple is known as the Seebeck effect. The complementary action is known as the Peltier effect. This occurs when a current is forced round the thermocouple circuit, giving rise to cooling at one junction and heat-ing at the other. When a current of several amperes at a low voltage is flowing the degree of cooling is considerable. This is the basis of thermoelectric coolers (Goldsmid, 1960). An ice-point apparatus for use with thermocouples can be made by using a thermoelectric cooler to cool a volume of water placed in a sealed metal bellows. When the water starts to freeze, the sudden diminution in volume causes the bellows to contract and trip a microswitch which cuts off the current to the cooler. The inflow of heat from the surroundings melts the ice, trips the switch and restores the current.

The law of the homogeneous circuit

An electric current cannot be sustained in a circuit consisting of a single homogeneous metal, however varying in cross-section, by the application of heat alone. Thus in a practical thermocouple, the thermoelectric e.m.f. will depend only upon the difference in the junction temperatures, and not upon the temperature gradient in the connecting wires.

The law of intermediate metals

The algebraic sum of the thermoelectric e.m.fs in a circuit consisting of any number of dissimilar metals is zero, provided that the complete circuit is at the same temperature. Hence any number of intermediate connections can be introduced into the circuit if they are all kept at the same temperature. Spurious e.m.fs may be generated if the temperature is not uniform.

The law of intermediate temperatures

The thermoelectric e.m.f. produced by any thermocouple made from homogeneous metals with its junctions at temperatures T_1 and T_3 is the algebraic sum of the e.m.f. of the thermocouple with one junction at T_1 and the other at any other temperature T_2 and the e.m.f. of the same thermocouple with its junctions at T_2 and T_3.

These laws combine to give the result that the thermoelectric e.m.fs generated in any circuit consisting of a number of dissimilar homogeneous metals are a function only of the temperatures of their junctions. If all but one of the junctions are kept at a constant reference temperature, the output of the thermocouple will be dependent upon the temperature of that junction alone.

SILICON DIODE TEMPERATURE SENSORS

The voltage drop developed across a forward biased silicon diode is temperature dependent. It varies at the rate of 2 mV/degC. Because of their small size, a silicon diode makes a convenient sensor for mounting in the axilla. A diode is supplied with a constant current via a series resistor from a 12-V source and the voltage drop across the diode is sensed with a d.c. operational amplifier, *Figure 13.4.* A

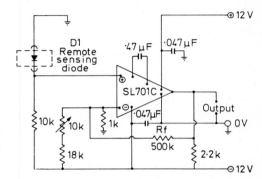

Figure 13.4. Operational amplifier circuit for use with silicon diode temperature sensor (after Griffiths and Hill, 1969)

backing-off circuit is provided so that the output meter of the amplifier can be calibrated, say, from 36–40degC. The technique is described by Griffiths and Hill (1969). The temperature coefficient of diodes from the same batch is reproducible.

THE CONSTRUCTION OF CLINICAL TEMPERATURE PROBES

The physical construction of a temperature-measuring probe is closely linked to the type of measuring element involved which in turn depends upon the application.

Thermocouples must be used when it is required to have a probe with a narrow, sensitive point (such as the tip of a slender needle) or a long, flexible probe. They are also suitable for skin temperature probes. Here the probe must possess minimal mass in order that errors arising from heat conduction to the probe are reduced. Their low thermal inertia also makes thermocouples very suitable for the recording of rapidly varying temperatures.

Considerable care must be exercised if thermocouples are to be operated at a distance from the temperature indicator. Any junction of dissimilar metals can give rise to artefact e.m.f. changes if the junction temperature changes. Special leads having similar e.m.f.-temperature characteristics to the thermocouple wires, but costing less, should be used. For this reason, it may be convenient to measure the temperature of patients at a central console by means of resistance thermometer coils. All probes and cables should be capable of being chemically sterilized. A number of them are designed to withstand autoclaving at 110°C.

A loop thermocouple probe for the measurement of the temperature of toes or fingertip is shown in *Figure 13.5(a)*; the loop diameter is 40 mm.

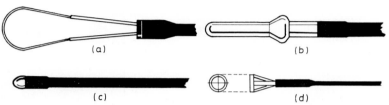

Figure 13.5(a) Loop thermocouple for the measurement of the temperature of the toes or fingertips (b) a typical rectal temperature probe (c) a human oesophageal temperature probe (d) a tracheal air temperature probe. (All figures reproduced by courtesy of Ellab Ltd.)

A typical rectal thermocouple probe is shown in *Figure 13.5(b)*. Its diameter is 5·5 mm its length 44 mm. The sheath is made from stainless steel. When suitably greased it slips easily into the rectum, but will not come out by itself because of the ball. A rectal probe with its temperature indicator is illustrated in *Figure 13.6*.

Typical needle probes would be mounted in 18–22 gauge needles (1·2–0·7 mm diameter) with lengths in the range 25–225 mm.

A human oesophageal probe is illustrated in *Figure 13.5(c)*. It has a 5·5 mm-diameter stainless steel sheath. The probe of *Figure 13.5(d)* measures the temperature of the air stream in the trachea. The thermojunction in the form of a fine cross is placed at the centre of a Nylon ring 7·2 mm in diameter. This construction gives a low thermal inertia and protects the junction from touching the sides of the trachea. The response is fast enough to follow individual breaths.

Thermistor beads for body temperature measurement are usually sealed into the tip of a glass tube. In this way the bead is protected by a thin layer of glass, but a rapid response is maintained. The probe tip can be placed in a patient's tidal air stream. For mounting in the axilla or rectum the thermistor assembly would be placed in a stainless steel sheath.

For use in the axilla, the temperature sensor can be mounted in a light plastic housing. The sensor is placed against the skin, and insulated on the opposite side with a piece of plastic foam. The assembly is held in place with a piece of adhesive plaster.

A technique for the recording of body temperature over a prolonged period is described by Tepas and Vianello (1966).

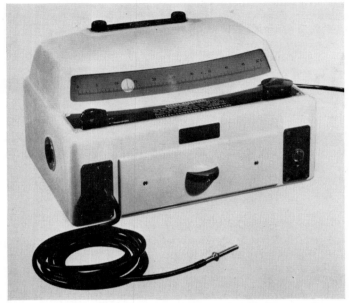

Figure 13.6. Rectal thermocouple probe and temperature indicator.
(Reproduced by courtesy of Sierex Ltd.)

THE MEASUREMENT OF TEMPERATURES DURING HYPOTHERMIA

A particular interest in the measurement of body temperature arises during hypothermic procedures. The concept of body temperature while adequate for most clinical purposes, is not sufficiently precise for induced hypothermia. Here there may exist considerable differences in temperature between various parts of the body. Since cardiac arrhythmia, the factor limiting the degree of cooling, appears to depend on the temperature of the heart itself there has been a number of studies carried out to see where an equivalent temperature could be measured.

Cooper and Kenyon (1957) showed that the temperature measured in the oesophagus at heart level is very close to that in the aorta

374

which may, however, differ from the rectal temperature by two or three degrees centigrade. The presence of faeces can also influence temperatures recorded in the rectum.

The oesophageal temperature is taken as an accurate indication both of the cardiac and cerebral temperatures. However, Whitby and Dunkin (1968) have shown the oesophageal temperature recorded in the anaesthetized and intubated adult depends upon the site at which it is measured. They found that the longitudinal variation in temperature is greater than the lateral and can be as much as 6degC. The lowest temperatures are found in the upper and middle thirds. Both longitudinal and lateral variations level out in the lower third. The lower fourth of the oesophagus is both the warmest and the most stable. To reach this area, thermocouple leads should be inserted at least 24 cm below the corniculate cartilages.

REFERENCES

Bracken, A., Broughton, G. and Hill, D. W. (1968). 'Safety precautions to be observed with cooled premixed gases.' *Br. med. J.* **2,** 715

Cooper, K. E. and Kenyon, J. R. (1957). 'A comparison of temperatures measured in the rectum, oesophagus and on the surface of the aorta during hypothermia in man.' *Br. J. Surg.* **44,** 616

Godin, M. C. (1962). 'A method of equalizing thermistors.' *J. scient. Instrum.* **39,** 241

Goldsmid, H. J. (1960). *Applications of Thermo-electricity.* London; Methuen

Griffiths, C. A. and Hill, D. W. (1969). 'Some applications of microelectronics to patients.' *Wld. med. Instrum.* **7,** 8.

Krog, J. (1954). 'Improved needle thermocouple for subcutaneous and intramuscular temperature measurements in man.' *Rev. scient. Instrum.* **25,** 799

Mackay, R. S. (1967). *Bio-medical Telemetry.* New York; Wiley

Norden, P. and Bainbridge, N. W. (1962). 'The use of unmatched thermistors for the measurement of temperature difference under varying ambient conditions.' *J. scient. Instrum.* **39,** 399

Richards, J. C. S. (1967). 'Sensitive thermistor thermometer.' *Electron. Engng.* **39,** 674

Scarr, R. W. A. and Setterington, R. A. (1960). 'Thermistors their theory, manufacture and application.' *Proc. Instn. elect. Engrs.* **107,** pt. B.

Scott, I. G. (1964). 'Linearization of the output of bridge networks.' *J. Scient. Instrum.* **41,** 458

Tepas, D. I. and Vianello, M. A. B. (1966). 'Method of recording body temperature for prolonged time.' *Aerospace Med.* **37,** 488

Trolander, H. W. and Sterling, J. J. (1962). 'Behaviour of thermistors at biological temperatures.' *I.R.E. Trans. biomed. Electron.* **BME-9,** 142

Whitby, J. D. and Dunkin, L. J. (1968). 'Temperature differences in the oesophagus.' *Br. J. Anaesth.* **40,** 991

14 – Counting Equipment for use with Radioactive Isotopes

A steadily increasing number of diagnostic tests are being performed with the aid of compounds labelled with radioactive isotopes. Normally, the bulk of the counting of samples *in vitro* will be performed in a special counting laboratory and the *in vivo* studies of the uptake and distribution of labelled compounds by means of a gamma camera or scanner will require a special room. Surgeons and anaesthetists are unlikely to be personally involved to any great extent with these techniques, but will find it useful to have some idea of what is involved when a particular test is requested. Counting equipment is used in the operating room for radiological protection monitoring during the implantation of radioactive sources for therapeutic purposes. Miniature Geiger counters or semiconductor detectors are used for counting in the vagina and rectum, and cerebral blood flow studies are performed with small Geiger counters and scintillation counters.

RADIOACTIVE ISOTOPES

Some of the elements can exist in different forms which have the same number of orbital electrons in their atoms, but different atomic weights. These are known as isotopes of the element concerned. Some isotopes are stable, while others are unstable and exhibit radioactivity. At random intervals the nuclei of the atoms of a radioactive isotope lose energy which is emitted in the form of a particle or gamma radiation. The most commonly encountered radioactivity in medical work is in the form of beta particles and gamma rays. There may also be low-energy X-rays associated with the decay.

Alpha particles

Alpha particles are emitted by some of the heavier elements and consist of 2 protons plus 2 neutrons. They have a very limited penetrating power (they are stopped by the outer layer of the skin) but because of the intense ionization they produce in tissue, they are very dangerous if ingested. They are not emitted by any isotope used in medical studies except for sealed sources of radium-226 and its daughter products contained in radium needles.

Beta particles

Beta particles are high-speed particles of the same mass as an electron emitted from the nuclei of atoms undergoing some forms of radioactive disintegration. Most beta particles are conventional negatively charged electrons. However, some elements such as gallium emit positrons which are similar to electrons but positively charged. An excess of neutrons within a nucleus may result in the spontaneous decay of a neutron into a proton and a negative electron. As a result, the nucleus concerned gains a proton, loses a neutron and gives off a beta particle. The nuclear mass is essentially unaltered by this process. A nucleus having a deficiency of neutrons may spontaneously change a proton into a neutron and a positron, the nuclear mass of the daughter element being virtually the same as that of its parent.

Gamma radiation

After emitting an alpha or beta particle, the atom may be in an excited state having an excess of energy. This is released, almost immediately in most cases, in the form of a gamma-ray photon— a quantum of electromagnetic radiation. Gamma radiation is similar to X-radiation, but more penetrating and having a shorter wavelength. It is emitted from the nucleus of an atom, unlike X-radiation which arises from energy changes occurring in the orbital electrons.

Electron capture

A positron can be emitted when a nucleus has an excess of protons. A competitive process exists which can also result in the change of a proton into a neutron. It is possible for a proton in the nucleus to capture an extra-nuclear electron from one of the inner electron shells of the atom, thus neutralizing the positive charge of the proton. This process is known as electron capture (E.C.). The electron is likely to be captured from the K-shell (the innermost electron

377

orbit) so that electron capture is also known as K-capture. The vacancy arising from the capture by the nucleus of an electron is filled by an electron moving in from another orbit. In doing this, X-radiation is emitted.

Annihilation and pair production

When a positron is emitted it will soon encounter a negative electron and the two will mutually annihilate. The positron-electron annihilation process yields two gamma-ray photons which move off in opposite directions. This gamma radiation is called annihilation radiation. It plays an important part in coincidence gamma camera techniques using positron emitters. After the injection of a gallium-labelled isotope into the patient the annihilation radiation can be detected by two gamma camera heads working in coincidence and situated on opposite sides of the patient.

If a gamma-ray photon has sufficient energy and is near a nucleus it may create a positron-electron pair. Each of these particles has a mass equivalent to 0·51 MeV, so that the gamma photon must have an energy in excess of 1·02 MeV for this process. The excess energy is given to the positron-electron pair in the form of energy of motion. Pair production predominates at high energies and is the reverse process to annihilation.

Internal conversion

A transition from one nuclear energy state to another can come about by means of a direct transfer of the excess nuclear energy to an orbital electron (usually in the K-shell). This electron is then ejected from the atom as a beta particle. Internal conversion electrons have well-defined energies.

Isomers

Some radioactive isotopes can exist in an excited state for an appreciable period of time before they lose energy by the emission of a gamma photon, and drop into a ground state. The excited state has associated with it a half-life, and the ground state can be either stable or unstable. Both the excited and the ground states have exactly the same number of protons and neutrons and are called isometric states or isomers. The excited state is also known as a metastable state. The short half-life of metastable states makes such isotopes attractive for *in vivo* applications. Examples are technetium-99m and indium-113m.

ENERGIES OF ALPHA AND BETA PARTICLES AND GAMMA RADIATION

The energies of both alpha and beta particles and gamma rays are expressed in terms of the electron volt. One electron volt is the energy that an electron would acquire if it were accelerated through a potential difference of one volt. Radioactive emissions have energies of the order of thousands or millions of electron volts. For example, two of the gamma rays from iodine-131 have energies of 360 and 640 keV, and the main gamma-ray energy of technetium-99 m is 140 keV.

Nuclides

An atom which has specific nuclear characteristics is known as a nuclide, for example, phosphorus of mass number 32 and atomic number 15. The mass number is the number of protons plus neutrons in the nucleus, while the atomic number is the number of orbital electrons in the atom. For simplicity, the mass number only is often quoted to identify the particular isotope, for example, P-32.

Half-life

Atoms of a radioactive element decay at random, the number decaying at any particular moment being determined on a statistical basis. The rate of decay of any particular atomic species is proportional to the number of those atoms present at that instant. This is a simple exponential decay curve of the form $N_t = N_0 . e^{-\lambda t}$ where N_0 is the number of atoms decaying per unit time at time $t=0$ while N_t is the corresponding figure at time t, λ is the decay constant for the element concerned, and e is the exponential (2·718). The time for the activity to decay by one half is known as the half-life, and is the physical half-life of the particular element. For iodine-131 it is 8 days. The half time $t_\frac{1}{2} = 0·693 . \lambda$.

Once the radioisotope has been administered to a living organism it is necessary to take into account the biological half-life of the isotope. This is because the isotope is eliminated from the organism by processes such as respiration, urination and defaecation. As a result of the clearance from the body the effective half-life of the isotope within the body is reduced. As an example, consider the case of human serum albumin labelled with iodine-131. The activity of the ^{131}I is diminishing with a half-life of about 8 days, while at the same time the iodine is being cleared from the body with a half-life of about 21 days. The two processes act in parallel so that the effective half-life of the iodine in the body becomes $1/T_{e\frac{1}{2}}=$ $1/T_{p\frac{1}{2}}+1/T_{b\frac{1}{2}}=5\cdot8$ days where $T_{e\frac{1}{2}}$ is the effective half-life, $T_{p\frac{1}{2}}$ is the physical half-life and $T_{b\frac{1}{2}}$ is the biological half-life.

The absorption of beta particles

When a beta particle passes close to a nucleus and is deflected by the field, the resulting velocity change produces electromagnetic radiation called Bremsstrahlung. This is similar to X-radiation but of a different origin. Bremsstrahlung production is high with absorbers having a high atomic number. For this reason, material used for absorption or shielding with beta particles should have a low atomic number.

A 3-MeV beta particle is stopped by about 6·5 mm of aluminium. In contrast, a 3-MeV alpha particle is stopped by about 0·015 mm of aluminium. Perspex of 0·5 inch thickness will also provide an effective shielding against beta particles. The absorption of beta particles depends mainly upon the number of electrons in their path. For materials having a low atomic number this is approximately proportional to the mass per unit area of the material (mg/cm²).

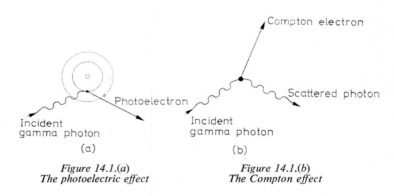

Figure 14.1.(a)
The photoelectric effect

Figure 14.1.(b)
The Compton effect

The interaction of gamma radiation with matter

Three competing processes act to take up the energy of the gamma photons.

The photoelectric effect transfers all the energy of the gamma ray to an electron in an inner orbit of an atom of the absorber, *Figure 14.1a*. This effect predominates at low gamma energies and with absorbers having a high atomic number.

380

The Compton effect occurs when a gamma ray makes an elastic collision with an electron. The gamma energy is shared with the electron, and another gamma ray of lower energy is produced and this travels in a different direction, *Figure 14.1b*. The Compton scattering can be repeated by the secondary gamma ray and continue for several collisions until so much energy has been lost that the final photon is absorbed by the photoelectric effect.

Pair production If the gamma ray has sufficient energy and is near a nucleus, it may create a positive-electron pair. Since each of these particles has a mass equivalent to 0·51 MeV, the gamma ray must have an energy in excess of 1·02 MeV for the process to happen. At medium gamma-ray energies, it is the Compton effect which predominates. Pair production becomes predominant at the higher gamma-ray energies and in absorbers with a high atomic number.

The curie

The unit of radioactivity is the curie. This was originally defined in terms of the disintegration rate of one gram of radium, but it is now also applied to both alpha and beta particle emitters. When used in this way, the value of the curie is taken to be $3·7 \times 10^{10}$ disintegrations per second. Thus a millicurie corresponds to $3·7 \times 10^{7}$ and a microcurie to $3·7 \times 10^{4}$ disintegrations per second. With some isotopes, for example phosphorus-32, it is possible to say that a microcurie of ^{32}P will emit $3·7 \times 10^{4}$ beta particles, on average, per second. With other isotopes this may not be so, depending upon the decay scheme. Manganese-52 gives off positrons in 35 per cent of its disintegrations and decays by electron capture in the remaining 65 per cent. Hence one microcurie of ^{52}Mn will emit only $0·35 \times 3·7 \times 10^{4} = 1·3 \times 10^{4}$ beta particles per second.

RADIATION DETECTORS
Ionization

The fact that the interaction of radioactivity with matter gives rise to ionization makes it possible to detect the presence of the radiation. When an atom is ionized it loses one or more orbital electrons to form a positively charged ion and negatively charged electron(s). This ion and electron constitute an ion pair. If the electrons can be attracted to a positively charged electrode and the positive ions to a negatively charged electrode then a current can be caused to flow in an external circuit. The magnitude of the current is proportional to the amount of radioactivity present between the electrodes. This is the operating principle of the d.c. ionization chamber which is widely used in radiological protection work.

The d.c. ionization chamber

An ionization chamber consists of a gas-filled chamber containing a pair of electrodes across which is maintained a potential difference of a few hundred volts. The radioactive source to be measured is placed either inside or close to the chamber. For use with beta particles a thin aluminium window must be provided in the chamber to allow the passage of the particles or photons from the sample. The polarizing voltage placed across the electrodes must be sufficiently high to collect all the ion pairs. The chamber current will then be proportional to the amount of radioactivity in the sample, *Figure 14.2*.

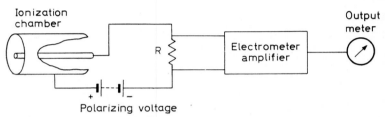

Figure 14.2. The use of a d.c. ionization chamber to measure the activity of a source

The number of ion pairs produced per beta particle is approximately given by dividing the average beta energy by 30, since about 30 eV is required to produce one ion pair. If this number is n and the geometrical efficiency of the chamber is E, then the chamber current

$$I = n.E.S. \times 3 \cdot 7 \times 10^{10}.1 \cdot 6 \times 10^{-19} \text{ amperes}$$

S being the source strength in curies; I is usually of the order of 10^{-10} A or less. It is measured either with a vibrating reed electrometer (Pavlensky, Swank and Grenchnick, 1947) or with a hybrid electrometer valve-transistor amplifier circuit. Portable pocket ion chambers are used to monitor personal radiation doses. Ion chambers of a standard construction are employed for the measurement of the activity of liquid isotopes for administration to patients. Hospital physicists widely use an ion chamber for this type of work which has been standardized by the National Physical Laboratory against known sources. For iodine-131 the chamber gives a current of approximately $10 \cdot 5 \times 10^{-12}$ A per millicurie of ^{131}I when 4 ml of the iodine solution is contained in a 5 ml ampoule placed inside the re-entrant portion of the chamber. The provision of a re-entrant thimble for the chamber enables liquid samples to be easily counted when they are in an ampoule, and also provides a good counting geometry.

The use of a guard ring

A material having a very high insulation resistance such as P.T.F.E. (polytetrafluoroethylene) is used as the insulation between the inner and outer electrodes of the ion chamber. The positive electrode (anode) is usually connected to the live input terminal of the electrometer and is kept at a potential close to that of earth. The positive pole of the polarizing voltage supply is also connected to earth, the negative pole of the supply being connected to the cathode of the chamber. The anode is thus positive to the cathode as required.

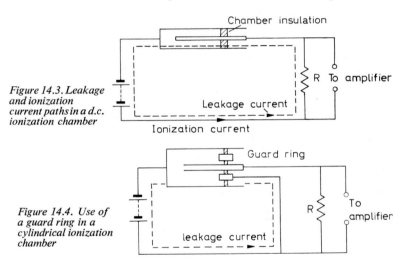

Figure 14.3. Leakage and ionization current paths in a d.c. ionization chamber

Figure 14.4. Use of a guard ring in a cylindrical ionization chamber

Any leakage currents occurring across the insulation of the chamber will be in parallel with the chamber current and will give rise to an increased voltage drop across the input resistor R of the electrometer, *Figure 14.3*, and thus to an error in the reading of activity. The effect of leakage currents can be minimized by the use of the guard ring technique. In this, the insulation is now divided into two parts, *Figure 14.4*, one part between the high-voltage electrode (cathode) and the guard ring electrode, the other lying between the guard ring electrode and the collector electrode (anode). As can be seen, the polarizing voltage is effectively applied across the first portion of the insulation, the second portion having almost no voltage across it. Thus leakage current from the anode is practically non-existent. Many commercial electrometers are provided with a third input terminal for connection to a guard ring electrode and also with a polarizing voltage of 200–300 V for use with an ionization chamber. Typically, the electrometer might require an input voltage of the order of 1 V, and this is developed by passing the chamber current through a high-value resistor. Three switched input resistors might be provided, 10^8, 10^9 and 10^{10} Ω, together with a 3 : 1 gain control on the amplifier.

Operating regions of ionization chambers

When there is zero potential difference applied across the electrodes of an ion chamber, the ions generated by incident ionizing radiation or particles are subject only to thermal motion and recombine before long. Only a small fraction of them will be collected at the electrodes. As the voltage across the electrodes is increased a greater proportion will be collected before recombining. When the electric field strength is about 10 V per cm between the electrodes nearly all the available ions will be collected, the chamber being saturated. The chamber is now said to be operating in the ionization region. If the polarizing voltage is increased still further, the ionization produced is increased as a result of a secondary effect, ionization by collision. The electric field strength is enough to accelerate the electrons formed in the chamber to attain sufficient energy so that they in turn can give rise to further ionization of the gas molecules. At first, the ionization produced is proportional to the number of original ionizing events, the current being multiplied by a constant factor. This is the proportional region. The proportional counter is operated in a counting mode, that is to say, a pulse of current is produced for each ionizing event, the magnitude of the pulse being proportional to the amount of ionization produced by that particular event. At still higher polarizing voltages, the multiplication produced by electron collisions approaches saturation and the pulses of current are multiplied to a constant final value, regardless of the initial amount of ionization. This is the Geiger region. All the pulses have virtually the same size irrespective of the number of primary ions produced in the initial ionizing event.

Ionization chambers are operated in two basic modes. With small time constants in the associated electronic equipment the chamber can be used in a counting mode in which it responds separately to each ionizing event. With a long time constant, the chamber operates in an integrating mode, collecting the ionization current over a relatively long period. Alpha particles, which produce an intense ionization can be assayed with either technique, but beta particles, electrons, gamma rays and X-rays give rise to relatively little ionization and require the integrating mode if a d.c. chamber is employed. Because of the amplification process, they can be counted with a chamber operated in the proportional or Geiger regions.

PROPORTIONAL COUNTERS

The design of the counter and the value of the polarizing voltage are chosen so that a high voltage gradient exists close to the positive anode. The primary electrons produced by the ionizing event can then be accelerated sufficiently to give rise to secondary electrons. The current pulse size is proportional to the initial amount of ionization, gas multiplication factors of 1,000 or more being possible. Proportional counter geometry usually takes the form of a cylindrical cathode with an axial fine wire anode. The cathode radius might be 1 cm and the anode radius 0·001 cm, with a polarizing voltage of the order of 1,000 V. The output pulses are of the order of several millivolts amplitude. For beta particle counting, methane gas is flowed through the body of the proportional counter. Argon is sometimes used as an alternative to methane, particularly for alpha particle counting because of its non-inflammability and the fact that it can be operated at a lower voltage. Weak beta-emitting isotopes such as sulphur-35 and carbon-14 can be placed inside the counter by means of an air lock, or introduced into the gas stream if they are in a gaseous or vapour form.

The counting equipment used with a flow-type proportional counter is shown in *Figure 14.5*. A cathode follower pre-amplifier feeds the chamber pulses into the main pulse amplifier. For proportional working, this must be a low-noise linear amplifier, the very stable gain required being in the range 50–1,000. It must also be a non-overloading type of amplifier, since large pulses from cosmic rays or a gamma-ray background can overload a conventional amplifier for an appreciable time causing counts to be missed (Fairstein and Hahn, 1965). A choice of differentiating and integrating time constants is provided for pulse-shaping purposes. When the counter is connected to the amplifier via a long cable, the capacitance may attenuate and distort the pulses. Under these circumstances the pre-amplifier should be placed close to the detector. The low output impedance of the pre-amplifier can drive the cable. In a proportional counter, radiation of different energies will produce output pulses of amplitude proportional to the isotope energy. A degree of energy selection is possible by following the pulse amplifier with a discriminator. This circuit enables a lower limit to be set to the pulse amplitudes which are fed into the counting equipment. Noise pulses can be rejected or a higher energy isotope counted in favour of a lower energy one. A more precise energy selection is made possible by the use of a pulse height analyser. In a single channel analyser both an upper and a lower energy level discriminator are used, so that only pulses having amplitudes lying between the levels are passed. The voltage or energy gap between the discriminator settings is called the channel width, gate or window.

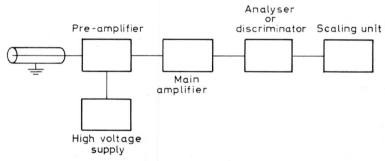

Figure 14.5. Counting equipment used with a proportional counter

The function of the scaling unit is to count down the pulses from the discriminator or analyser so that they can be displayed on a series of digital displays. These are usually run on a decade system showing units, tens, hundreds, thousands and ten thousands of counts. With a fast scaler the resolution time is about one microsecond and it is not usually necessary to make a correction to the observed counts for the dead time of the scaler. Many scalers incorporate a counter/timer operated from a tuning fork, or for reduced accuracy, from the mains frequency. With this arrangement the time taken to record a definite number of counts can be indicated, or else the number of counts given which occur within a definite time interval. Instead of a scaler, a ratemeter is often used. This is a circuit which continuously indicates on a meter and recorder the mean value of the rate at which pulses from the discriminator or analyser are fed into it. As has been mentioned previously, there is no control over the rate at which atoms of a radioactive isotope decay, so that the instantaneous count rate varies in a random fashion, the variations being marked at low count rates. The rate-meter accepts the incoming pulses and shapes them to a standard profile after which they are caused to charge a capacitor which has a resistive leak in parallel. The mean level of the voltage to which the capacitor charges reflects the mean count rate, and this is indicated on the output meter and recorder. The longer the time constant of the capacitor-resistor combination the more damped (smoothed) will be the output. If a steady pulse rate is applied suddenly to the ratemeter this will indicate approximately two thirds of the rate in a time equal to one time constant and 99 per cent in five time constants. A range of time constants can usually be switched in, the longer time constants being used at the lower count rates. A typical count rate range would be from 10 to 10,000 counts per second covered in steps of $\times 3$ and $\times 10$. A loudspeaker is often fitted to provide an audible indication of the count rate or rate change.

Ratemeters fitted with a 10 mV or 100 mV potentiometric recorder are particularly useful when changes in count rate with time have to be recorded, as for example when taking renograms. The speed of response of the recorder and its chart speed should be commensurate with the time constant of the ratemeter and the changes in count rate. When the count rate is constant apart from the inevitable statistical fluctuation, a more accurate estimate can be obtained from the digital output of a scaler.

Extra high tension (EHT) voltages of the order of 500 V are frequently available from ratemeters or scalers to operate halogen-quenched Geiger counters. Higher voltages for other forms of Geiger counter, proportional counters and scintillation counters are provided from a separate general purpose EHT unit. This might be able to provide up to 3 mA at 3,000 V. A high voltage stability is called for when supplying the dynodes of scintillation counter photomultiplier tubes.

GEIGER COUNTERS

The Geiger-Müller counter consists of a cylindrical cathode, usually one or two centimetres in diameter, and an axial wire anode. The cathode is often made from copper. This assembly is placed inside

387

a tubular glass envelope containing a gas or mixture of gases, which is easily ionized, at a pressure of a few tens of centimetres of mercury absolute. In mechanical construction it is similar to a proportional counter, but the gas filling and pressure are different. In addition to the gas which is ionized, there is also a quenching vapour. The pressure is sub-atmospheric in order to avoid the use of very high polarizing voltages.

The principal component of the counter filling is one or more of the inert gases, often argon or neon. Once the discharge between anode and cathode had been initiated by an ionizing event, it would continue, the only way of stopping it being to lower the anode voltage below the limit required to sustain a discharge. In practice, the counter contains an organic vapour such as ethyl alcohol or a halogen such as bromine vapour. The quenching agent acts by absorbing the free electrons and also by releasing the energy of metastable argon atoms. The operating voltage of a Geiger counter with organic vapour quenching is of the order of 1,000 V. Some of the vapour is dissociated each time a count is recorded so that the counter has a limited life, of the order of 10^8 counts. Bromine, however, is not used up, so that halogen-quenched counters have a longer life. They also operate at a lower voltage, typically 400–800 V. The reactive nature of bromine limits the choice of the materials available for the electrodes. Chrome-iron and stainless steel are suitable. The current pulse produced in a halogen-quenched tube is high, so that a high value of anode load resistor is used to limit the current, no quenching probe being used. Most halogen-quenched tubes give an output pulse of several volts, sufficient to operate a ratemeter or scaler without amplification. A Geiger counter ratemeter for use in the operating room is described by Kemp (1969). A discriminator is used to pass the Geiger pulses while rejecting noise pulses.

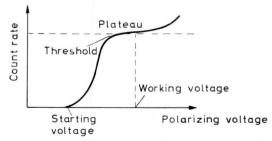

Figure 14.6. Voltage-count rate characteristic of a Geiger counter

The operation of Geiger counters

The variation of the count rate recorded by a typical Geiger counter when the polarizing voltage is altered is shown in *Figure 14.6*, the counter being irradiated with a constant flux of radiation. Below the starting voltage, no counts are recorded. The count rate rises rapidly to the threshold voltage above which there is a count rate plateau which is where the counter is normally operated. The rate is then little dependent on changes in polarizing voltage. The slope of the plateau is expressed in terms of a percentage of the count rate per volt, and should be less than 0·1 per cent per volt for a counter in good condition.

In order to operate the counter with a minimum background count, it is normally placed inside a lead shield or lead castle. This is equipped with shelves to hold sources in planchettes with a defined counting geometry, and also for holding sheets of aluminium or other absorbers between the window of the counter and the source. For counting beta particles an end-window type of counter is commonly used, the window being made of mica.

Dead time

While it takes less than a microsecond to collect the free electrons produced by each ionizing event in a Geiger counter, the positive ions formed move much more slowly. Initially they form a sheath around the wire anode. This positive ion space charge acts to reduce the field below the value necessary to maintain the discharge. The counter remains inoperative until the positive ions have moved sufficiently far away from the wire. This time can be of the order of several hundred microseconds, and can vary from counter to counter and between types of counter. In order to rationalize the situation it is usual to make use of a quenching probe. This unit applies a negative voltage pulse to the anode of the counter and holds it below the maintenance value for 200, 400 or 800 microseconds as required. Once the paralysis time t seconds is known, then the observed count rate can be corrected for the counts lost during the paralysis period. If the observed count rate is N_o per second, the corrected count rate N is given by $N + N_o(1 - N_o t)$ counts per second. The effect can be seen in the following table.

TABLE 14.1

$t \mu s$	N_0 counts/min	N counts/min	Per cent error if correction not made
400	1,000	1,007	0·7
400	10,000	10,715	6·7
400	20,000	23,070	13·3

The dead time of a fast scaler would be one microsecond or less, so that for a count rate of 1,000 per second the error would only be 0·1 per cent and for 10,000 counts per second it would be 1 per cent. For many purposes the error can be neglected.

Miniature Geiger counters

The metabolism of some forms of tumour is greater than that of the surrounding tissue and there is a consequent enhanced uptake of radioactive phosphorus-32 which is a pure beta emitter. Small Geiger counters have been developed which can be used in the rectum for counting activity in the prostate gland or implanted in breast tumours. One of the smallest counters is the type MIN by 20th Century Electronics Ltd. This is less than one inch long with a diameter of 2 mm and a gas volume of about 0·03 cm^3. The cathode is made from thin (0·003 in) stainless steel and the active anode length is 8 mm, the gas filling being an argon-neon-halogen mixture. The nominal working voltage is 500 V, the plateau length being 100 V with a slope of 0·15 per cent/V. The background count of the counter alone is less than one count per minute and the charge produced per ionizing pulse is about 10^{-9} coulombs. The sensitivity for ^{32}P is approximately 0·25 counts per second per millimicrocurie per millilitre.

SCINTILLATION COUNTERS

Scintillation counter systems are very widely used in medicine, particularly for the *in vitro* and *in vivo* counting of gamma-emitting isotopes. The use of liquid scintillators has made possible the routine counting of soft-beta emitters such as tritium and carbon-14 *in vitro*.

When ionizing radiation enters certain substances known as scintillators minute flashes of light are produced. The light arises from the recombination and de-excitation of ions and excited atoms produced along the path of the radiation. For gamma counting the scintillator usually consists of a crystal of sodium iodide activated with about 0·5 per cent of thallium iodide. If an anthracene crystal is used, the method can be applied to beta-particle counting. The flashes of light are observed with a sensitive photomultiplier tube. Because it is hygroscopic, the crystal is usually mounted in a sealed aluminium container having a glass window on the side which is in contact with the face of the photomultiplier. These surfaces must make a good optical contact and this is achieved by placing a film of silicone oil or clear grease between them.

For *in vitro* counting, particularly of liquid specimens, the crystal is provided with a 'well' into which the sample in a standard plastic container is introduced. In order to reduce the background counts, the crystal-photomultiplier assembly is placed inside a heavy cylindrical lead shield fitted with a lead lid as shown in *Figure 14.7*. For *in vitro* work, for example counting over a kidney, the crystal-photomultiplier assembly is mounted in a lighter shielding so that it can be held in an adjustable stand and offered up to the patient.

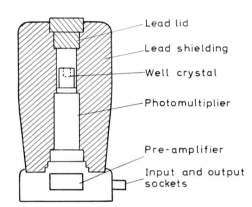

Lead lid

Lead shielding

Well crystal

Photomultiplier

Pre-amplifier

Input and output sockets

Figure 14.7. Well-type scintillation counter assembly

The front portion of the housing, between the patient and the crystal, is designed to act as a collimator for the gamma rays concerned. The collimator is usually a lead block one to two inches in thickness containing one or more holes. These may be drilled parallel to the axis of the crystal, or they may be drilled at an angle so that if projected they would intersect at a point on the axis a specified distance in front of the crystal. The latter type of collimator gives a focusing action so that only gamma rays from a certain depth in the patient should be detected if scattering is neglected. Three common types of collimator are illustrated in *Figure 14.8*.

Light photons from the scintillator produce photoelectrons from the bi-alkali photocathode of the photomultiplier tube. These electrons are then accelerated to the first of a series of electrodes or dynodes, the potential difference between the cathode and first dynode being of the order of 150 V. The dynodes are made from a low work function material such as beryllium-copper alloy. Having acquired an additional 150 eV of energy each electron incident upon the first dynode releases from it a few secondary electrons. These in

391

turn are accelerated to the second dynode which is a further 150 V positive and the process repeats. After a chain of 10 dynodes has been traversed, the number of secondary electrons collected at the final anode will be of the order of 10^5 or 10^6 for each primary photo-electron. An anode load resistor is connected between the anode and the stabilized high-voltage supply, so that the arrival of a burst of electrons produces a negative-going pulse across the resistor, and this is fed to an amplifier. The total time taken in the passage from photocathode to anode is less than one microsecond so that much higher counting rates can be achieved than is the case with Geiger counters. A cathode-follower pre-amplifier is often mounted in the scintillator-photomultiplier housing in order that the output pulses can be fed into a coaxial cable.

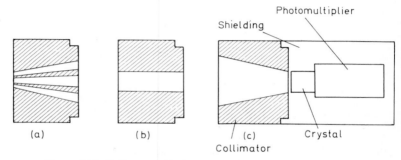

Figure 14.8. Collimators (a) focusing (b) parallel bore (c) wide angle

The two main processes in medical isotope work which give rise to scintillations within the crystal are the photoelectric effect and Compton scattering. These differ in one respect. The photoelectric effect completely absorbs the energy of the incident gamma ray so that the resulting photomultiplier output pulse is proportional to the gamma energy. This is an important characteristic of scintillation counters. As with gas proportional counters the amplitude of the output pulse is proportional to the energy of the incident radiation. The counter can thus be used as an energy spectrometer. The relationship between energy and pulse height is subject to statistical variation, so that a mono-energetic gamma ray becomes represented by a relatively broad band of pulse heights. With Compton scattering, however, the incident gamma ray only gives up a portion of its energy, so that the output pulses form a continuum of values up to that amplitude produced by the photoelectric effect. This is illustrated in *Figure 14.9* which shows a typical spectrum of a scintillation counter output for a mono-energetic gamma source. In the simplest case, pulses of amplitude less than the photopeak of interest can be rejected by means of a discriminator circuit. When an isotope has more than one photopeak or more than one isotope is involved, then a pulse-height analyser is used. By sweeping the voltage level of the

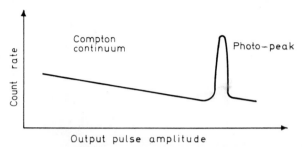

Figure 14.9. Typical spectrum of a scintillation counter output for a mono-energetic gamma emitter

pulse-height analyser window in synchronism with the chart movement of the recorder attached to the output ratemeter, it is possible to plot the spectrum of the gamma-ray energies of a given radioactive isotopes. This arrangement is known as a gamma-ray spectrometer. The normal electronic equipment used with a scintillation counter is similar to that used with a proportional counter *Figure 14.5*. A typical well-counter system is shown in *Figure 14.10*.

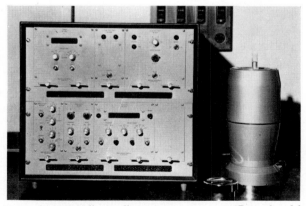

Figure 14.10. Well scintillation counter system. (Reproduced by courtesy of Nuclear Enterprises Ltd.)

Adjustment of a scintillation counter

Apart from setting the time constant of any associated ratemeter, there are four adjustments to be made: high voltage setting, pulse-height analyser threshold voltage, analyser channel width and amplifier gain. A reasonable procedure which can be followed to arrive at the optimum settings is as follows.

(1) Set the amplifier gain to about mid-scale.

(2) Select an analyser channel width of about 0·5 V.

(3) Set the analyser threshold to about mid-scale.

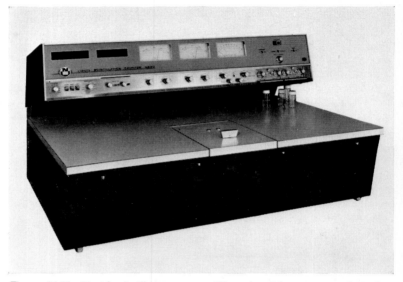

Figure 14.11. Liquid scintillation counter (Reproduced by courtesy of Nuclear Enterprises Ltd.)

(4) With the counter looking at a fairly active sample of the isotope of interest, the high voltage is gradually raised until the count rate passes through a maximum.

(5) Set the high voltage at the value which gives the maximum count rate.

(6) The threshold voltage is then increased in 0·5-V steps from a few volts below its previous setting to a few volts above it, a count being taken at each setting.

A graph is plotted of count rate against threshold voltage, and the optimum setting for the analyser determined to take in the photopeak concerned. There may be more than one photopeak. In many cases it may be preferable to work with the principal peak, but an alternative peak may have to be used in order to avoid overlap when more than one isotope is present in the sample. Higher count rates can be obtained with wider analyser windows, but if a well-defined photopeak is present, the count rate/background count ratio is usually highest when the window width is such as just to contain the peak. In general, the aim is to maximize the fraction S^2/B where S is the sample count rate and B the background count rate.

Liquid scintillation counters

Samples containing weak beta emitters such as carbon-14 and tritium can be counted efficiently by mixing the sample with a liquid scintillator so that the scintillator is in intimate contact with the short-range betas. Counting is performed with a one-inch diameter photomultiplier. A typical liquid scintillator would be a mixture of specially purified xylene, naphthalene, activators and a wavelength shifter. The temperature of the scintillator is stabilized by passing mains water or refrigerant through the counting head unit cooling jacket. A turntable or endless belt arrangement is often employed so that a large number of samples can be passed automatically, in turn, over the counting head and the count rate printed out, *Figure 14.11.*

SEMICONDUCTOR DETECTORS

In recent years there has been a great deal of development work carried out on solid-state semiconductor radiation detectors since these can be made small and robust and some types have a very good energy resolution and are thus useful for radiation spectroscopy. A useful review of semiconductor detector technology is that of Dearnaley and Northrop (1963). One interesting device is a needle counter for *in vivo* beta-particle counting. It consists of a small p-i-n type semiconductor element mounted on a silicon base at the tip of a thin-walled stainless steel needle. The wall thickness of that part of the needle where the detector element is located is only 0·05 mm, so that beta particles with energies down to about 150 keV can be measured. The counting tip of the needle is 10 mm long by 1·1 mm in diameter, this being followed by a shaft 1·5 mm in diameter and 30 mm long. With the counter immersed respectively in a phosphorus-32 solution and a mercury-203 gel, the sensitivities are quoted as 1100 counts per minute/microcurie/millilitre P-32 and 100 counts per minute/microcurie/millilitre²⁰³Hg. The needle detector works into a charge sensitive low-noise pre-amplifier which is a hybrid with an electrometer tube input stage, the input resistor being 22 MΩ. It can supply a bias voltage to the detector in the range 0 and ± 300 V. The detector can be sterilized at a maximum temperature of 125°C with an applied voltage of 5 V.

CHOICE OF A COUNTER

Beta particles

A Geiger counter is very suitable for the counting of solid specimens. A one inch diameter counter fitted with a 2 mg/cm² mica window to let through beta particles is often used. It employs bromine quenching. (It might be mentioned that for a given element, the thickness of a window can be estimated in terms of mass/unit area since density=thickness×unit area.)

For counting beta-emitting liquid samples, either halogen or organic vapour quenched counters are available mounted inside a test tube which holds the sample (Veall, 1948). This gives a good counting geometry with the counter inside the liquid. The wall thickness is about 30 mg/cm² so that this method is only possible with the higher energy beta particles. The efficiency of a Geiger counter for beta particles is almost 100 per cent for particles which enter its sensitive volume. This efficiency must be multiplied by a geometrical factor to allow for the proportion of radiation from the source which reaches the counter. Typical overall efficiencies for the test tube type of Geiger counter are 10 per cent for ³²P, 1 per cent for ¹³¹I and less than 0·01 per cent for ³⁵S.

For the measurement of isotopes with weak beta particle energies such as those from carbon-14 (155 keV), tritium (13 keV) and sulphur-35 (167 keV) liquid scintillation techniques are attractive. Typical efficiencies are for counting tritium in whole blood with hyamine using a xylene-naphthalene scintillator, 17 per cent and for counting a carbon-14 organic solution with the same scintillator, 95 per cent.

Gamma rays

The counting efficiency of an ordinary Geiger counter for gamma photons is low, usually less than 1 per cent. Some improvement in efficiency can be achieved by employing a construction such as a wire mesh which will increase the area of the cathode surface per unit volume of the counter since this will increase the number of secondary electrons liberated into the gas from the cathode. The cathode should also be made from material having a high atomic number, such as copper or lead. For counting volumes of the order of 2 litres of urine containing an isotope such as [131]I a ring of 6, 8 or 12 Geiger counters can be placed around the container (Veall and Vetter, 1952).

Scintillation counting is attractive because its efficiency may be as high as 50 per cent or more. Thallium-activated sodium iodide is the most efficient and widely used scintillator for gamma counting. Its high atomic number means that there is a large ratio of photoelectric to Compton effect which is desirable for selecting photopeaks. The resolution time can be made less than one microsecond.

Apart from the efficiency of a particular type of counter other factors must be taken into consideration when making a choice. These include the background count rate, the volume of sample that can be handled, the amount of sample preparation needed, the time taken and the cost of the apparatus. In some cases a Geiger counter working at a lower efficiency might be preferable to a scintillation counter which has a higher efficiency but can only hold a small amount of sample. In the majority of cases where a sample emits both beta particles and gamma radiation, it is better to count the gamma photons. This follows because no sample preparation may be involved and larger volumes of sample can be used without the need to correct for self-absorption of beta particles in the sample. For both potassium-42 and sodium-24 it is better to use a liquid Geiger counter and to count the beta particles rather than to count the gamma ray photons with a scintillation counter (Tothill, 1966).

For the routine determination of blood volumes and renal function on a limited scale a simple well counter fitted with a pulse height analyser and counter timer is adequate. However, in the determination of glomerular filteration rates, for instance, it is often necessary to count for 1000 seconds. As the number of samples builds up, this becomes very tedious. An automatic counting assembly becomes essential if the throughput of work is to be maintained. In one arrangement, the sample vials are placed in numbered trays which are loaded into a paternoster system, the contents of each tray being extracted, vial by vial, and loaded into a well counter for gamma counting. They can also be loaded into a beta particle counting head. Each sample can be counted for three different isotopes for either a pre-determined count or a pre-determined time, and automatic background subtraction can be performed. The results of the counting are printed up on a teleprinter and punched on paper tape for computer analysis.

Coincidence counting

A coincidence unit receives pulses on two inputs from the amplifiers associated with a pair of counters. It will produce a single output pulse if the pair of input pulses arrive (coincide) within a certain time period, that is to say, the separation of the input pulses must be less than that period. This is typically variable from 3 to 100 nanoseconds by means of a ten-turn control.

The coincidence method can be used to count a beta emitter in which there is a simultaneous gamma emission with each beta, for example, gold-198. Let there be N disintegrations per second, and two counters be used. It is assumed that one counts beta particles only, the other counting gamma-ray photons only. Let N_1 be the beta count rate, e_1 the counter efficiency, g_1 a term which takes into account the geometry of the detector, and B_1 its background count. Then $N_1 = N.g_1.e_1 + B_1$ and similarly for the gamma counter $N_2 = N.g_2.e_2 + B_2$. On switching in the coincidence unit, the coincidence rate $N_3 = N.g_1.e_1.g_2.e_2$. In practice allowance must be made for a contribution from gammas on the beta channel and from betas on the gamma channel together with an allowance for accidental coincidences. From the equation, e_1g_1 and e_2g_2 can be found and thus N_3 calculated. Coincidence counting reduces background arising from random noise pulses produced in the photomultiplier and chemiluminescence and phosphorescence arising in the sample.

Counting a mixture of two isotopes with a scintillation counter

Consider the case of counting, one at a time, two isotopes contained in a sample. If the elements concerned are A and B it is assumed that B will give a count rate when the analyser is set on the photopeak for A and similarly A will give a response when the analyser is set for the photopeak of B. Before counting the mixture a sample of A alone is counted followed by a sample of B alone. It is found that isotope A will have a count rate of A_a in A's window and A_b in B's window. Isotope B will have a count rate of B_b in B's window and B_a in A's window. The ratio A_b/A_a is the fraction of the count rate of isotope A as observed in A's window that passes through B's window. B_a/B_b is the fraction of the count rate of isotope B, as observed in B's window that passes through A's window.

On counting the mixture of A and B the observed count rates for each are A_o and B_o. Corrections have to be made to reduce these observed values to the corresponding true values A_t and B_t which would be without overlap.

$$A_t = A_o - \frac{B_a}{B_b}\left[\frac{B_o}{1-\left(\frac{A_b}{A_a}\right)\left(\frac{B_a}{B_b}\right)}\right] \text{ and } B_t = B_o - \frac{A_b}{A_a}\left[\frac{A_o}{1-\left(\frac{A_b}{A_a}\right)\left(\frac{B_a}{B_b}\right)}\right]$$

The denominator in these expressions is usually close to unity since at least one of the fractions A_b/A_a or B_a/B_b will be small. Hence

$$A_t = A_o - (B_a/B_b)B_o \text{ and } B_t = B_o - (A_b/A_a)A_o$$

If $A_a = 1,000$ counts per second in A's window and $A_b = 100$ counts per second in B's window while $B_b = 3,000$ counts per second in B's window and $B_a = 600$ counts per second in A's window then $A_b/A_a = 1/10$ and $B_a/B_b = 1/5$. When the mixture is counted it is found that in A's window there are recorded 1,000 counts per second as against 800 counts per second in B's window. Thus $B_t = 800 - (1/10).1000 = 700$ counts per second and $A_t = 1000 - (1/5).800 = 840$ counts per second.

The counting of gamma-emitting isotopes in vivo

In the simplest types of experiment a collimated scintillation head is placed over the organ concerned, such as the thyroid gland or a kidney. A one inch, or more usually, a two inch diameter crystal is used. If only one isotope such as ^{131}I is administered to the patient, then a pulse-height analyser is not required, a simple discriminator being satisfactory. This arrangement forms the basis of the radio-isotope renogram, in which the passage of ^{131}I-labelled Hippuran is followed through the kidneys. One detector is placed over each kidney, and there may be a third over the heart to record the blood level of isotope. Using operational amplifiers this blood level is continuously substracted from the kidney curves in order to produce a sharper trace. With this simple apparatus much can be learnt concerning renal function and the presence of a possible obstruction.

THE RADIOISOTOPE SCANNER

When it is required to map out the distribution of a labelled compound in a particular organ or body site, the scintillation detector head can be moved in a zig-zag fashion backwards and forwards over the area concerned. At the same time a mechanical linkage causes a printing head to trace out the same motion across a chart paper. The detector is usually either a three- or five-inch diameter crystal situated behind a focusing collimator. At pre-set intervals during the scan, the printing head makes a mark on the chart which is characteristic of the count rate at that moment, the position of the mark on the chart corresponding to the location in the patient where the activity is being measured. An elegant arrangement makes use of colour printing. The detector is rapidly moved over the portion of

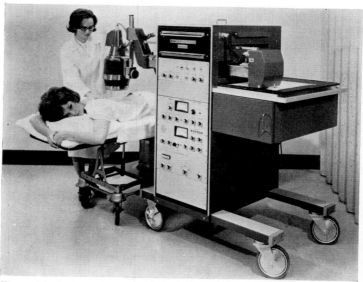

Figure 14.12. Radioisotope scanner. (Reproduced by courtesy of Picker Corporation)

interest of the patient's body and the maximum count rate established. This is then divided into perhaps six ranges each being associated with a different colour print. As each count rate is recorded, it is allocated to one of the groups and the colour printed. In this way a coloured map is built up showing the distribution of the isotope. Each complete scan takes a period of the order 15–30 minutes, so that a considerable time is required to make a complete anterior posterior and lateral scan. A colour scanner is shown in *Figure 14.12*. In some other forms of scanner, the patient can sit up instead of always having to lie under the head. Some scanners will also move the patient's couch in a zig-zag fashion under the fixed head rather than move the head.

THE GAMMA CAMERA

The mechanical motion of the head sets a limit to the time required to complete a good resolution scan. This limitation has been removed in the gamma camera (Anger 1967). This is basically a camera working with gamma radiation rather than with visible light. In its most common form, the camera head contains a twelve inch diameter half inch thick crystal of sodium iodide. On the patient's side of the crystal can be fixed various collimators. A pin-hole collimator is used for thyroid gland studies, otherwise parallel-hole collimators two or three inches thick are employed. These have perhaps 1,000 holes. Coupled to the other side of the crystal by a carefully shaped Perspex light guide is a matrix of 19 three inch diameter photomultipliers. Each has its own high-voltage supply adjustment. During the initial setting-up phase a collimated source of an isotope such as ^{203}Hg, which has a single photopeak, is placed over each photomultiplier in turn and the high-voltage adjusted to equalize the pulse heights produced from each tube. The output pulses from each tube are fed into a resistor weighting network. When a gamma ray passes through the collimator and gives rise to a scintillation in the crystal the light is fed to all the 19 photo-multipliers by the light guide. The pulses from the tubes are summed by the resistor network in such a way that the contribution from any individual tube is proportional to its distance from the place in the crystal where the scintillation was produced. In fact two pulses are output from the network, an X-pulse and a Y-pulse corresponding to the co-ordinates of the scintillation. The origin ($X=0$, $Y=0$) is taken as the centre of the crystal face. The X and Y pulses are applied to the X and Y deflector plates of a display cathode-ray tube. The energy or Z-pulse from the photomultipliers is passed through an analyser and caused to unblank the cathode-ray tube beam. Thus for each scintillation, a corresponding spot of light is produced on the screen, its position matching that of the scintillation in the crystal. A Polaroid camera is used to photograph the build-up of perhaps 50,000 dots on the screen and in this way a map is available of the distribution of activity. With a short half-life (6 hours) isotope such as technetium 99m, doses of the order of 5 millicuries can be administered to the patient. Gamma camera pictures can then be taken in as little as 20 seconds while the patient holds his breath. It is possible to count technetium (140 keV) in the presence of ^{131}I (360 keV).

The head unit can be raised or lowered and rotated by electric motor drives (*Figure 14.13*). Using four additional pulse height analysers working in two crossed pairs two areas can be selected on the crystal face so that only gamma rays falling within $(X_1+\Delta X_1,\ Y_1+\Delta Y_1)$ and $(X_2+\Delta X_2,\ Y_2+\Delta Y_2)$ are counted. This system can be used for counting over a patient's kidneys to give a

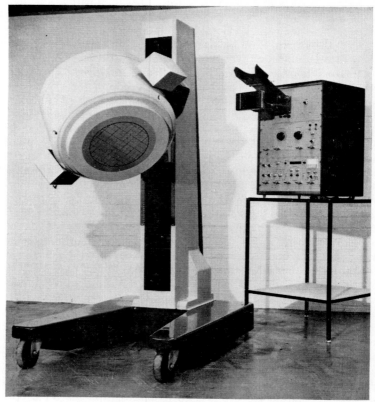

Figure 14.13. Gamma camera. (Reproduced by courtesy of Nuclear Enterprises Ltd.)

renogram, or for checking on the uniformity and linearity of the head characteristics (Constable and Hill, 1969). The facility for being able to monitor the activity from two separate areas has been elegantly exploited in the plotting of renograms from both moieties of a duplex kidney (Constable and Werry, 1972). In the latest technology, the X, Y and Z pulses from the gamma camera head are digitized by fast analogue-to-digital converters, and stored on-line in a digital computer. The computer can be programmed to map out iso-activity areas and to analyse the build-up and decay of activity in a more sophisticated fashion than is possible by a visual inspection of a sequence of polaroid pictures of the camera displays. This approach has been used to follow the uptake of pertechnetate by brain tumours and the following of a bolus of pertechnetate as it passes through the heart.

The use of off-line computer processing has enabled corrections to be made for distortions introduced by the collimator and a lack of uniformity of the complete camera head as determined from isotope phantom studies (Spector *et al.*, 1972). It is also feasible to use smoothing techniques to weight the activity found at any co-ordinate point on the display in terms of the activity found at neighbouring co-ordinates. These approaches can be helpful in delineating small 'cold' areas such as, for example, in trying to detect tumours of the parathyroid glands. They are also being extensively applied to nuclear scanner displays. A useful account of computer techniques for smoothing, resolution recovery and transformation for display variation in relation to radioisotope scans is that of Pizer (1971). The use of Fourier and other transformation techniques for the spatial filtering of scans is also described by Cyckowski *et al.* (1971) and Brown *et al.* (1971). The performance of the focusing collimators used in scanners can be assessed in terms of the modulation transfer function (Cradduck, 1971). When a scanning system scans an object the radioactivity within which is varying in a sinusoidal manner, the output from the scanner will also be sinusoidal but with a different amplitude. The ratio of the output modulation to the input modulation is a measure of the modulation transfer coefficient at that particular spatial frequency and a plot of the variation of this ratio against spacial frequency constitutes the modulation transfer function. The spatial frequencies are expressed in terms of lines per centimetre.

RADIOLOGICAL PROTECTION EQUIPMENT

Excessive exposure to ionizing radiation can give rise to serious damage to tissues, the effects of which may not be apparent for some years. Since radiation is silent and colourless some form of instrument is required in order to be able to indicate the dose rate and the total dose received over a given time. The calibrations would normally be in millirads per hour for dose rate and the accumulated dose in rads or millirads. The rad is the unit of röntgen absorbed dose. It is defined as the quantity of ionizing radiation which produces an energy absorption of 100 ergs per gram, and it applies to all types of radiation.

Film badges

The most common method of measuring general exposure to the body makes use of the fact that a photographic film becomes blackened upon exposure to ionizing radiation. After development of the film, a densitometer is used to measure the degree of blackening. A calibration is found by exposing films from the same batch to known doses of radiation from an X-ray set. The film has a sensitive emulsion on its front surface and a less sensitive emulsion on the reverse side. It is wrapped in paper having a density of 30 mg/cm^2 in order to cut off photons having energies less than about 20 keV and beta particles below about 200 keV. The plastic film holder has an open aperture as well as areas containing plastic filters and various metal filter combinations. It is possible to estimate the amount and character of the incident radiation to an accuracy of about ± 20 per cent for doses greater than 20 millirads.

Quartz fibre electroscopes

Miniature fountain-pen size electroscopes using a gilded quartz fibre as the moving element are also widely used to measure personal doses. The electroscope is first plugged into a charging unit and this charges up the small ionization chamber. To the inner electrode of the chamber is attached the quartz fibre in the form of a hairpin movement. When charged the fibre takes up a position corresponding to zero on the instrument's scale. As the chamber receives radiation it discharges causing the fibre to move across the scale calibrated in millirads. Typically, the charging voltage is 150 V, the range 0–200 mr with an electrical leakage rate equivalent to 3 mr in 8 hours. When the instrument is placed in the charger a small lamp allows the scale to be read.

Radiation monitors

In the United Kingdom, by law, all users of radioisotopes must have available a calibrated monitor. The simplest type consists of a thin side-wall Geiger counter probe with a battery-operated ratemeter and loudspeaker. An aluminium cover can be placed over the tube to distinguish beta particles from gamma rays. Two ranges are normally provided, 0–50 and 0–5000 counts per second. This type of monitor is useful for hunting for lost sources and checking for contamination in laboratories. For quantitative measurements an accurately calibrated ionization chamber type of dose meter is required.

STATISTICS OF COUNTING

When a definite amount of radioactive material is counted, the count will vary slightly each time counting is performed, even though the half-life of the isotope may be so long as to exert a negligible influence on the count rate over the time of counting. If a histogram is plotted of the counts obtained it will be found that these are distributed about the mean value as shown in *Figure 14.14* which corresponds to a Poisson distribution. The Gaussian approximation, often referred to as the normal distribution is used in counting statistics. It is only necessary to use a Poisson distribution curve when the number of counts recorded is less than about 30.

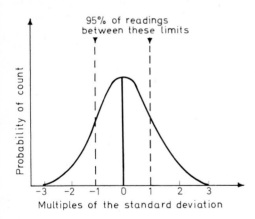

Figure 14.14. Gaussian distribution of counts from a sample

If the standard deviation of the mean of the observations is calculated it is found that 68 per cent of the observations can be expected to lie within plus or minus one standard deviation of the mean, while 95·5 per cent lie within plus or minus two standard deviations. It is a convenient property of the Poisson distribution that the standard deviation equals the square root of the mean value. For a count of 10,000 the standard deviation is 100 so that 95·5 per cent of all count readings would be expected to lie within 9,800 and 10,200. Even if the count of 10,000 were not very representative it could not make a difference of more than one or two per cent to the value assumed to be the mean. It would also not affect the important result that 68 per cent of the counts will be expected to lie within plus or minus 1 per cent of the mean.

The quantity (s.d./mean)×100 per cent might be thought of as a percentage error associated with the statistical nature of the measurement. Thus a count of 100 has a possible statistical error of 10 (10 per cent), a count of 10,000 has a statistical error of 100 (1 per cent) while that for 1,000,000 has an error of 0·1 per cent. A suitable strength of source and counting time must be chosen to reduce the statistical error to the required level.

In normal practice, a source is only counted once or a few times, so that an accurate mean count is not available. There is a 68 per cent chance that a single count measurement will differ from the mean by less than one standard deviation. The chance of its deviating by more than two s.ds is 4·5 per cent and only one in four hundred chance that it will lie outside three s.ds from the mean. Hence it is necessary to record a total of 10,000 counts (irrespective of the time taken) to reduce the random error to less than 1 per cent on a 1 in 400 basis.

In many practical cases one is concerned with the difference between two count rates, for instance, sample and background. The two counts are both subject to statistical variations. The standard deviation of the difference of two counts is equal to the sum of the squares of the standard deviations of the individual counts. If N is the count for (sample+background) and in the same time the background count is B, then the sample count is $(N—B)$. The individual standard deviations are $N^{\frac{1}{2}}$ and $B^{\frac{1}{2}}$ so that the standard deviation of $N—B$ is $(\sqrt{N^2}+\sqrt{B^2})^{\frac{1}{2}}=(N+B)^{\frac{1}{2}}$. The count rate of the sample is given by

$$\frac{(N—B)}{t} \pm \frac{(N+B)^{\frac{1}{2}}}{t}$$

where t is the time taken for counting.

If the sample count rate is about ten times that of the background, the effect of the latter on the accuracy can be ignored. It is never necessary to count the background for longer than the sample.

REFERENCES

Applications of radio-isotope techniques
There are now so many applications for radioactive isotopes in the literature that only a small selection is included in order to give some indication of the possibilities.

Instrumentation (general)

Birks, J. (1953). *Scintillation Counters*. Oxford; Pergamon

Boag, J. W. (1963). 'Radiological quantities and units, their inter-relationships and conditions of use.' *Physics Med. Biol.* **7**, 409

Dearnaley, G. and Northrop, D. C. (1963). *Semiconductor Counters for Nuclear Radiations*. London; Spon

Eaves, G. (1964). *Principles of Radiation Protection*. London; Iliffe

Faires, R. A. and Parks, B. H. (1964). *Radioisotope Laboratory Techniques*. 2nd ed. London; Newnes

Fairstein, E. and Hahn, J. (1965). 'Nuclear pulse amplifiers—fundamentals and design practice.' *Nucleonics* **7**, 56

Hoffer, P. B., Beck, R. N., Lembares, N., Charleston, D. B., and Gottschalk, A. (1971). 'Use of lithium-drifted germanium detectors for clinical radionuclide scanning.' *J. nucl. Med.*, **12**, 25

Kandiah, K. (1968). 'Nuclear instruments over the last fifty years.' *J. scient. Instrum.* **1**, 369

Kemp, L. A. W. (1969). 'A compact battery-operated ratemeter employing "bootstrapping" to eliminate cable capacitance effects.' *Physics Med. Biol.* **14**, 133

Pavlesky, H., Swank, R. K. and Grenchick, R. (1947). 'Design of a dynamic condenser electrometer.' *Rev. scient. Instrum.* **18**, 298

Tothill, P. (1966). 'Measurement techniques for the clinical application of radioisotopes.' *Medical Monograph No.* 2. Amersham, England; Radiochemical Centre

Veall, N. (1948). 'A Geiger-Müller counter for measuring the beta-ray activity of liquids and its application to medical tracer experiments.' *Br. J. Radiol.* **21**, 347

— Vetter, H. (1958). '*Radioisotope Techniques in Clinical Research and Diagnosis*.' London; Butterworths

Gamma cameras

Anger, H. A. (1967). 'Radioisotopes cameras.' In *Instrumentation in Nuclear Medicine*. p. 485. Ed. by G. J. Hine. New York; Academic Press

Constable, A. R. and Hill, D. W. (1969). 'Quantitative assessment of the characteristics of a gamma camera without the use of a multi-channel analyser.' *Physics Med. Biol.* **14**, 139

Downham, M. C., and Evans, R. G. (1971). 'Economic analysis of scintillation camera useage in nuclear medicine facilities.' *Radiology*, **101**, 643

Freedman, G. S. (1972). 'Gamma camera tomography.' *Radiology*, **102**, 365

Kulberg., G. H., Van Dijk, N., and Muehllehner, G. (1972). 'Improved resolution of the Anger scintillation camera through the use of threshold preamplifiers.' *J. nucl. Med.*, **13**, 169

Spector, S. S., Brookeman, V. A., Kylstra, C. D., and Diaz, N. J. (1972). 'Analysis and correction of spatial distortions produced by the gamma camera.' *J. nucl. Med.* **13**, 307

Scanners

Brown, D. W., Kirch, D. L., Ryerson, T. W., Throckmorton, A. J., Kilbourn, A. L., and Brenner, N. B. (1971). 'Computer processing of scans using Fourier and other transformations.' *J. nucl. Med.*, **12**, 217

Brownell, G. L. and Aronow, S. (1967). 'Radioisotope scanning.' In *Instrumentation in Nuclear Medicine.* p. 381. Ed. by G. J. Hine. New York; Academic Press

Cradduck, T. D. (1971). 'Modulation transfer function and its application to radioisotope scanning.' In *Advances in Medical Physics*, p. 164, Ed. by J. S. Laughlin, (2nd Int. Conf. Med. Physics) Boston.

Cykowski, C. B., Kirch, D. L., Polhemus, C. E., and Brown, D. W. (1971). 'Image enhancement of radionuclide scans by optical spatial filtering.' *J. nucl. Med.*, **12**, 85

Pizer, S. M. (1971). 'Resolution recovery in radioisotope scans.' In *Advances in Medical Physics*, p. 297, Ed. by J. S. Laughlin, (2nd Int. Conf. Med. Physics) Boston

Applications
Blood flow

Cosgrove, M. D., Evans, K. and Raphael, M. J. (1968). 'The use of xenon-133 to measure renal blood flow in patients.' *Br. J. Surg.* **55**, 245

Holzman, G. B., Wagner, H. N., Ilo, M., Rabonowitz, D. and Zierler, K. L. (1964). 'Measurement of muscle blood flow in the human forearm with radioactive krypton and xenon.' *Circulation* **30**, 27

Bone

Krishnamurthy, G. T., Walsh, C., Winston, M. A., Weiss, E. R., and Blahd, W. H. (1972). 'Comparison of fluorine-18 bone studies obtained with rectilinear scanner and scintillation camera equipped with high-energy diverging hole collimator.' *Radiology*, **103**, 365

Mishkin, F. S., Reese, I. C., Chua, G. T. and Huddlestun, J. E. (1968). 'Indium 113m for scanning bone and kidney.' *Radiology* **91**, 161

Spencer, R., Herbert, R., Rish, M. W. and Little, W. A. (1967). 'Bone scanning with Sr-85, Sr-87 and F-18.' *Br. J. Radiol.* **40**, 641

Brain

Subramanian, G., McAfee, J. G., Bell, E. G., Blair, R. J., O'mara, R. E., and Ralston, P. H. (1972). '99m-Tc labelled polyphosphate as a skeletal imaging agent.' *Radiology*, **102**, 701

Croll, M. N., Brady, L. W., Faust, D. S., Kazem, I, Antoniades, J. and Tatem, H. R. (1968). 'Comparison brain scanning with mercury-203 and technetium-99m.' *Radiology* **90**, 747

Handel, S. F., Powell, M. R., Wilson, L. B., and Emot, K. J. (1971). 'Scintiphotographic evaluation of response of brain neoplasms to systemic chemotherapy.' *J. nucl. Med.*, **12**, 292

Krishnamurthy, G. T., Mehta, A., Tomiyashu, U., and Blahd, W. H. (1972). 'Clinical value and limitations of 99m-Tc brain scan.' *J. nucl. Med.* **13**, 367

Loken, M. K., Wigdahl, L. O., Gilson, J. M. and Staab, E. V. (1966). 'Mercury-197 and mercury-203 chlormerodrin for evaluation of brain lesions using a rectilinear scanner and scintillation camera.' *J. nucl. Ned.* **7**, 209

Foetus

Sy, W. M., Rosen, H., Griffin, N. E., Fink, H., Vasicka, A., Lorber, S. A., and Solomon, N. A. (1972). 'Radiation dose in a human fetus following use of Hg-197.' *Radiology*, **103**, 139

Haematology
Eckelman, W., Richards, P., Hauser, W., and Atkins, H. (1971). 'Technetium-labelled red blood cells.' *J. nucl. Med.*, **12**, 22
Lajth, L. G. (1961). *The use of Isotopes in Haematology*. Oxford; Blackwell
Szirmai, E. (1965). *Nuclear Haematology*. New York; Academic Press

Heart
Bennett, K. R., Smith, R. O., Leman, P. H., and Hellems, K. (1972) 'Correlation of myocardial 42K uptake with coronary arteriography. *Radiology*, **102**, 117
Burke, G., Halko, A., and Peskin, G. (1971). 'Determination of cardiac output by radioisotope angiography and the image-intensifier scintillation camera.' *J. nucl. Med.*, **12**, 112
Chwojnik, A., Torreggiani, G. and Donato, L. (1966). 'Improved technique for measuring coronary blood flow by Rb-86 single injection method.' *J. nucl. Biol. Med.* **10**, 89

Liver
Groth, C. G., Brown, D. W., Ceaverland, J. D., Cordes, D. J., Brettschneider, L. and Starzl, T. E. (1968). 'Radioisotope scanning in experimental and clinical orthoptic liver transplantation.' *Surgery Gynec. Obstet.* **127**, 808
Rollo, F. D. and DeLand, F. H. (1968). 'The determination of liver mass from radionuclide images.' *Radiology* **91**, 1191
Saba, T. M., Kaplan, E., and Graham, L. (1972). 'Hepatic phagocytic, metabolic and blood flow evaluation by dynamic scintigraphy.' *J. nucl. Med.* **13**, 300

Lungs
Poe, N. D., Swanson, L. A. and Taplin, G. V. (1967). 'Physiological factors affecting lung scan interpretations.' *Radiology* **89**, 661
West, J. B. (1966). 'The use of radioactive materials in the study of lung function.' *Medical Monograph No.* 1. Amersham, England; Radiochemical Centre

Pancreas
Eaton, S. B., Potsaid, M. S., Lo, H. H. and Beaulieu, E. (1967). 'Radioisotope "subtraction" scanning for pancreatic lesions.' *Radiology* **89**, 1033
Hatchette, J. B., Shuler, S. E., and Murison P. J. (1972). 'Scintiphotos of the pancreas: analysis of 134 studies.' *J. nucl. Med.*, **13**, 51
Rodriguez-Antunez, A., Filson, E. J., Sullivan, B. H. and Brown, C. H. (1966). 'Photoscanning in diagnosis of carcinoma of the pancreas.' *Ann. int. Med.* **65**, 730

Pituitary
Fergusson, J. D. and Phillips, D. E. H. (1962). 'A clinical evaluation of radioactive pituitary implantation in the treatment of advanced carcinoma of the prostate.' *Br. J. Urol.* **34**, 485
Straffon, R. A., Kiser, W. S., Robitaille, M. and Dohn, D. F. (1968). '90-Yttrium hypophysectomy in management of metastatic carcinoma of prostate gland in 13 patients.' *J. Urol.* **99**, 102

Placenta
Johnson, P. M., Sciarra, J. J. and Bragg, D. G. (1966). 'Placental localiza-tion with radioisotopes—results in 86 verified cases.' *Am. J. Roentg.* **96,** 677
— Chao, S., and Reilly, J. A., (1972). 'Placental imaging with 113m in results in 100 patients.' *Radiology* **103,** 359

Prostate
Haskin, M. E., Wagner, M. L., Ivker, M. and Widmann, B. P. (1959). 'The early diagnosis of prostatic malignancy by the use of P-32.' *J. Urol.* **85,** 99
Johnson, G. S., Wade, J. C., Murphy, G. P. and Scott, W. W. (1968). 'Zinc-65 and Zinc-69m studies in the dog, monkey and man.' *J. surg. Res.* **8,** 528

Renal studies
Cohen, M. B., Pearman, R. O., Mims, M. M. and Blahd, W. (1963). 'Radioisotope photoscanning of the kidneys in urologic disease.' *J. Urol.* **89,** 360
Constable, A. R., and Werry, Diana, M. (1972). 'Simplified regional renography applied to the duplex kidney.' *Br. J. Radiol.,* **45,** 377
Hauser, W., Atkins, H. C., and Richards, P. (1971). 'Renal uptake of 99m-Tc iron ascorbic acid complex in man.' *Radiology,* **101,** 637
Ross, J. C., Edwards, E. C., Kulke, W. and Haggart, B. G. (1963). 'Recovery of renal function as demonstrated by the radioisotope renogram.' *Br. J. Urol.* **35,** 394
Secker-Walker, R. H., Shepherd, E. P., and Cassell, K. J. (1972). 'Clinical applications of computer-assisted renography.' *J. nucl. Med.,* **13,** 235

Spleen
Burdine, J. A. and Legeay, R. (1968). 'Spleen scans with 99m technetium labelled heated erythrocytes.' *Radiology* **91,** 162
Hermann, G. and Custer, R. P. (1966). 'Splenic scintiscans with meri-soprol Hg-197. A new radioactive pharmaceutical agent.' *J. Am. med. Ass.* **195,** 1015

Stomach
Calderson., M., Sonnemaker, R. E., Hersch, T., and Burdine., J. A. (1971). '99m-Tc human albumin microspheres (H.A.M.) for measuring the rate of gastric emptying.' *Radiology,* **101,** 371

Thyroid
Ben Porath, M., Hockman, A. and Gross, J. (1966). 'A comparison of iodine-125 and iodine-131 as tracers in the diagnosis of thyroid disease.' *J. nucl. med.* **7,** 88
Hurley, P. J., Strauss, H. W., Pavoni, P., Langan, J. K. and Wagner, H. N. (1971). 'The scintillation camera with pinhole collimator in thyroid imaging.' *Radiology,* **101,** 133.
Sanders, T. P. and Kuhl, D. E. (1968). 'Technetium pertechnetate as a thyroid scanning agent.' *Radiology* **91,** 23

Urine
Veall, N. and Vetter, H. (1952). 'An apparatus for the rapid estimation of tracer quantities of radioactive isotopes in excreta.' *Br. J. Radiol.* **25,** 85

Index

Acid base balance,
  heart surgery, during, 232
  temperature coefficient of blood
    affected by, 232
Acid base balance measurements,
  buffer solutions for, 232
  computers for, 251
  electrodes for, 224, 226–233
    glass, 227
    pH meter, 230
Alpha particles, 377
  detection, 385
  energy of, 379
Amplifiers,
  (*see also* Pre-amplifiers)
  blood flowmeters, for, 139, 147
  chopper type, 79
  Clark electrodes, for, 245
  ECG, 340
  filters, 7
  impedance pneumographs, for, 120
  incorporating photo-isolator stages, 341
  low-level output from, 16
  nerve and muscle stimulation, for, 56
  parametric, 13–15
  performance requirements, 5
  pneumotachograph, for, 113
  proportional counters, in, 385
Amplitude distortion in recording systems, 52
Anaesthesia, spirometry in, 129, 130
Anaesthetics, use with diathermy apparatus, 341

Anal incontinence, electrical stimulators for, 321
Anal plug, for bladder stimulation, 321
Angina pectoris, 322
Aorta,
  blood flow in, 144, 149
  pressure in, 264
Axilla, temperature in, 373

Babies, respiration monitoring in, 121
Beta particles, 377
  absorption of, 380
  choice of counter for, 396
  detection, 385
    coincidence counting, 398
  energy of, 379
  needle counter, 395
  proportional counters, 385
  scintillation counters, 390, 395
Bladder stimulators, 312
Blood, acid-base balance, 232
  carbon dioxide content, 238
  carbon dioxide tension
    (*see* Carbon dioxide tension)
  gas tensions in, 208
  halothane analysis, 215, 216, 217
  handling of samples for CO_2 electrode, 236
  methoxyflurane in, 215
  optical density, 354
  oxygen content of, 246
  oxygen saturation of, 348
    (*see also* Oximetry and oximeters)

Blood—*continued*
 definition, 357
 pulmonary, 362
 oxygen tension in
  (*see* Oxygen tension)
 temperature coefficient, acid base
  state affecting, 232
 transmission of light through, 350
Blood flow, mathematical expression,
 148
Blood flow measurement, 134–170
 a.c. field flowmeters, 139
 catheter-tip thermistor flowmeters,
  149
 catheter tip velometers, 145
 direction, 163
 d.c. field flowmeter, 138
 electromagnetic flowmeters, 134
  applications of, 144
  calibration of, 143
  hydraulic occluders, 142
  zero flow adjustment, 141
 flowmeter heads, 134, 135, 137
 patterns, 136
 sensitivity of instruments, 137
 size of, 143
 thermal-type flowmeters, 146–150
  conductivity, 149
  dilution, 146
 thin-film resistance thermometers,
  161
 'transformer effect signals', 139
 ultrasonic meters, 150–154
  Doppler shift, 151
 venous occlusion plethysmography,
  155–161
Blood loss, replacement of, 57
Blood pressure recording, 3
 capacitance manometers in, 72
 computers in, 59
 finger-cuff methods, 104
 indirect methods, 96–104
  accuracy of, 104
  automatic, 100
  De Dobbeleer's system, 101
  double-cuff, 98
  Flanagan and Hull's system, 102
 integrators in, 114
 Parkinson's disease, in, 100
 pressure transducers in, 90

 silicon-diaphragm pressure transducers in, 82, 83
 strain gauge transducers for, 86
Blood vessels, stress transducers, 95
Blood volumes, estimation, 397
Body fluids, pH of, electrode systems
 for, 226
Body temperature,
 measurement of, 365–375
  during hypothermia, 374
  endoradiosondes, 368
  metal resistance thermometers,
   367
  resistance thermometers, 365
  silicon diode sensors, 371
  temperature probes, 372
  thermistors, by, 366
  thermocouples, 369
Boter's electrode, 180
Brachial artery, blood pressure recordings in, 98
Brain,
 midline identification, 154
 regional blood flow, 283
 tumours, 403
Breast tumours, 390
Bremsstrahlung, 380

Carbon dioxide, analysis, 205, 217, 218
 breath, in, 200, 201, 202, 213
 content of whole blood, 238
 expired air, in, 200
 infra-red, 204
 mass spectrometry, 207, 211
Carbon dioxide tension,
 electrode systems, 224, 230, 233–240
  calibration of, 236
  dynamic response, 238
  handling of blood samples, 236
  mode of action, 234
  read-out, 237
  response time, 235
  temperature effects, 237
Carbon monoxide measurement, infra-
 red, 201, 202
Cardiac arrhythmias,
 analysis of, 57, 289
 storage of display, 24
Cardiac catheterization, recording
 systems, 31

Cardiac catheters,
  damping, 88
  fibre optic bundles in, 87
  miniature, 89
  pressure transducers in, 86
    frequency response, 94
    resonance effects, 88
  safety precautions, 337
  small diameter, 88
  strain gauge pressure transducers on, 86
Cardiac output,
  definition, 257
Cardiac output measurement, 4, 159, 182
  computer, by, 59, 261, 263
  electrical impedance technique, 275
    accuracy of, 279
  ECG in conjunction with, 271
  indicator dilution methods, by, 257–275, 354, 360, 362
    calculations, 260, 262
  thermal dilution technique, 273
Cardiac pacemakers, 297–312
  atrial-triggered, 301
  bio-electric energy sources, 309
  circuits, 302
  complementary pair, 304, 305
  developments in power sources, 310
  electrical hazards, 306
  electrode arrangements for, 298
    electrolytic disintegration of, 306
  external, 299
  implanted, 297, 300
    bio-electric energy sources of, 309
    external rate control, 301
    reliability of, 308
  inductive type, 305, 306, 307
  long-term, 299
  'on-demand', 301
  radioactive sources of energy, 311
  reliability of, 308
  short-term, 298
  'thin-film' construction, 308
  use of diathermy and, 343
Carotid sinus nerves, stimulation, 322
Catheter-tip transducer for oxygen tension measurement, 245
Catheter-tip velometer, 145
Catheter-type oxygen electrodes, 249

Cathode ray tubes,
  astigmatism, 18
  direct-view bistable storage, 24
  display systems, 3, 6, 16, 17–25
    double beam, 20
    multi-trace, 21
    raster, 21
    storage oscilloscopes, 24
  post-deflection acceleration, 18
  principles, 17
Cation electrodes, 240
Children, measurement of cardiac output in, 259
Chloroform, analysis, 216, 217
Circulation studies, mercury strain gauges in, 84
Clark electrode, 242, 244, 249
Coincidence counting, 398
Collimators, 391, 392
Colorimeters, 346
Compton effect, 381, 392, 397
Computers, controlling mass spectrometry, 213
  decision making by, 61
  dye dilution methods and, 261, 263
  gamma camera, with, 403
  interpreting acid-base parameters, 251
  medical records, in, 63
  patient monitoring, in, 57–67
  spirometry, in, 126
  terminology employed, 63
Coronary arteries, blood flow measurements, 145
Coronary care units, patient monitoring, 3
Counting equipment for radioactive isotopes (see under Radioactive isotopes)
Curie, 381
Cyclopropane, safety precautions, 341

De Dobbeleer's double cuff system, 101
Defibrillators, 288–296
  a.c., 288
  concept of delivered energy, 295
  d.c. 289, 290
    checking performance of, 294
    energy stored in, 295
    portable and battery operated, 291
    routine inspection, 295

Defibrillators—*continued*
  synchronized, 292
  double square pulse, 293
Densitometers, 346
  dichromatic, 354
  dye dilution studies, in, 360
  fibre optics, 360, 362
  monochromatic, colorimetry, in, 346
  use of oximeter as, 360
Diathermy apparatus, 327–345
  burns from, 332
  cardiac pacemakers and, 307, 343
  electrical interference from, 334
  explosive anaesthetics and, 341
  safety precautions, 327, 332, 333
  spark-gap, 327
  thermionic valve, 330
  use of screened rooms, 335
Diethyl ether, safety precautions, 341
Display systems, 16–32
  cathode ray tube, 3, 6, 16, 17–25
    double beam, 20
      multi-trace, 21
      post-deflection acceleration, 18
      raster, 21
    choice of, 2
    computer, 61
    recorder, 25
Dye dilution methods,
  calculations, 260
  calibration of densitometer, 262
  cardiac output measurement by, 257–275, 354, 360, 362
  dichromatic densitometers for, 354
  shape of curve, 260
  use of, 258

Ear oximeters, 358
Electrical impedance,
  associated with cardiac activity, 265, 281
  transthoracic, in pulmonary oedema, 281
Electrical impedance technique,
  measurement of cardiac output by, 275
  accuracy of, 279
Electrical interference, from diathermy sets, 334
Electrocardiograms, 2, 3, 284
  amplifiers for, 340

common mode rejection ratio, 189
electrodes for, 171, 175–182
  adhesive chest, 179
  AVL lead measurement, 188
  Boter's, 180
  distortion effects, 188
  floating, 180
  high impedance effects, 186
  impedance pneumographs and, 120
  insulated, 181
  jellies and creams, 278
  Kahn's, 180
  motion artefacts, 177, 180
  multipoint, 175
  spray-on, 181
  use with impedance pneumographs, 115
in conjunction with cardiac output measurement, 271
mains interference, 189
pre-amplifiers for, 7, 13
radio, 176
recording channels, 6
recording systems, 20
  blood pressure measurement and, 97
storage of traces, 24
use to control defibrillators, 292
Electrodes, 171–195
  bladder stimulators, for, 317
  blood flowmeters, for, 137
  calomel reference, 229
  carbon dioxide, 230
  carbon dioxide content of whole blood, for, 238
  carbon dioxide tensions, for, 233–240
    calibration of, 236
    dynamic response, 238
    handling of blood samples, 236
    mode of action, 234
    read-out, 237
    response time, 235
    temperature effects, 237
  cardiac pacemakers, for, 298, 306
  cation, 240
  choice of, 171
  contact impedance, 171, 184, 190
  defibrillators, for, 288
  desirable characteristics, 171

Electrodes—*continued*
diathermy apparatus, for, 330
ECG, 171, 175–182
  adhesive chest, 179
  AVL lead measurement, 188
  Boter's, 180
  distortion effects, 188
  floating, 180
  high impedance, effect of, 186
  impedance pneumographs and, 120
  insulated, 181
  jellies and creams, 178
  Kahn's, 180
  motion artefacts, 177, 180
  multipoint, 175
  spray-on, 181
  use with impedance pneumographs, 115
EEG, 171, 172, 174, 182–183
electromyography, for, 183–184
electro-oculograms, for, 172
endocardial, 300
garments for use with, 191
impedance, 182
intracellular, 240
membrane potential, 225
myocardial, 343
oxygen tension,
  catheter-type, 249
  Clark, 242, 249
pH measurements, for, 224, 226–233
  glass electrodes, 227
  pH meters, 230
pessary, 318
  choice of material, 320
plethysmography, for, 186
polarization over-voltage, 174
polarographic,
  oxygen tension, for, 241
  tissue oxygen tension, for, 248
potential, 225
reversible, 172, 174
silver-silver chloride, 173
skin interface, 172, 190, 225
skin potential response, 172
surface, 183
voltage from, 172
Electroencephalograms, 2, 284
amplifiers for, 4
causing fibrillation, 340

computer analysis, 59
diathermy interference to, 334
electrodes for, 171, 172, 174, 182–183
Electromanometers, comparison with mass-spring analogue, 93
Electromanometry, 91–95
Electromyograms, 2
electrodes for, 183–184
recording channels, 6
Electron,
  annihilation, 378
  capture, 377
  pair production, 378, 381
Electron capture detector, 216
Electronic pessary, 318
Electro-oculograms, 2
electrodes for, 172
Electroretinograms, 2
Electroscopes, 404
Endoradiosondes, 74
thermistor, 368
Eye, abnormalities of, 155

Fibre optics,
  principle, 361
Fibre optic bundles in cardiac catheters, 87
Fibre optics oximeters and densitometers, 360,
Film badges, 404
Filters, 7
Finger-cuff measurement of systolic pressure, 104
Fingertip temperature, 373
Flame ionization detector, 214
Flanagan and Hull's double cuff system, 102
Fleisch head, 109
Flow can, 108
Foetal heart beat, ultrasonic measurement, 152, 153
Foot, blood flow in, 161
Forced expiratory volume, 127, 128
Forced vital capacity, 127
Fuel cells, 249

Galvanometers,
  blood flow meters, for, 138
  characteristics of, 32–40
  damping, 32, 35
  linearity aspects, 38

Galvanometers—*continued*
  pH meters, for, 230
  pencil, 6, 29, 32
Gamma cameras, 401
Gamma radiation, 377
  Compton effect, 381, 392, 397
  detection, 385
    choice of counter, 396
    coincidence counting, 398
    counting *in vivo*, 399
  energy of, 379
  interaction with matter, 380
  pair production, 381
  photoelectric effect, 380
  scintillation counting, 390
Gamma ray spectrometer, 393
Gas and vapour analysis and analysers,
    196–223
  gas chromatography, 213–220
    electron capture detector, 216
    flame ionization detector, 214
    thermal conductivity detector
      (katharometer), 217
  gas-discharge nitrogen meter, 207
  infra-red, 200
    calibration, 220
  lasers in, 205
  Luft type, 203, 206
  magnetic wind, 197, 199
  mass spectrometers, 207–213
    computer controlled, 213
    quadrupole, 210
  measurement of refractive index, by,
    206
  non-dispersive type, 202
  paramagnetic, 197
  preparation of standard mixtures,
    218
  thermal conductivity analysers, 199
Gas chromatography,
  electron capture detector, 216
  flame ionization detector, 214
  gas analysis, in, 213–220
Gas flow,
  measurement, 108–118
    Wright respirometer, 129, 130
  patterns, 112
Gas meters, dry displacement, 115–118
Gas volumes, measurement, 115, 118
Gauge factor, 78
Geiger counters, 387

  choice of, 396
  components of, 388
  dead time, 389
  miniature, 390
  operation, 389
  radiation monitors, in, 404
Geiger region, 384
Glomerular filtration rate, 397

Haemoglobin concentration, 347, 348
Haemoglobinometer, 347
Halothane, analysis in blood, 215, 216,
    217, 220
Halothane meter, ultra-violet, 206
Heart (*see also* under heading Cardiac)
  ejection rate, 277
  impedance changes associated with
    activity, 281
  internal pressure measurements, 74
  stroke volume,
    beat-by-beat changes in, 264, 279
    Kubicek's equation, 281
    pulse contour methods, 265
  ventricular output, 151
Heart muscle, contractile force, 95
Heart rate, 3, 120
Heart sounds, recording of, 363
Heart surgery, 283
  acid base balance in, 232
Heart valves, disease of, ultrasonic
    diagnosis, 155
Hydraulic occluders in blood flow
    meters, 142
Hypothermia,
  acid base balance during, 232
  body temperature during, 50, 374

Indicator dilution methods,
  cardiac output measured by, 257–275
    dye methods, 258, 272
    radioactive indicators, 266, 279
  dichromatic densitometers for, 354
  principles of, 257
  use of, 258
Indocyanine green in dilution methods,
    259, 272, 273, 279
Infra-red gas analysers, 200–206
  calibration, 220
Ink-jet recorders, 40–45
  behaviour of fluid, 43
  intensity modulation, 45

Ink-jet recorders—*continued*
  tangent error, 45
Inks for recorders, 46
Intensive care units,
  computers in, 62
  safety precautions, 336
  temperature monitoring in, 365
Ionization, 381
Ionization chambers, 382
  operating regions, 384
  use of guard ring, 383
Isomers, 378

Kahn's electrode, 180
Katharometer, 199, 217
Korotkoff sounds, 96
Krogh spirometer, 128
Kubicek's equation for cardiac stroke
  volume, 281

Lambert-Beer law, 346, 348, 358
Lasers, gas analysis, in, 205
Limbs, blood flow in, 147
Lithium-iodine cells for pacemakers,
  310
Lithium-nickel cell for pacemakers,
  310
Liver disease, ultrasonic diagnosis, 155
Luft non-dispersive infra-red gas
  analyser, 203, 206
Lungs,
  comparison of ventilation between
    left and right, 123, 124
  oxygen saturation, 362
Lung function studies,
  infra-red gas analysers in, 204
  pneumotachographs in, 113

Magnetic wind, 197, 199
Manometers,
  calibration systems, 87
  capacitance, 72
    blood pressure recording by, 73
  design of, 92
  electro-, 91–95
    comparison with mass-spring
      analogue, 93
  optical de-focusing pressure, 75
  pneumotachograph heads, with, 110
Mass spectrometry,
  computer controlled, 213

gas and vapour analysis, in, 207–213
  quadrupole, 210
Maximum expiratory flow rate, 127
Medical records, use of computers, 63
Membrane potential, 225
Meniere's disease, 155
Mercury strain gauges, 84
Methoxyflurane in blood, 215
Microphones for phonocardiography,
  8
Minute volume, 111, 112
Monitoring (*see* Patient monitoring)
Muscle contractions, recording, 80
  (*see also* Myography)
Muscle stimulators, 55
  constant-current, 57
Myocardial stimulation, 298
  (*see also* Cardiac pacemakers)
Myocardium, contractility, 278
Myography,
  isometric, 80, 95
  strain gauge, 10

Nernst equation, 225
Nerve stimulators, 55
Newborn,
  respiration monitoring in, 121
Nitrogen,
  concentration in breath, 213
  gas discharge meter, 207
  infra-red analysis, 200
  mass spectrometry, 207
  tension in blood, 209
Nitrous oxide,
  analysis, 110, 217, 218
    infra-red, 201, 202
  tension in blood, 209
Nitrous oxide-oxygen mixtures,
  measurement of, 207
Nuclides, 379

Obstetrics, ultrasonics in, 152, 153, 155
Oesophagus,
  temperature of, 373, 374
Operating theatres,
  safety in
    (*see under* Safety precautions)
  ventilation, 341
Optical absorption,
  principles of, 346

Oscillotonometer for blood pressure recording, 98
Oximetry and oximeters, 346
  basic theory of, 348, 350
  components of, 353
  dichromatic transmission, 354
  ear, 358
  electrical systems of, 354
  fibre optics, 360
    pressure transducer combined with, 363
  reflection, theory of, 357
  transmission, 359
  two-wavelength, 259
  use as densitometer, 360
Oxygen,
  catheter-tip transducer, 245
  concentration in breath, 213
  content of whole blood, 246
  mass spectrometry, 211
  paramagnetic analysers, 197–199
  saturation of blood, 348
    definition, 357
    pulmonary, 362
Oxygen analysis, 217
  mass spectrometry, 207
Oxygen–nitrous oxide mixtures, measurement of, 207
Oxygen tension in blood, 209
  continuous recording, 251
  electrode systems for, 224
  electrodes for, 241
    catheter-type, 249
    response time, 244
    tissue, in, 248

pH measurements,
  buffer solutions for, 232
  electrode systems for, 224, 226–233
    glass, 227
    pH meters, 230
pH meters, 230
  calibration of, 231
Pacemakers (see Cardiac pacemakers)
Paper chart records, 2
Parathyroid gland tumours, 403
Parkinson's disease, blood pressure recordings in, 100
Patient monitoring 3–4
  anaesthetic agents and, 341
  computer systems for, 57–67

multi-bed, 61
electrocardiography, 177, 179
  garments for electrodes and transducers, 191
  impedance matching of components of system, 4
  multi-trace displays in, 21
  phonocardiography, 9
  safety precautions for, 336
    earth-free mains supply, 336
    isolation transformers, 338
  stroke volume changes, 265
  temperature measurement, 365, 366
Peltier effect, 370
Pencil galvanometers, 6, 29, 32
Pen motor recorders,
  damping factors, 34
  error-correction, 39
  frequency response, 34
  linearity aspects, 38
  moving coil and moving-iron, 29
  orders of instruments, 51
  role of friction, 35
Phonocardiography,
  pre-amplifiers and microphones for, 8
Photoelectric effect of gamma radiation, 380
Piezo-electric bimorph pacemakers, 309
Piezo-electric crystals,
  blood flow meters, in, 150
Piezo-electric effects,
  strain gauges and, 80
Placenta,
  ultrasonic localization, 154, 155
Plethysmography and plethysmographs, 155–161
  air-filled, 161
  calibration, 158
  capacitance plethysmograph, 156
  electrical impedance, 159
  electrodes for, 186
  mercury-in-rubber strain gauge, 157
  venous occlusion, 155–161
  water filled plethysmograph, 156
Pneumographs,
  electrical impedance, 115, 118, 186
  applications of, 121
  calibration of, 121

Pneumographs—*continued*
post-operative patient monitoring, 121
ventilation studies, in, 123, 124
Pneumotachograph, 108
calibration of, 110
connected to lung ventilators, 111
drift in, 113
Fleisch head, 109
integrating, 111
Positrons, 378
Potentiometric recorders, 47
Pre-amplifiers, 1, 4–5
(*see also* Amplifiers)
carrier-type, 12–13
chopper-type, 5, 10–12
differential, 5
ECG, 6, 7, 13
phonocardiography, for, 8
push-pull action, 5
raster-type cathode ray tube oscilloscope, for, 23, 24
resistive and reactive transducers, for, 10
scintillation counters, in, 392
transistorized, 7
Pressure transducers, 10, 13, 70–87
blood pressure measurement with, 72, 82, 83, 86
display of, 90
site of, 90
catheter-tip, 86
combined with fibre optic oximeter, 363
damping, 94
frequency response, 94
linear variable-differential transformer, 76
silicon-diaphragm, 81
strain gauges, 77–87
unbonded strain gauge, 84
variable capacitance, 72
variable inductance, 74
venous pressure, for, 91
Pulmonary artery,
blood flow in, 144, 145, 154
passage of catheters in, 89
Pulmonary oedema, detection by transthoracic impedance, 281
Pulse pressure, relations to heart stroke volume, 266

Quartz fibre electroscopes, 404

Radiation,
detection, 381–385, 404
choice of counters, 396
coincidence counting, 398
collimators, 391, 392
d.c. ionization chambers, 382
Geiger counters, 387
scintillation counters, 390–395
detectors,
semiconductor, 395
use of guard ring, 383
protection equipment, 403–405
statistics of counting, 405
Radioactive isotopes, 376
coincidence counting, 398
counting equipment for, 376–410
counting mixtures, 398
detectors (*see* Radiation, detection)
half-life, 379
nuclides, 379
proportional counters, 385
protection equipment, 403–405
statistics of counting, 405
Radioactive sources for pacemakers, 311
Radioisotope scanner, 399
Radiological protection equipment, 403–405
Radio pills, 74, 368
Recorder systems and recorders, 25–32
amplifiers, performance requirements, 5
amplitude distortions, 52
choice of, 1, 3
circular-chart, 46
criteria for faithful reproduction, 52
error-correction system, 39
frequency response, 52
hot-stylus, 6, 26, 35
role of friction, 35
impedance matching of components, 4
ink-jet, 40–45
behaviour of fluid, 43
intensity modulation, 45
tangent-error, 45
inks, 46
moving-coil, 29
moving-iron pen motors, 29

Recorder systems (*continued*)
    orders of instruments, 51
    paper chart, 2
    pen-arm, 26
    pen-motor,
        frequency response, 34
        linearity aspects, 38
        role of friction, 35
    phase distortion, 53
    photographic, 29
    poor frequency response, 54
    potentiometric, 47–50
    slow-response, 45–47
    step function testing, 54
    strip or roll chart, 45
    transient response, 53
    ultra-violet, 29
    X-Y recorders, 50
Rectal temperature, 373
Refractive index measurement in gas
        analysis, 206
Renal function,
    radioactive methods, 50, 397, 399,
        402
Respiration,
    measurement, 114-115, 125
        babies, in, 121
        impedance electrodes, by, 182
Respiratory distress syndrome, 282
Respiratory flow patterns, 112
Respiratory patterns,
    impedance changes for, 122
Respiratory volume,
    measurement by impedance, 275
Respirometer,
    Wright, 129, 130
Rheoencephalography, 283

Safety precautions,
    operating rooms, 327
    patient monitoring, 336
Scintillation counters, 390–395
    adjustment of, 394
    choice of, 397
    liquid, 394, 395
    mixture of isotopes, 398
Seebeck effect, 370
Semiconductors, 57
    radiation detectors, in, 395
    strain gauges, in, 80
Serum albumin, ^{131}I labelled, 379

cardiac output measured with, 266,
        279
Shocked lung syndrome, 282
Signal conditioners, 71
Silicon diode temperature sensors, 371
Skin potential response of electrodes,
        172
Skin temperature, 372
Spectrometer,
    gamma ray, 393
Sphygmomanometer, 96–98
    automated, 97
Spinal cord dorsal columns,
    stimulation of, 322
Spirometry, 125–130
    anaesthesia, in, 129, 130
    computers, use of, 126
    continuous flow, 129, 130
    frequency response, 128
    Krogh, 128
Splenic artery,
    blood flow in, 144
Strain gauges, 77–87
    bonded, 78
    mercury, 84
    mercury-in-rubber, 157
    resistive, 12
    semiconductor, 80
    silicon bonded, 80
    unbonded, 84, 86
Stress and strain,
    definitions, 77
Stress incontinence, 312
    electronic pessary for, 318
Strip or roll-chart recorders, 45

Temperature of body,
    measurement of, 62, 365–375
        during hypothermia, 50, 374
        endoradiosondes, 368
        metal resistance thermometers, 367
        resistance thermometers, 365
        silicon diode sensors, 371
        temperature probes, 372
        thermistors, by, 366
        thermocouples, 369
Temperature probes, 372
Temperature sensors, 10
    silicon diode, 371
Thermal   conductivity   detector
    (Katharometer), 217

Thermal dilution technique for cardiac output, 273
Thermistors,
blood flow meters, in, 149, 150
body temperature measurement by, 366
endoradiosondes, in, 368
respiratory rate measurement, in, 114
thermal dilution technique, in, 274
Thermocouples, 369–371, 372
laws of, 370
Thermometers,
metal resistance, 367
recorders for, 49
resistance, 365
thin-film resistance, 161
Thermostromuhr, 149
Thoracic surgery, 283
Thyroid gland,
radioactive studies, 401
Tidal volume measurement, 118, 125
Toes,
temperature of, 373
Transducers, 1
blood vessel stress, for, 95
definition, 70
diaphragms, 72
frequency response, 70
garments for use with, 191
pressure (see Pressure transducers)
principles, 71
sensitivity, 70
signal conditioners and, 71
variable capitance, 72
variable inductance, 74
Transformers,
isolation, 338

Trichloroethylene analysis, 216, 217
Tumours,
Geiger counters implanted in, 390
radio sensitivity of, 248

Ultrasonics,
blood flow meters, 150–154
foetal heart beat measurement by, 152, 153
obstetrics, in, 152, 153, 155
surgical applications, 154–155
Ultra-violet halothane meters, 206
Urinary incontinence,
electronic stimulators for, 297, 312
'demand' type, 320
pessary type. 318
neurogenic, 317
Urine,
measurement of velocity, 146

Veins,
blood flow in, 146, 147
Vena cava,
blood flow in, 145
Venous plethysmography,
mercury strain gauges in, 84
Venous pressure, measurement, 62, 90
Ventilation,
between left and right lungs, 123, 124
Ventricular fibrillation,
cardiac catheters causing, 337, 340
defibrillators causing, 289
defibrillators for, 292
diathermy causing, 343
ECG machine causing, 340

Whelpton and Watson integrator, 113
Wright respirometer, 129, 130